QUALITATIVE RESEARCH IN HEALTH

An Introduction

CAROL GRBICH

SAGE Publications

London • Thousand Oaks • New Delhi

Copyright © Carol Grbich 1999

First published 1999
by Allen & Unwin
9 Atchison Street
St Leonards NSW 1590
Australia

SAGE Publications Ltd
6 Bonhill Street
London EC2A 4PU

SAGE Publications Inc
2455 Teller Road
Thousand Oaks, California 91320

SAGE Publications India Pvt Ltd
32, M-Block Market
Greater Kailash – I
New Delhi 110 048

British Library Cataloguing in Publication data

A catalogue record for this book is
available from the British Library

ISBN 0 7619 6103 8 (hbk)
ISBN 0 7619 6104 6 (pbk)

Library of Congress catalog record available

Typeset in 11/15pt Goudy by DOCUPRO, Sydney
Printed in Singapore by South Wind Productions

Contents

Preface

This book seeks to provide a broad but comprehensive overview of current debates and issues as well as the practicalities of conducting qualitative research. It will be of most interest to those planning to enter or already in the health industry—doctors, nurses, physiotherapists, occupational therapists, medical records and other administrators, orthoptists, prosthetists, health promoters, educators and evaluators—because the examples given come from health. Qualitative researchers from the disciplines of sociology, education, social work and all other areas that use qualitative approaches should also find it interesting and useful.

My aim is to present a comprehensive selection of the major methodologies and techniques of qualitative data collection, interpretation and presentation. I have taken an even-handed approach to allow readers to make their own decisions as to the appropriateness of each approach. Continual emphasis is placed on the dynamic nature of qualitative research, with particular reference to each researcher's capacity to add to the changing nature of techniques and debates through their own published works.

The book consists of four parts, which follow the general order of the research process. *Part One, Theory and Design*, explores theoretical and conceptual frameworks and any implications these may have for the research design. *Part Two, Techniques of Data Collection*, and *Part Three, Methodological Approaches*, are difficult to separate, since methodological approaches often impose particular frameworks that influence data collection. These two parts examine the dominant and emerging techniques used for collecting data, and the increasingly diverse methodological approaches that inform these techniques. *Part Four, Interpretation, Analysis and Presentation of Data*, examines methods of analysis and appropriate interpretation of data, once data collection is under way. It also addresses the important, final issues of presentation and display.

Issues and debates pertaining to key areas of qualitative research are examined throughout the text. Arguments for choosing either quantitative or qualitative orientations and for using qualitative computing packages are explored, as are arguments pertaining to 'validity', 'objectivity' and 'reliability'.

I anticipate that this text will provide readers with sufficient knowledge to choose and undertake qualitative research approaches in a well-informed manner. Lists of further readings relevant to particular methodologies, techniques and debates are provided at the end of each chapter, while there is a complete bibliography at the end of the book.

Part One
Theory and design

Part One comprises three chapters. It aims to provide an historical overview; a general introduction to issues of definition; a description of certain theorists' positions and the potential for application of their theories; and an exploration of the contentious debates surrounding research design. Chapters 1, 2 and 3 are necessarily superficial, as they are an attempt to introduce readers to the many debates surrounding qualitative research. These early chapters are designed to whet readers' appetites to seek more in-depth information in the later chapters, and to consult the further readings offered.

Chapter 1 explores textbook definitions, historical trends and current orientations in health research in an attempt to answer the question: *'What is qualitative research?'* Detailed examples illustrate what is involved in qualitative research. There is also a brief discussion of the divisions between proponents of qualitative and quantitative approaches, and their claims for locating 'truth'. Although there is considerable variation within the two approaches those favouring quantitative approaches see reality as external, measurable and controllable, while those favouring qualitative approaches see it as complex, multifaceted and constructed by individuals. The chapter ends with an exploration of recent theoretical innovations and their implications for qualitative research. The principle of uncertainty, chaos theory and the advent of postmodernism receive special attention in this regard.

Chapter 2 looks at four general approaches to the use of theory/concepts in qualitative research:

- *Theory/concept-driven approach:* A particular theoretical position is used to drive the research design, data collection and interpretation. This is examined in detail.
- *Theory/concept-generating approach:* Particular theoretical positions lightly underpin the process and inform the outcomes. This is briefly outlined.

- *Postmodern or poststructural approaches:* These share an emphasis on deconstructing representations of social reality. These are presented for discussion.
- *Feminist approaches:* These are not theoretical positions, but have been included because their underpinning principles have had a strong influence on current directions in qualitative research.

Chapter 3 examines the historical debates and current dilemmas surrounding research design:

- How are qualitative researchers viewing 'validity', 'reliability', 'objectivity' and 'subjectivity'?
- To what extent is generalisability possible?
- What are the ethics of interviewing or observing vulnerable people, in particular children, people who are older and those with disabilities?
- How can researchers 'manage' funding and other agencies on whom the results of her/his study will impact?

I do not pretend to answer all these questions, but do provide an in-depth exploration of the arguments for and against particular approaches.

1 Qualitative research: an introduction

This chapter explores the various debates surrounding the questions: 'How is qualitative research defined?' and 'Where can "truth" be located in social research?' I plan to conduct a brief exploration of textbook definitions, historical trends and current orientations within health research in an attempt to answer these questions within the context of the broader question:

What is qualitative research?

An initial search through a selection of existing texts indicates a diversity of definitions of the term *qualitative research*. These range from an emphasis on the 'methods and techniques of observing, documenting, analysing and interpreting attributes, patterns, characteristics and meanings of specific, contextual or gestaltic features of phenomena under study' (Leininger, 1985, p. 5), through approaches 'which seek to uncover the thoughts, perceptions and feelings experienced by informants' (Minichiello et al., 1995, p. 10), to the view that 'inquirers do not "discover" knowledge from behind a thick one-way mirror; rather it is literally created by the action of inquirers with the "object" (construct) inquired into' (Guba, 1996, p. x).

This variety of definitions indicates that even within qualitative approaches there are differences in emphasis between those who believe that there is a world 'out there', which can be accessed through the use of particular techniques, and those who believe that this world is socially constructed by the researcher and other participants (Kellehear, 1993). The first group believes that the researcher can participate in, and document, the 'outer' world with minimal intrusion. The second group believes that the perceptions of the researcher and other participants in the 'socially constructed' world are intricately interwoven.

Similarly, there tend to be two ways of gaining access to 'phenomena', 'informants' and 'worlds', whatever their definition. The first focuses primarily on methods or techniques. The second emphasises a paradigmatic approach, in which a particular way of seeing the world also has theoretical, and therefore methodological, implications for the research being undertaken.

Methods-based approaches

Authors taking a predominantly *methods-based approach* include Michael Patton (1990), who focuses on the techniques of interviewing, observation and documentation to show what qualitative data looks like, and Matthew Miles and Michael Huberman (1984), who emphasise rigorous procedures of data collection and analysis. These authors view reality largely as being 'out there', so that a researcher, by careful application of these techniques, should be able to access it and report on it in a fairly objective manner.

Paradigmatic approaches

Norman Denzin, Egon Guba and Yvonna Lincoln take the *paradigmatic approach*. They contrast the naturalistic (qualitative) paradigm with the scientific or positivistic (quantitative) paradigm. The *positivistic (quantitative)* paradigm holds the mechanistic view that knowledge is concerned with 'facts' and the observed world, and that social laws underpin the development of the human species (Auguste Comte, 1969 [1830]). Denzin, Guba and Lincoln identify several key differences between the qualitative and quantitative approaches. The *naturalistic (qualitative)* paradigm portrays reality as a multiple, constructed, interdependent whole that cannot be broken down into measurable segments. Equally inseparable is the interactive relationship between the knower (the inquirer) and the known (the object of the inquiry) and the presumption that all events, phenomena and situations are bound by time and context so that generalisations are rarely possible (Lincoln and Guba, 1985). Quantitative investigations are based on concepts of 'cause', 'effect' and 'objectivity'. Such concepts are thought to be minimally applicable to entities that appear to be in a constant state of change, affected by the researcher, context and theoretical perspectives, which in turn influence research design, choice of methods and the interpretation of findings.

There is an emerging trend within the paradigmatic tradition that attempts to capture the historical and multidisciplinary complexities of research within overarching theoretical paradigms that join schools of theories. These schools propound specific *world views* that have implications for data collection and interpretation. Denzin and Lincoln's four paradigms (1994, p. 109) are examples of this trend:

- *positivist*, in which 'reality' is viewed as being external to the researcher;
- *postpositivist*, which propounds that knowledge about 'reality' can only be approximated, but can be sought through rigorous approaches such as 'grounded theory';
- *critical*, which focuses on the critique of economic structures, and emphasises emancipatory outcomes; and
- *constructivist*, in which individual constructions of 'social reality' are the focus.

The last three paradigms fit within the qualitative tradition. Paradigm-based approaches have both advantages and disadvantages.

Advantages of paradigm-based approaches

The advantages of paradigm-based approaches lie in the systematisation of knowledge. Placing different orientations into separate boxes achieves a sense of order and control, and provides a way of managing, highlighting and contrasting varying approaches.

Disadvantages of paradigm-based approaches

The disadvantages of paradigm-based approaches lie in oversimplification. This is evident when the qualitative and quantitative paradigms are examined.

A general overfocus on techniques gives the impression that *qualitative* research is simply a matter of identifying a research question and gathering information through interviews, documents and observation. When this data collection is rounded off with the location and interpretation of emergent or recurring themes, the research question appears to be answered. This simplified process dramatically minimises crucial issues such as the conceptual or historical origin of the questions posed, researcher bias, and the interpretive framework/s within which emergent themes can test existing theories or develop new ones.

Equally, the *quantitative* approach appears to be limited to hypothesis testing, variable control and statistical analyses. This does not take into account the variation that has now become evident through the changes in theoretical physics.

The paradigmatic approach thus emphasises simplistically the differences rather than the similarities and shared concerns, further promoting the polarisation of qualitative and quantitative research. Some writers believe that the two paradigms are antithetical: that they are so far apart in purpose that they should never be combined. This stance belies 'reality', however, because the two are often included in the same study.

Lengthy debate has also taken place about grouping theories that have similar world views and methodological implications into qualitative paradigms such as those developed by Guba and Lincoln. On the one hand, similar positions are brought together. On the other, the tendency towards singularity and conformity means a loss of the richness of individual perspectives, resulting in oversimplification, distortion and rigidity (Atkinson, 1995). There is often such a great diversity of views within a particular paradigm in some cases that the usefulness of this approach must be questioned.

Dynamic approaches

The focus on techniques and the emphasis on paradigms reflect two aspects of the qualitative spectrum, within which the researcher's position can be seen to vary. The researcher may at some stage see him/herself as separate from the reality under exploration, then later see his/her role as integral to, and impacting on, the construction of processes, meanings and outcomes of the research investigation. In short, it is essential to encompass the evident diversity and the researcher's dynamic approach in any answer to the question, 'What is qualitative research?' Any definition will only provide a cine shot of the state of the art at a given moment.

This shows that qualitative approaches are complex and varied, allowing the researcher to study a situation from a range of positions and perspectives to find out how people interact in, experience and define contexts within cultures. These explorations should enable researchers to investigate organisational structures, to describe patterns of behaviour and processes of interaction, and to reveal the meanings, values and intentions of people's life experiences. Qualitative approaches also have the capacity to allow assessment of the researcher's subjective experiences and impact on the setting.

Historical trends

It is difficult to pinpoint historical changes in qualitative approaches with any clarity. The most an author can hope to achieve is to indicate dominant trends within an era. These trends, however, are not limited by chronological boundaries. Earlier trends persist, making it easy to trace the genesis of current trends. Despite this, two broad eras are readily identified.

Era 1 (pre 1965) covers a period dominated by ethnographic and participant observation studies, including anthropological research on tribal groups and investigations of urban cultures such as prisons, medical schools, street youth, diverse communities, hospital wards, massage parlours and nudist beaches. These studies were often longitudinal. Data were gathered over a certain period, with emphasis placed on social process, rigorous data collection and the testing of theories, or the development of new conceptual or theoretical frameworks to explain the situations under investigation.

Era 2 (post 1965) is characterised by a vast diversity of approaches and continuing debate and change, particularly with regard to such issues as the researcher's role and the rigour of data collection. The women's movement, with its emphasis on the location of power—Does it lie mainly within structures or with individuals?—and the advent of postmodernism, have both contributed to the changes. Feminists have been particularly vocal in querying the position of the objective 'neutral' researcher, and the relative value of 'objective' versus 'subjective' research. These debates provide the researcher with options, ranging from a central to a decentred position, and from distant non-involvement to collaboration or actual participation in the research process. An emphasis on outcomes has arisen from the issue of the researcher's accountability in disturbing the settings of distraught or vulnerable people. Desirable outcomes take the form of empowering participants through knowledge transmission, or through social action facilitated by the researcher.

Validity and reliability

The terms 'validity' and 'reliability' have come under question. Should multiple data sources and a tight design be valued above the intensive exploration of one person's expert opinion? Does a study become more 'reliable' if the views of 200 or 2000 people are collected, rather than of two? What is 'validity'? Whose version of 'truth' is being represented, and how? The postmodern rejection of the grand theory as a singular explanation of 'reality', in favour of multiple perspectives and the development of small-scale contextual theoretical explanations, adds greater complexity to this debate. The further assertion that language reflects discursive practices embedded in history, rather than current reality, has led to the interpretation and reinterpretation of texts in the process of deconstructing past influences. Given this turmoil, what does a qualitative research study look like?

Research orientations

There are three main approaches to qualitative research: field-based, action-based and library-based. These form the bases of Chapters 5–8 of this text. They are briefly presented here as 'ideal types' or 'aspects' that can be conveniently grouped for the purpose of demonstrating trends. All three are differentiated more by their major purposes than by theoretical perspectives or techniques.

The main purpose of *field-based research* is to collect original data from participants, through interviews and/or some form of observation. Textual data may also be included. The majority of qualitative research is carried out in this way.

Action-based research attempts to bring about change through an evaluation of a situation. The researcher achieves her/his aims by means of intervention, by working with people to help them change their environment, or by providing sufficient information to enable them to take responsibility for changes in their own life situations.

The main purpose of *library-based research* is to investigate and analyse information, which tends to be stored in libraries, institutions or private collections in the form of journals, diaries, letters, newspapers, case notes, legal, political and medical documents, books, photos, film, videos and television programs.

The areas of exploration that have tended to dominate health research within the above approaches are the organisation, operation, interaction, experiences and meanings of people within cultures, phenomena, structural processes and historical changes. The following examples demonstrate some design possibilities within these categories.

Cultures

A *culture* is generally defined as a group of people with shared knowledge, beliefs, values and ways of living. Cultural explorations can range from longitudinal anthropological studies of the health practices of a large cultural group, such as a tribal or community group, to investigations of the culture of a hospital ward, seen from the perspectives of administrators, health professionals and patients. An investigation of the lifestyle of a group of drug-addicted homeless youth in an inner city suburb is another example. Requirements for identification as a 'culture' generally include some shared beliefs or feelings of identity, and a common location also tends to be involved. Jan Reid's exploration (using interviews and observation) of the healing practices of the Yolngu people of Yirrkala in the Northern Territory of Australia (Reid, 1983) is an example of a longitudinal cultural study. Reid investigated the extent to which western medicine had been adopted and adapted, and how social change had impacted on the traditional belief systems and health care practices of this community. Her findings indicated that at that time the causes of serious illness and death were still explained within traditional indigenous frameworks, even though western medicine and biomedical explanations were sought for a variety of ills. The traditional frameworks often involved sorcery, which demanded the skills of traditional indigenous healers.

Phenomena

Investigations of phenomena tend to focus on individual experiences, such as loneliness, marginalisation or the stigma incurred in a particular situation. Examples are the debilitation of old age and the contraction of the HIV virus.

Minichiello (1992) used an interview approach to collect the narratives of carefully selected groups from different living situations in an exploration of the interpretation, experiences and strategies developed by gay and bisexual men to help them cope with becoming HIV positive. The diversity of experiences in moving from a state of good health to a career of illness, and the accompanying renegotiation of expectations, life choices and priorities, were investigated in depth. Responses and strategies were very individual, but it was clear that such societal concepts as 'deviant' sexuality and the 'stigma' attached to the AIDS virus were often important factors in who disclosed what information to whom, and at what point in time.

Structural processes

An example of a structural process could be the medico-legal investigation of work-damaged people, seen from the perspective of bureaucrats' experiences (policy effectiveness) or clients' experiences (positive and negative, and how they make sense of the process) or both. The evaluation of large scale departmental or institutional restructuring could be another research area.

Grbich and Sykes (1989) investigated policy change in their exploration of the impact of integrating severely intellectually disabled young people into the community, regular secondary-school classes and the workforce. A random sample was drawn from a total population of these people. Their views and those of parents, school and work personnel were canvassed through formal interviews and observed interaction in a variety of contexts. An analysis of policy documents was also included. The findings indicated that:

- All parents viewed support services as minimal.
- There was poor communication between health professionals and parents.
- Families in this situation were marginalised at all societal levels.
- 'Integrated' students in regular schools experienced segregation.
- The 'special' educational and workforce systems were also segregated from the mainstream.
- These people, particularly women with intellectual disabilities, had restricted access to community living, educational programs and the workforce.

Many recommendations were made for change after these results were placed against the ideals and intentions of normalisation and integration policies. Reference will be made to this research project throughout this text to highlight various aspects of qualitative research for health professionals.

Historical changes

Archival research involves the analysis of documents or stories from times past, such as health policies covering the last 200 years, newspaper clippings revealing shifts in public opinion regarding the AIDS virus (Aroni, 1992), or the search for changing discourses in the abortion debates.

Hepworth and Griffith's (1990) poststructuralist study of the medical documentation of the condition anorexia nervosa is an example of this form of research. They identified five discourses apparent since the late nineteenth century:

- *Femininity*, which brands women as creative, emotional, deviant and mad. Women's unpredictable behaviour is seen as relating to the female psyche, which is driven in turn by reproductive capacities and mental perversity;
- *Medical*, which involves the search via scientific medicine for physical or organic causes. Food refusal is viewed as a pathological condition: a manifestation of a

psychological condition requiring confinement and scientific medical interventions.

- *Clinical*, which focuses on prescriptive treatments and the quality (moral power) of relationships (doctor–patient, or family–patient).
- *Discovery*, which makes the link between medical and psychiatric orientations in developing the term 'anorexia nervosa'.
- *Hysteria*, which provides the link to femininity and the psycho-medical framework through the notion of hysteria.

These discourses were examined further in terms of theories relating to power, language, ideology and punishment for women.

Why categorise?

It is obvious that dividing health research into the four areas of cultures, phenomena, structural processes and historical changes is simply a technique for illustrating variety. Most studies contain aspects of more than one category. An exploration of a culture may include an examination of historical, economic, legal and political processes, as well as the social structures that influence interpersonal interaction and individual experiences of various phenomena. Categorising may be used as a tool in the attempt to locate 'truth' in a research project, but the location of this elusive concept has always been contentious and seems destined to remain so.

In pursuit of the elusive concept 'truth'

The major goal of all social research is to discover, understand and communicate the *truth* of situations. This begs the difficult question, 'What is truth?' How do we know if or when we have discovered it? Pursuing the most accurate location and description of 'truth' requires an exploration of the fall and subsequent resurgence in popularity of qualitative research approaches. The following brief history outlines the major thoughts about 'truth' from the earliest recorded descriptions of time and space, to current theories and philosophies.

Prior to medieval times, qualitative views dominated. Descriptions of time and space were comprehensible; that is, they made sense to most people, in terms of both their own daily perceptions and the generally accepted and shared symbols of the time.

A new view of 'truth' had emerged by the Middle Ages, however, due to the rise of universities and the middle classes. This view emphasised precision, quantification and physical phenomena (Crosby, 1997, p. 58). Its focus was on logic and mathematics. Rationalist views, which involved precise definitions and meticulous, logical and routine reasoning, became dominant. Empirical knowledge, derived from observation and experience, was rejected in favour of intellectual thought about the world. This shift resulted in the view that intellectual knowledge, or 'truths', were absolute and accessible only to those of high status, who used them to control those of lower status. Such 'truths' as were passed down required unquestioning faith from the masses, particularly in relation to religious principles and explanations. It was said that the plague, for example, was visited upon individuals through the medium of the 'evil eye' as retribution for past sins, rather than through lack of sanitation, which an empirical approach might have suggested.

Frustration with these explanations and the power they gave to particular religious authorities led scientists to view mind and body as separate entities. This separation was termed 'the Cartesian duality'. It was attributed to seventeenth-century scholar René Descartes (1968 [1637]) and rested on the assumption that a physical world of a higher order existed. This world was linked to, but separate from, subjective interpretations, emotions, reflection and consciousness. 'Truths' were self-evident and observable, leaving no room for doubt. 'Reality' could be reduced, controlled and measured by reason, logic and mathematical means to provide accurate predictions of future events.

Opposition to this view arose between the seventeenth and twentieth centuries. Philosophers Immanuel Kant (1974 [1781]) and John Stuart Mill (1906 [1843]) asserted that mind and body were not separate. They believed that they were inextricably interlinked, so that the process of measuring 'reality' must necessarily involve ideas, perception, decision making and intellectual analysis, all of which could be affected by contextual and psychological factors. Wilhelm Dilthey (1976) went further. He questioned the appropriateness of measurement in situations where documenting individuals' understandings of life's experiences might be a better method of obtaining the views and constructed meanings of the self and others. His view was that these individual understandings needed to be placed in context so that aspects of freedom and choice could be assessed.

Despite these attempts to validate subjectivity in the search for 'truth', the classical science/positivist view had become widely accepted by the early nineteenth century. This was a system of philosophy that recognised only observable phenomena, objective relations and the laws determining them. The French scientist Pierre Laplace went so far as to suggest that scientific laws could provide the knowledge to predict all incidents in the universe, including human behaviour. The belief that the methods of logic on which classical physics was structured could be applied to social phenomena became one of the major tenets of positivism. Consequently, all knowledge could be expressed only by referring to observable, measurable, predictable and generalisable realities in an objective value-free manner, based on an assumption of linear causality (cause–effect).

Nineteenth-century philosophers further questioned the applicability of classical science methods to social, cultural, economic and political aspects of society on the grounds of relativity. They argued that knowledge relating to human action could only be 'relatively true', as it depended on the changing relationship between individual and society, and was therefore bounded by context and time. The duration, continuance, comparativeness and recurrence of incidents in such circumstances must inevitably be unpredictable. The continuing debate about the opposing views of 'truth' suggested the existence of a variety of 'truths' that needed different approaches for clarification. Is 'truth' a reality 'out there', awaiting the development of sufficient levels of knowledge to enable comprehension? Or is it a set of socially constructed or consensually evolved beliefs and meanings, which may be limited by powerful discourses? These views have been further challenged by David Bloor (1991) from within the sociology of knowledge. Bloor took an opposing view to Pierre Laplace, asserting that sociological approaches have the capacity to investigate and explain the content and nature of scientific phenomena, including mathematics and logic. The principles that would be utilised in such investigations include causality, impartiality, symmetry and reflexivity.

'Truth' in the twentieth century

Two major research approaches, quantitative and qualitative, were identified as a result of the nineteenth-century debates about the source of 'truth'. Despite the previously discussed challenges to the quantitative view, this orientation has been particularly persistent and has dominated twentieth-century research methodology. Quantitative researchers presume that there is a singular material 'reality' that exists independently 'out there'. 'Truth' can be found by applying the proposition that measurable influences (independent variables) affect measurable outcomes (dependent variables) in a cause–

effect manner. These variables can be expressed numerically and processed by statistical analysis to determine relationships between phenomena.

As was mentioned earlier, the practice of qualitative research demonstrates considerable variety. Most qualitative researchers believe that 'truth' lies in gaining an understanding of the action, beliefs and values of others, from within the participant's frame of reference. This frame is believed to have been socially and historically constructed, and to be delimited by the researcher's views, context and time. However, some qualitative researchers believe that in the search for 'truth' hypotheses can be developed and tested; relationships between entities can be demonstrated; variables can be identified and controlled; and descriptive statistics can be used to display outcomes. Other qualitative researchers see truth lying in the reality constructed by the interaction of the researcher and the researched.

Quantitative–qualitative debate

John Smith and Louis Heshusius (1986) pinpointed three stages in the quantitative–qualitative debate from the nineteenth century to 1986. These were conflict, détente and cooperation. Each stage had a corresponding dominant position, from which theorists argued for or against the 'validity' of quantitative or qualitative research. Gretchen Rossman and Bruce Wilson (1985) identified these positions as purist, situationalist and pragmatist.

Conflict, which was the accepted position from the late nineteenth century to the 1970s, involved polarisation. The *purist* view asserted that both techniques (quantitative and qualitative) derived from different theoretical positions, which in turn had specific and separate methodological implications. The two positions from which the methodologies had emerged were seen as fundamentally different, divided at the core by notions of objectivity and subjectivity.

Détente emerged during the late 1970s. It featured *situationalist* theorists, who moved away from describing the 'good' and 'bad' aspects of the two approaches. They focused instead on procedural issues and comparable criteria for examining them. The philosophical differences tended to submerge beneath the view that the two approaches were parallel research tools. Earlier conflicts between internal 'validity' and credibility, dependability and 'reliability', consistency and confirmability, and 'objectivity' (neutrality) and 'subjectivity', became accepted as variations of the same concept.

Cooperation, the third stage, emerged in the early 1980s. It is characterised by the *pragmatist* notion of compatibility. This stage is marked by an enthusiasm to develop criteria that will enhance the 'rigour' of qualitative research, enabling it to earn greater 'credibility' and recognition as a legitimate tool. *Epistemological* differences (ways of thinking pertaining to particular claims of knowledge) appear to have been forgotten in the process. The increasing popularity of grounded theory in health research is related to this enthusiasm for 'rigour' of qualitative research. Matthew Miles and Michael Huberman's text on qualitative analysis (1984, p. 21) contains an assertion that the development of 'valid' qualitative methods would allow them to become 'scientific' in the positivist sense of the word. The development of 'theory-generating' computer packages in the mid 1980s can also be attributed to this third stage of the debate.

Smith and Heshusius (1986) concluded their historical overview with the contention that the contrasting scientific and naturalistic positions could only be reconciled trivially at the level of method, and that qualitative approaches were in considerable danger of becoming a procedural variation of quantitative inquiry. The view that qualitative methods are merely procedures or techniques, separate from the epistemological positions that influence question conceptualisation, data collection and interpretation, has been one of the major facilitators of the idea of compatibility. The maxim of using 'the best tool for the job' has also been a contributing factor. This again reduces 'tools' to mere practical techniques, divorced from any theoretical origins. Despite these expressed concerns, 1990s evaluators are still seeking to identify commonalities in the values and approaches of the two paradigms (Reichardt and Rallis, 1994).

The 1990s

The concerns featured in the above debates are still evident. They have led to different ways of utilising both approaches in an attempt to gain the advantages of combining both forms of data collection without compromising their different derivations. In general, the aim is either to seek convergence of data (terminating at some point to provide reinforcement of common findings), which is said to enhance 'validity', or to establish a more complete picture of a phenomenon by combining different perspectives.

One recent attempt to combine both forms of data collection (Pradilla, 1992) was based on a parallel methods approach, in which the results of two similar but separately located studies were triangulated. *Triangulation* entails overlapping the results at several points to enhance reliability. The *quantitative study* used a researcher-developed, pretested, factor-analysed questionnaire to investigate students' perceptions of their academic supervisors. (In a *factor-analysed* questionnaire, the analysis is the product of a series of factors in arithmetical order.) Results featured academic skills, personal caring and being a good person (socio-emotional skills); meeting dynamics; problems with advice; and level of knowledge. The *qualitative study* used interviews that were analysed through concept modelling to locate types of supervisors, what they do, how they do it, and the rapport between supervisor and student. (*Concept modelling* involves linking various concepts under one umbrella to emphasise a particular perspective or interpretation.) Pradilla pointed to the consistency of results (both sets of which were computer assisted), and thus to the potential of convergent triangulation.

Other documented research has attempted to gain a broader view through the triangulation of two sets of data (quantitative and qualitative) on the same question, taken from the same respondents in a single study. One such project (Prein, 1992) investigated links between women's professional career decisions and their private family biographies. The qualitative approach (interviews) found that family factors such as husbands' views and children's needs had the main impact on decision making. The quantitative data (cluster analysis and the development of contingency models) indicated that the particular profession, *not* family factors, was the major casual component. Thus the researchers viewed the results of the two sets of data as being completely contradictory.

Another study (Mason, 1994) used two data sets, one quantitative and one qualitative, to investigate the same topic. The topic explored what people thought they should do for their relatives. A large scale survey of 978 respondents (quantitative data set) was undertaken to provide a broad picture. Then 120 semi-structured face-to-face interviews were undertaken (qualitative data set) to investigate different aspects of meaning on the topic. In this case, the purpose of using dual data sets was not to attempt triangulation, but to use varied approaches to gain information on different levels of meaning.

Several other approaches have been trialed in combining qualitative and quantitative research (Cresswell, 1994). *Simultaneous triangulation* involves answering the quantitative and qualitative questions at the same time in the study and analysing them separately. *Sequential triangulation* involves alternating quantitative and qualitative data sets, and interweaving survey questionnaires and experimental designs with qualitative data. Again, separate analysis occurs. Sequential triangulation aims to document convergent findings that provide the study with elaboration or extension. Another as yet untried, iterative approach to dual data collection is one in which the researcher sets up separate quantitative and qualitative designs for the same project and moves from one technique to the other, clarifying findings progressively.

This approach shares similarities with one tried in the exploration of conditions affecting depression among Afro-Americans in a southern United States community (Dressler, 1991). Open-ended ethnographic interviews were used to collect data initially. The results were used to construct quantifiable survey instruments. Analysis of these was followed by the collection of life histories and case studies to aid interpretation of the quantitative results.

Current situation

Recent changes indicate that in some countries there is now greater acceptance of qualitative approaches as stand-alone techniques of data collection. Institutions that control funding for medical research have attempted to develop ethical guidelines for the assessment of qualitative research projects (see Australian Health Ethics Committee, 1996). On the one hand, this indicates an acceptance of this form of research within an area previously almost totally dominated by scientific methods. On the other, it highlights the powerful position held by medicine in attempting to control guidelines and to define and limit the boundaries of what is, in effect, a dynamic research approach. Regardless of these potential limitations, the development of ethical guidelines would appear to be a major step forward in legitimising qualitative research as an epistemologically based and separate approach, as opposed to its less legitimate position of 'end-on' tokenism to quantitative approaches seen in previous times.

In addition to the quantitative versus qualitative debates, the demands of 'uncertainty', 'chaos', 'postmodernism' and 'poststructuralism' have served to undermine many previously accepted assumptions in the search for 'truth', and have further complicated current debates.

Uncertainty

Around 500 BC, Aristotle asserted that any examination of natural events was futile because the act of human interference produced distorted results. Physicist Henri

Poincaré pointed to a similar problem at the turn of the twentieth century. He observed that the minutest change in the initial conditions of an experiment could produce very great differences in the final outcome, making accurate prediction impossible. In 1926 another physicist, Werner Heisenberg, added his *Principle of Uncertainty* to Aristotle and Poincaré's views.

Heisenberg's uncertainty principle

Heisenberg warned that the act of measurement disturbs the object that is being measured, causing a different action to that which existed prior to measurement. He derived this conclusion from his attempts to accurately measure subatomic particles with the aim of predicting their future positions and velocity. A certain amount of light was required to determine a particle's position. This light disturbed the particle, changing its velocity so that neither speed nor position could be measured accurately. In view of this, it can be argued that greater accuracy in the control and measurement of one variable tends to lessen the accuracy in the control and measurement of other variables. This, in turn, tends to lessen the accuracy of prediction regarding aspects of the object being examined.

When developing quantum mechanics based on the uncertainty principle, Heisenberg later indicated that the *quantum state* (a combination of position and velocity) could only produce, at best, several approximate outcomes rather than a single predictable one. This uncertainty questions the possibility of accurate predictions based on measurement, and confronts scientific determinism as applied to social, and some physical, phenomena.

Hawthorne experiments

Seven experimental projects carried out between 1924 and 1932 at the Western Electric Company in Hawthorne, Chicago (Roethlisberger and Dickson, 1964) further substantiated 'uncertainty'. The purpose of this research was to trial the impact of certain changes on worker productivity. These changes included variations in illumination, supervisory styles and working conditions. The two independent variables were:

*   pauses for rest; and
*   the duration of working hours.

Results indicated that, regardless of manipulation of the independent variables over time, there was a persistent and continuing increase in the productivity of the small groups of workers being tested. These increases appeared to bear no direct or measurable relation to the independent variables.

Various analyses of these experiments (Parons, 1974) have attempted to locate extraneous variables that could have produced this result. It has been suggested that any one of the following may have been the culprit:

- the improved working conditions of the experimental group, including a better-lit environment;
- five rather than 100 workers;
- a sympathetic rather than an autocratic foreman;
- freedom to talk during worktime;
- rests or half-days off; or
- that greater motivation was achieved by working as a small cohesive group on a piecework basis, where improved productivity would result in higher salaries.

Many researchers prefer to reject these suggestions in favour of the conclusion that the Hawthorne experiments demonstrate one of two things:

- the effect of intruding an experimental situation into an environment; or
- that the experiment itself—the effect of being part of a select team, 'on show' in a special environment—facilitated the increased output.

This research not only cast further doubt on the predictive capabilities of empirical data, but also pinpointed the problem of *reductionism*, in which a higher order phenomenon is explained in terms of a lower order phenomenon. The rigid control of a limited number of variables made it difficult to assess or explain the multiplicity of other variables that may have been impacting on the situation and therefore affecting the measuring of human behaviour.

Fuzzy logic

The view of variables as precise all-inclusive concepts has also been challenged by the advent of *'fuzzy set'* theory (Zimmerman, Zadeh and Gaines, 1984; Zimmerman, 1991). This is a mathematical approach based on the theory of *graded concepts*, in which everything is perceived as a matter of degree. *Fuzzy logic* focuses on the concept of a linguistic variable and its application to approximate reasoning. This approach recognises that phenomena are rarely just black or white, but are complex, having different degrees of membership in a number of sets. This membership may also vary.

A colour, for example, may appear to have aspects of red, orange, purple or black in different contexts.

This approach has links with the concept of *possibility* rather than probability. It is used when the complexity of a system means that precision and significance will tend to become mutually exclusive, making the use of probability inappropriate. Fuzzy logic has been used in artificial intelligence, decision theory and the management of uncertainty in expert systems. It has also been used to program washing machines to judge the degree of dirt and the quantity and type of clothes, so that the machine can automatically select the best water level and washing cycle.

Chaos

More recently, the theoretical physics notion of chaotic boundaries to the universe has had implications for researchers attempting to impose orderly explanations on such disorderly phenomena as human beings.

Patton (1990) has derived several implications for qualitative inquiry from *chaos theory*, including the proposition (extended from uncertainty) that once the researcher enters a setting he/she may change it forever. Other implications are that:

- Minute and seemingly unconnected events may make a critical difference to (much later) outcomes.
- No concepts are value neutral.
- We must learn to appreciate disorder as a normal state without attempting to pattern it into orderly categories.

Further indications from models of chaotic simulation confirm that:

- Predictability and determinism, previously viewed as synonymous, are no longer linked.
- Chaotic systems are not entirely made up of chaotic elements.
- Chaotic systems are complex, interdependent and diverse.

Predictability and determinism

Experiments show that sensitive dependence on initial conditions (for example, the *Butterfly Effect*) may provoke instability, leading to a multiplicity of unpredictable outcomes. Small differences in input may very rapidly become large differences in output, as is shown by our inability to predict weather patterns beyond the short term.

This tendency also means that generalisability is not possible. No matter how close you get to reproducing the initial conditions of an experiment, replication of outcomes may not occur. Similarly, unpredictability and indeterminism are not linked, and uniqueness of existence and incompatibility are not necessarily antagonistic.

Chaotic systems: elements

Order and disorder can coexist. Fluctuation, interaction and change can create order out of disorder and vice versa in an ad hoc manner. The Lorenz Attractor, which shows the geometric regularity of an orderly pattern of concentric circles evolving from three continuously changing variables, is the perfect example of order within disorder. Pendulum desk toys, which create stable and unstable patterns in a creative and unpredictable manner, are examples of the order–disorder continuum.

Chaotic systems: complexity

Change is continuous and discontinuous, evolutionary and revolutionary, ordered and disordered. The greater the complexity, the greater the potential diversity. All of this information must be considered when applying chaos theory to people. This application involves an acceptance of individual behaviour as erratic, group behaviour as unpredictable, and the link between internal dialogue, values, beliefs, emotions, external pressures and action as both existent and non-existent.

Mathematical models of chaos (Thompson, Thompson and Hocking, 1992) were applied to three years of a telecommunications industry's occupational accidents, which consisted of 30 000 incidents. Researchers found little or no indication of relevant variables or causal factors for the intensity, frequency and severity of accidents, age or sex of participants, work activity, accident type or time of day. They concluded that, although some underlying deterministic factors were noted but not identified, simple two-dimensional modelling could be used only to make qualified short-term predictions. They also suggested that a system in a chaotic state is likely to be more resilient to change and random shocks (Hocking and Thompson, 1992), and might therefore have lower accident costs than an environment that is continually being forced into an inherently unstable state of equilibrium.

Postmodernism and poststructuralism

Reflections of 'chaos' can be observed in postmodern and poststructural theories. 'Truth' is again questioned as discussion centres on the assertions that:

- There is no single 'reality' or universal 'truth' for any situation.
- Objectivity is impossible, and measurable 'reality' can only exist at the simple short term level; therefore only subjectivity has value.
- Language cannot represent 'reality', although it has been used to control it with labels and categories.
- Influences on the construction of behaviour, expression and understanding are located in discursive practices that lie within larger historical and theoretical discourses, originally imposed to maintain individual or group power.

Contradiction, multiplicity of perspectives and deconstruction—which involves searching back through the discourses to unravel the history, power and knowledge bases, and biases of particular 'truths'—dominate postmodern and poststructural thought. They have far-reaching implications for research.

Changes over the last century have been quite dramatic. Theories of relativity, uncertainty and chaos, as well as postmodern and poststructural positions, have challenged the basic principles of classical science. This questioning has served to highlight qualitative approaches and to position them so that the importance of their contribution to the identification and location of 'truth' in social research has gained greater acceptance.

Summary

This chapter has presented a brief history of the qualitative–quantitative research debates in an attempt to provide the reader with enough background information to enable her/him to formulate some answers to the question, 'What is qualitative research?' The following summary pulls the main points together as a lead-in to the next chapter, which deals with the use of theoretical/conceptual frameworks in the qualitative research process.

Qualitative research has generally been approached from either a methods-based (techniques) or paradigmatic (with methodological implications) perspective. Both approaches have limitations. Researcher position has also differed, from 'objective', in which 'reality' is viewed as being 'out there', to 'interactive', in which the dominant view is one of joint construction of social meaning.

Qualitative research is also dynamic. It is generally library, field or action based. It has been used in the health area to examine intention, social construction and meaning in cultures, phenomena, structural processes and historical changes, using the techniques of interviewing, observation and document analysis.

The principle of 'uncertainty', the theories of 'chaos', postmodernism and poststructuralism, and the compatibility of quantitative and qualitative data, are issues that impact on all research. These issues have served to question scientific approaches. They have also illuminated qualitative research's capacity to provide important insights into different perceptions of 'reality' in the search for 'truth' in social research.

Further readings

General

Bell, C. and Encel, S. (1990) *Inside the Whale*. Sydney: Pergamon Press.

Burgess, R. (ed.) (1988) *Conducting Qualitative Research*. Studies in Qualitative Methodology, 1. London: JAI Press.

——(1990) *Reflections on Field Experience*. Studies in Qualitative Methodology, 2. London: JAI Press.

——(1992) *Learning About Fieldwork*. Studies in Qualitative Methodology, 3. London: JAI Press.

——(1994)*Analysing Qualitative Data: Experiences and Issues Regarding (Ethnographic) Research*. Studies in Qualitative Methodology, 4. London: JAI Press.

——(1995) *Computing and Qualitative Research*. Studies in Qualitative Methodology, 5. Greenwich: JAI Press.

Denzin, N. (1989) *The Research Act: A Theoretical Introduction to Sociological Methods*, 3rd edition. New Jersey: Prentice Hall.

Denzin, N. and Lincoln, Y. (1994) *Handbook of Qualitative Research*. California: Sage.

Gleick, J. (1988) *Chaos: Making a New Science*. London: Heineman.

Hawking, S. (1988) *A Brief History of Time: From Big Bang to Black Holes*. London: Bantam.

Lincoln, Y. and Guba, E. (1985) *Naturalistic Inquiry*. California: Sage. (Chapter 1 provides an extensive discussion on paradigms: the pre positivist, the positivist and the post positivist eras. In addition to this, Egon Guba's 1990 text *The Paradigm Dialog* and Section 1 of Denzin and Lincoln's 1994 text (above) are essential reading for the debate on the paradigming of theoretical perspectives.)

Roethlisberger, F. and Dickson, W. (1964) *Management and the Worker: An Account of a Research Program Conducted by the Western Electric Company, Hawthorne Works, Chicago*. Cambridge: Harvard.

Quantitative versus qualitative

Brannen, J. (1992) Combining qualitative and quantitative methods: an overview, in J. Brannen (ed.), *Mixing Methods: Qualitative and Quantitative Research*, pp. 3–38. Brookfield: Avebury.

Cresswell, J. (1994) *Research Design: Qualitative and Quantitative Approaches*. California: Sage.

Silverman, D. (ed.) (1997) *Qualitative Research: Theory, Method and Practice*. London: Sage.

2 Theory in research: approaches to the use of theoretical perspectives

This chapter examines various approaches to the use of theoretical/conceptual frameworks in qualitative research. It is necessary to answer some key questions relating to research and theory before examining these frameworks, to ensure that they are understood within the overall research context. The first question that needs an answer is:

What is theory, and why is it necessary?

Several smaller questions make up this large question. The first of these, which is very important in qualitative research, is: 'When does a piece of work warrant the label "research"?'

Again, by seeking the answers to smaller questions within this, we should reach a suitable answer. We must also ask: 'Is it sufficient to elicit the opinions of a few key people regarding a particular issue, and to consolidate and interpret their responses from the researcher's perspective? What about the collection and display of one person's life history in their own words, or the administration of a questionnaire and the collation and display of responses to a particular issue?'

If such undertakings are to merit the label *research*, they must meet the following requirements:

- Data collection of some description must occur.
- Some form of framework derived from an/some identifiable theoretical tradition/s must also be present.
- Collected data must be placed within this framework/s for analysis and interpretation.

Simply collecting and presenting data without identifying the framework within which the design, collection and interpretation have occurred will attract the criticism that the researcher is confirming her/his own unexplained biases. Even when biases are explained, the outcome runs the risk of attaining the Monty Pythonesque position in which one's own limited perceptions provide a narrow interpretation of events: 'This is my theory and it's my very own'.

Having established the necessity for some form of theoretical underpinning, it is time to answer the larger question 'What is theory?' The *Shorter Oxford English Dictionary* (1973, p. 2281) defines theory as 'a scheme or system of ideas or statements which has been held as an explanation or account of a group of facts or phenomena'.

In more detail, *theory* is derived from the exploration of phenomena, the identification of, and interrelationships between, concepts surrounding phenomena and the subsequent development of a framework within which some comments can be made.

Levels of theory

There are three levels of theory:

- micro;
- middle range; and
- grand.

Micro theory

Micro theory consists of a set of hypothetical theoretical statements about narrowly defined phenomena. These statements are derived from interpretations of interrelated concepts. Some would argue that micro theory is not legitimate theory in its own right, but simply a set of propositions, models or hypotheses providing the basic building blocks of theory.

Middle range theory

Middle range theory is used to guide inquiries regarding limited aspects of social organisation and action. It is characterised by the inclusion of:

- concepts such as status, role, power and socialisation;
- variables of substantial size and cohesiveness, such as sex or class; and
- statements that derive from a combination of concepts and variables.

Middle range theory develops an overarching position through considerable research at the micro level. The germ theory of disease provides a good example. This position can be tested empirically, yet is sufficiently general to be applicable to a range of phenomena. Concepts are operationalised, but the ultimate result is the production of statements of empirical regularity, or propositions that then require grand theories to explain them.

Grand theory

Grand theory is a comprehensive approach involving the production of explanations for uniformity of social behaviour, social organisation and social change (Merton, 1968, chapter 2). Grand theories are counterintuitive. They give a new slant, make sense of puzzling aspects of existence, and generate new ways of thinking and interpreting (Giddens, 1993, p. 729). Grand theories comprise definitions, concepts, variables, statements and, very importantly, theoretical formats that address issues, theoretical strategies and various analytical forms of classification. These forms of classification consist of two parts: *propositional formats*, which link variables, and *modelling schemas*, which clarify the issues that individual theories must address.

Grand theory is characterised by abstractness and wide applicability. Karl Marx's (1971 [1893–4]) theory of social stratification and economic organisation is a well-known grand theory. It can be used to examine all economies based in capitalism. (Capitalism is a formal class-based economic system in which those possessing capital use it to control the production of goods and services for profit.)

Theoretical/conceptual approaches

There is considerable variety in the manner in which theoretical/conceptual frameworks can be used when undertaking research. The view that qualitative research is dynamic means that particular approaches are not static. Any researcher adopting and adapting these, then publishing the outcomes in peer-refereed journals, can add to the possible interpretations of a particular approach and its theoretical/conceptual underpinnings.

The basic aim of qualitative research is to gain a thorough understanding of particular phenomena within certain contexts. The design undertaken will depend on the question to be explored and will be strongly or lightly influenced by the chosen theoretical underpinnings. If the research is theory/concept driven, for example, the influence on question focus, design and interpretation will tend to be considerably stronger than if minimal underpinnings are being used to encourage uncontaminated themes to emerge from the data.

Four broad approaches have been chosen to clarify the range of possibilities within qualitative research:

- theory/concept-driven;
- theory/concept-generating;
- postmodern/poststructural; and
- feminist.

The latter is not generally recognised as a theoretical approach in its own right, but I am including it here for its important contribution to qualitative research processes. All four approaches will be discussed in relation to different theorists and health research projects.

Theory/concept-driven and theory/concept-generating research

Theory/concept-driven research

The researcher who uses the theory/concept-driven approach needs to familiarise him/herself with the theorist/s whose views seem most relevant to the research topic. If the topic involves the medical profession's increasing control over definitions of health and illness, Michel Foucault's (1971, 1973) views on the surveillance of bodies in the construction of 'normality' may be one starting point. Karl Marx's (1971 [1893–4]) views on profitable industries under capitalism may be another. If the research topic is concerned with changes in health delivery, Max Weber's (1966) discussion of bureaucracy and the concepts of economic rationalism and resource allocation may be relevant. Drawing out implications for the research topic and refining the study's major questions follow this critical exploration of the chosen theoretical perspectives. As the investigations proceed, the emergent findings are compared with these theoretical and conceptual positions. A critical debate as to their capacity to illuminate the research question should then ensue.

Theory/concept-generating research

The theory/concept-generating approach generally draws on perspectives from the interpretativist/interactionist position, adopted by theorists such as Max Weber,

George Mead, Erving Goffman and Jürgen Habermas. Arguments and concepts from a range of other theorists are also often used. The researcher's initial intention is either to explore an area where minimal research has been undertaken, or to conduct an in-depth exploration of a particular aspect of a topic. She/he must avoid the trap of allowing previous researchers' and theorists' ideas to dominate the study's design, analysis and interpretation. This can be achieved by undertaking the initial literature review very lightly, merely to alert the researcher to previous outcomes, or by not undertaking it at all. The idea is that the researcher enters the field without overdirection, enabling her/him to see the evolving issues more clearly.

The major problem with this approach is that the researcher may simply reiterate his/her biases. The researcher needs a sound knowledge of both the area under investigation and the possible theoretical or conceptual frameworks that may impinge on it, if he/she is to carry out effective theory/concept-generating research. This solid background knowledge need do no more than lightly underpin the design. Its major contribution is to make the researcher aware of areas that need careful consideration.

There are specific guidelines as to how some theory/concept-generating approaches should be undertaken. *Grounded theory* is one example, in which a rigorous process of coding and theoretical memo development occurs from the start of data collection. A constant comparative process of movement between grounded data and existing theoretical/conceptual frameworks is undertaken to shed light on the situation under observation. The final discussion, however, should be a critical dialogue between the data, the emergent theoretical propositions and relevant theoretical/conceptual frameworks.

The major types of theory/concept-generating research are:

- ethnography;
- phenomenology;
- grounded theory;
- memory work;
- historical research;
- evaluation; and
- action research.

These are discussed in more detail in Chapter 7.

Approaches used in health research

Health researchers have adopted and adapted theory/concept-driven and theory/concept-generating research approaches drawing primarily on the ideas of eight theorists, namely: Karl Marx, Emile Durkheim, Talcott Parsons, Michel Foucault, George Mead, Erving Goffman, Max Weber and Jürgen Habermas. Although these theorists come from the disciplines of sociology, history, philosophy and psychology, they have all presented ideas that are relevant to health research.

Focus on social controls: Marx, Durkheim, Parsons and Foucault

Marx, Durkheim, Parsons and Foucault have focused on those societal structural organisations that facilitate harmonious coexistence and system equilibrium by enforcing patterns of thinking and behaviour. Karl Marx is perhaps the best known of these theorists.

Marx (1818–83)

Karl Marx saw all social activity as being influenced by the basic needs of food, shelter and clothing. Social change was therefore prompted by issues relating to these needs and fuelled by conflict among interest groups in the struggle for power and control. Marx (1971 [1893, 1894]) examined *social stratification* (the hierarchical structures of society) from an economic perspective, in which social relationships were based on work or production modes. Societies were viewed as having two levels: the *infrastructure*, which formed the economic base; and the *superstructure*, with its institutional overlays of law, medicine and religion, which motivated and directed people towards 'work' as an ideal. A two-class system was also seen to exist, where *class* was defined as a group of people sharing the same relationship to the means of production. The dominant class (the bourgeoisie) controlled or privately owned the means of production in a market-regulated system. The workers (working class/*proletariat*) owned only their labour, which they sold in exchange for wages. Exploitation of the proletariat formed the basis of this relationship. The term *alienation* was used to describe involvement in work over which workers had no control. Poor health, high levels of injury, industrial pollution and minimal quality control of products could be expected within this system.

Some workers showed individual resistance to such an oppressive system by adopting stigmatised or marginal identities, which minimised their labour contribution, or by developing the skills and knowledge that enabled them to confront the system. Marx predicted that once the proletariat developed class consciousness/group awareness of their exploitation, and the internal conflicts of their position became *manifest* (obvious) rather than *latent* (hidden), they would rise up, take collective action, overthrow the bourgeoisie and redistribute resources to create a classless (*communist*) society. This form of *competitive capitalism* was particularly applicable to the nineteenth-century industrialised society.

Economic systems have undergone a more recent change to a system that neo-Marxists label *monopoly capitalism*. Ownership and control of capital have become separate activities. A new group, the managerial class, has emerged to control production. Other changes include greater class mobility, the move towards a common culture, and the intervention of the state in providing the infrastructure for creating and maintaining a healthy workforce. Health services, education, workplace legislation, wage control, taxation to fund social services and price controls are examples of this. There is some debate as to the 'true' aims of these interventions. Have they been implemented solely to support the bourgeoisie's efforts to maximise profits, or are they an attempt at genuine social reconstruction and protection of the proletariat?

Writers have pointed to a new development following the neo-Marxists. This is the rise of the 'service class', a group that provides social and health services. Carl Offe (1985) states that this group responds to changing system needs within the capitalist framework. Areas affected include child care, aged care and home nursing, services that were previously supplied by families. The 'service class' also facilitates the transfer of surplus labour by providing new areas of work. The growing numbers within this sector are predicted to produce their own pressure for survival and expansion.

Implications for health research

This brief overview of Marxist approaches indicates a number of implications for health research, in particular that:

- The capitalist system is exploitative, creating particular ills for which other exploitative subsystems, such as health, become necessary (Renaud, 1975).

- The delivery of the health system is shaped by profit requirements (Navarro, 1976).
- Doctors acquire wealth within this system through a range of sources, such as overservicing, the overuse of medical technology and the establishment of private hospitals.
- Doctors' position of control in a hierarchical division of health labour (Willis, 1989; Wearing, 1996) has enabled the medicalisation of such social events as birthing and dying (Mishler, 1984), and control of certain knowledge bases, diagnoses, drugs, certificates and reports regarding workplace injury. These latter tend to target the 'careless worker' rather than poor working conditions, enabling employers to extract the maximum profit (Zola, 1978; Waitzkin, 1981).
- The further down the class hierarchy individuals are, the less access they will have to power and control. Combined with poor nutrition, breakdown of social relationships and 'alienation', this will ensure a lower standard of health (Navarro, 1976; Turner, 1984; McKeown, 1988; Burdess, 1996).

Criticisms

Marxist positions have been criticised for failing to recognise individual and group action taken against the 'capitalist system'. Consumers, trade unions and professional organisations have all worked to counternegotiate aspects of the capitalist health system.

A second criticism is the Marxists' failure to recognise different forms of capitalism and their particular political (O'Connor, 1977) and socio-cultural (Habermas, 1976) factors.

Durkheim (1858–1917)

Emile Durkheim emphasised *structural controls*, seeing individuals responding to social constraints and changes within a *cause–effect* type of framework. He also saw these individuals as complex beings in a state of *tension*, caught between two orientations. On the one hand, they were individual and distinct organisms; on the other, they were social beings. This tension was viewed as problematic and volatile. Durkheim focused on what he termed the *collective consciousness* when looking for ways by which individuals became social beings. He saw 'collective consciousness' as existing within and beyond human beings. Its role was to promote a properly functioning society through constraining human action, and regulating desires by confining them to socially acceptable purposes.

The social disintegration that accompanied the industrial revolution influenced Durkheim's ideas. He took particular interest in people's separation from their small-town geographic origins and their consequent separation from the values, norms, expected behaviours and support systems previously reinforced by stable kin and friendship groups. His work on suicide, published in 1897, described his attempts to correlate actual incidents of suicide with demographic factors such as age, sex, family background and religion. He found that Protestants were more likely than Catholics to commit suicide—not entirely surprising, because Catholics regard suicide as a sin—and that unmarried men and people without families were the most likely to commit suicide.

Durkheim noted four contradictory *structural/moral forces* that he saw impacting upon individuals and thereby determining outcomes. These were:

- *egoism*, where society is not cohesive enough to influence all its members, resulting in considerable autonomy;
- *anomie*, where there is insufficient collective force among social groups, resulting in some individuals experiencing isolation, aimlessness and uncertainty during periods of economic and social change;
- *altruism*, when society is too highly integrated and individuals are overcontrolled, so that their goals become separate from themselves and are dictated to them by religious, political and social institutions; and
- *fatalism*, or extreme regulation, where the repressed individual looses all power to act independently.

Durkheim believed that individuals could be completely healthy only when a *balance* existed among these four forces. This balance occurs when people are attached to social goals but not so committed to them that personal autonomy is lost, and when there are sufficient social controls and supports in times of change to prevent people from becoming isolated.

In relation to health, an excess of egoism can be a source of stress. If balanced with altruism, however, harmony will occur. Excessive altruism plus fatalism, unbalanced by other aspects, can remove any desire for survival from the collective consciousness. This may happen as a result of religious or cult ceremonies, for example.

Criticisms

Steven Lukes (1985) and Steve Taylor and Clive Ashworth (1987) provide detailed critical analyses of Durkheim's views. These authors take issue with the notions of causality, motivation, collective consciousness and the limited generalisability of models that were heavily influenced by the upheaval of the industrial revolution. Despite this, researchers have used Durkheim's work to support links between suicide and social isolation, depression, low self-esteem, minimal resources and the lack of support groups, in the contexts of family and economic breakdown (Brown and Harris, 1978; Hassan, 1983).

Parsons (1902–79)

Talcott Parsons viewed society as comprising four systems:

- *cultural* (knowledge);
- *social* (roles and positions);
- *personality* (beliefs, feelings); and
- *physiological* (organic body).

Parsons (1951) saw society's needs as being fulfilled *externally* by economic production and political power, and integrated *internally* by social control (both legal and medical) and mechanisms of socialisation. These *mechanisms of socialisation* include the processes of becoming social through conforming to social norms, taking appropriate roles in one's society and ensuring the transmission of culture between generations.

Parsons (1978) saw illness as one area where individual action required particular control if societal equilibrium was to be maintained. Illness was viewed as both organic and socio-cultural, resulting from the following factors:

- bacterial invasion and the body's inability to cope;
- internal pathological processes, such as tumours; or
- a breakdown of an individual's capacity or desire to conform to the expectations of society by staying healthy (Parsons, 1978, pp. 69–70).

Sick role

The last of these points encompassed Parsons' (1978) particular concern for the individual's capacity for consciously or unconsciously motivated illness, which was viewed as a form of deviance. An important factor in maintaining a stable society was the condition that the sick role was only entered under legitimate circumstances.

Uta Gerhardt's (1989) work led to the perception that ill people occupied one of two groups: those experiencing 'incapacity' or those experiencing 'deviance' (something viewed as beyond the norm for a particular culture). *Incapacity* was viewed as a failure to keep well, resulting in the negative achievements of passivity, dependence and emotional disturbance. The sick role provided a niche where those experiencing incapacity could withdraw and recuperate with the help of the medical profession. Those experiencing *deviance* were seen as being motivated towards a positive achievement of ill health, via regression, to an emotional state of dependency resembling that of early childhood. The predisposition to illness through accident or psychosomatic disorder that is noted in the deviance model is thought to be linked to the stress caused by too rapid change, such as industrialisation, urbanisation, technologisation and computerisation.

Rights and obligations

Whatever the pathway, the sick role involves certain reciprocal rights and obligations to which patients and health personnel must conform. The patients' rights include the right to legitimately withdraw from work and family responsibilities without loss of salary or position, and the right to receive no blame for suffering illness. Patients' obligations are to seek and follow professional advice and to recover as quickly as possible. The health professionals' obligations are to place the patient/client's welfare above all else and to use the highest standards of professional care. Cooperation, trust, and access to the (sick) body and complete information are necessary precursors to proper professional care. Health professionals have a right to these essential elements in fulfilling their obligations.

Criticisms of the sick role

The concept of the sick role has been criticised for overemphasising conformity (Wrong, 1961) and for failing to acknowledge the individual's capacity to resist societal expectations (Garfinkel, 1967), as illustrated by patients and staff constantly bending institutional rules, thereby creating new social arrangements. The sick role also concentrates on social reproduction rather than social production (Giddens, 1976), because in reality consultation with health professionals is far from automatic (Scambler, 1987; Zola, 1978). When this does occur, drug compliance is only 50 per cent (Walton, 1980). Issues of power, hierarchy or the status of patients within public and private systems (Cartwright and O'Brien, 1976) are not taken into account by Parsons' ideal portrayal of health professional–patient relations. There is no acknowledgment of the dominance of doctors' material interests (Merton, 1968), and inadequate discussion of issues of personality and emotional involvement in the exchange. The sick role has also been challenged on the grounds that it is applicable only to short term acute illness. Parsons (1978) has countered this by arguing that the same processes apply to chronic illness and, although the outcome is not recovery, drugs can minimise symptoms and enable some participation in mainstream society.

Relevance for health research

Parsons' (1951, 1978) work has particular relevance for current health research, both through the concept of the sick role and in areas where medical authorities have the power to define patients' symptoms as genuine or otherwise, in order to control access to compensation or insurance payouts.

Foucault (1926–84)

Michel Foucault was interested in tracing the historical links between knowledge and power, and what he perceived to be the increasing global and individual *surveillance and control* of bodies by medical institutions and clinical personnel. He viewed society as comprising three forms of power:

- *sovereign power* (monarchy, law, justice);
- *disciplinary power*, which filtered out via the arteries of major institutions (medicine, for example) into the capillaries of all levels of society; and
- *bio-power* (using the control of bodies to regulate behaviour).

Sovereign power

Foucault saw sovereign power as absolute power that comes from the monarchy and is implemented through the judicial system of law. There have been four historical types of sovereign power:

- the feudal monarchy;
- the large scale administrative monarchy;
- the court system that reinforces royal power; and
- parliamentary democracy (Foucault, 1980, p. 103).

Sovereign power operates to maintain a stratified class system with the monarchy as head. The court system, as well as individuals at all levels, network and allow the circulation of power via the consolidation of ideology. Any moves by the public to set up or influence the current system are defused by incorporating them as part of the institutions of state. For example, some indigenous health and legal services started as independent organisations but became government funded. Following this, their activities became subject to monitoring and review, control and limitation.

Disciplinary power

Disciplinary power operates simultaneously with sovereign power, and is the means by which time and labour are extracted from peoples' bodies. It puts people under continual surveillance (monitoring or watching over) rather than inflicting ritual punishments through sovereign power. Prisons, hospitals, schools and workplaces all carry out surveillance. Foucault uses the metaphor of the Panopticon to explain the technique of disciplinary regulation. The Panopticon is a circular prison with a central watchtower where a watcher can observe all the cells. These cells have glass panels on both the inner and outer walls, allowing light through and making it impossible for prisoners to avoid the watcher's 'gaze'. The design also encourages prisoners and guards to 'gaze' upon each other. This structure has been used to demonstrate the potential for internalisation of modes of behaviour through continual surveillance of self and other, using peer evaluation and self-appraisal. These powerful surveillance 'technologies' are used to produce docile bodies and to maintain hierarchies of power. This process has been developed further by the advent of computer-processed information.

Bio-power

Foucault also highlighted bio-power as an important control tool. This focuses on the regulation of bodies as a means of regulating whole populations. He viewed doctors as medical surveillance agents, encroaching on patients' lives through the use of techniques such as body monitoring and 'confession'. *Confession*, in which doctors encourage patients to divulge ethically protected information, resembles the way priests gain information in the confessional. Medical 'confessions' often produce information that enables doctors to direct moral conduct as well as body function.

Normality

Health professionals' rituals of body monitoring also lead to the construction of beliefs regarding *normality* and *abnormality* (Foucault, 1971, 1973). These *discourses* (verbal and written explanations of implicit belief systems) of scientific knowledge become widely internalised through '*capillary action*'. Health professionals become conductors of powerful 'norms' that affect people's monitoring of themselves and others. Societal regulation of the wider population, through the development of state administrative structures such as clinics, hospitals and mental asylums, can then enforce this cyclical process of 'normalisation', leading to population control.

Derived assumptions

Foucault made two major assumptions from his explorations of knowledge and power. These related to the power of language and the 'clinical gaze'.

Foucault's (1980) first assumption was that knowledge is limited by what our *language* and its culturally associated discourses allow us to see. Medical terminology provides a good example: it limits views of illness to a particular scientific framework. Since we can only 'know' disease through language, what we define as a 'disease' is the outcome of a socio-historical process. The individual is hedged in by the discursive practices of specific fields of power. The discourse of 'medicine' is used to establish power relations and ritual processes of examination between health professional and client.

The second assumption was that medical power (the '*clinical gaze*') has allowed doctors to define 'reality', 'normality' and 'deviance', thus enforcing a 'norm' of action and behaviour (Foucault, 1973). People who fail to meet particular criteria of 'normality' are constrained by medication or institutionalised for processing or reprocessing. Doctors who use their medical power to pass judgement on their patients'/clients' 'normality', and treat them accordingly, become part of an extensive network of regulating agents who are particularly aligned with those who hold sovereign power, such as legal judges.

Criticisms

Foucault's work has been criticised for its inability to fully recognise creative, autonomous individuals who have the capacity to use counter discourses and negotiation to resist the health profession's authority. His work also fails to acknowledge the variety of attitudes and interactions within the health profession itself. Despite these concerns, Foucault provides a provocative analysis of the rise of medical control and its power to limit individual action.

Summary of Marx, Durkheim, Parsons and Foucault

Together with Marx, Durkheim and Parsons, Foucault has identified some of the structural, historical, economic, political and medical processes of control that ensure minimal deviation from the 'norm'. Their views have been criticised for excessive concentration on:

- processes that produce stability and order; and
- the maintenance of certain structures.

This has created difficulties in explaining situations of rapid change and autonomous action taken by groups of people.

Focus on the capacity for autonomous action: Mead, Goffman, Weber and Habermas

In contrast to Marx, Durkheim, Parsons and Foucault, theorists George Mead, Erving Goffman, Max Weber and Jürgen Habermas, whose ideas have been used in health debates, view societal institutions as historical, cultural entities that influence rather than direct action. They emphasise the belief that real power lies in the hands of people who undertake social action within particular contexts. These people are in a constant process of creating and recreating definitions and meanings during negotiation with institutional representatives. This constant creation and recreation lead to potentially unpredictable outcomes, dependent upon each participant's resources (relative power). Outcomes may, however, be dominated by the reproduction of existing scenarios.

Mead (1863–1931)

George Mead and Erving Goffman both viewed people as creative, autonomous beings who use interpersonal processes, such as socialising and the need to consider others' views, to provide a *balance* between maintaining stability of order and implementing change.

Mead made use of the 'I' and 'me' aspects in his writings. The 'I' is the innovative and creative aspect of self that responds to the attitudes of others. The 'me' aspect comprises 'the organised set of attitudes of others which one himself (sic) assumes'

(Mead, 1934, p. 175). *Self-awareness* occurs when we can distinguish 'I' from 'me'. Mead's emphasis here is on *social constraint*. An example of this in the health context is the way in which interaction between the patient/client and the health professional is viewed as a process of *reflexiveness* (Mead, 1934, p. 134). This process means that the patient/client is confronted with a '*societal reaction*', in which:

1   A professional diagnosis is made.
2   Significant others, such as family and friends, form their own interpretations of the diagnosis.
3   The client takes these responses into account within him/herself, and comes to see him/herself as others do.

Goffman (1922–83)

In more general contexts, Erving Goffman's ideas focus on the negotiation of order within *frames*, where participants arrive at a *working consensus* regarding their meeting. Interaction within institutional and societal frameworks is thus viewed as a fairly active *game* (Goffman, 1959, pp. 107–192). All roles involve situated performances that are 'played at' as well as 'played'. These performances may or may not be sincere. The games involve *strategies* with an emphasis on mutual assessment of moves, resources (information, power, eloquence), the operational code being used, style of play, resolve (how far will the other go), game worthiness and integrity (adherence to agreed upon interests). Assessment is made on the basis of verbal and non-verbal expressions 'given off' and 'communications transmitted' (Goffman, 1959, pp. 107–192).

Goffman assumed that people have many different aspects to their personalities and that these are revealed to different people at different times. His exploration of this aspect of *presentation of self* through the management of impressions emphasised the dramaturgical view of interaction, where actors perform as if on stage. Their motivation is to present themselves in as positive a light as possible, so that they fit into the current norms of society and thus avoid labels.

Stigma and labelling

Goffman's work on stigma clarified the effect on people of certain illness labels, particularly those such as leprosy, AIDS and mental illnesses, which mark people as socially unacceptable. Individuals experiencing certain illnesses often adopt coping strategies to avoid *stigma*. These include covering up symptoms, presenting themselves as being as close to the 'norm' as possible, and controlling information about, or avoiding discussion of, the condition.

Socially produced value judgements or labels (Becker, 1963) attached to certain health experiences have the capacity to marginalise people. Stigma is produced when powerful persons such as doctors apply labels to individuals. This stigma is continually emphasised in the interaction between the labelled person and others, to the point where the view of that person as socially deviant may become entrenched. This view has been accepted as a major aspect of mental illness (Scheff, 1966).

One particularly pertinent study in this area involved eight researchers attempting to discover what it was like to be a patient in a psychiatric institution (Rosenhan, 1973). The research team gained admission to 12 psychiatric institutions in five States on the east and west coasts of America. The only aspects of the researchers' life experiences that were falsified for this study were their names and occupations. Each person made an appointment at a different hospital, and all complained of the same symptoms. Each said that she/he was hearing voices, in particular the words 'hollow', 'empty' and 'thud'. All were admitted and all but one labelled 'schizophrenic'. The exception was diagnosed as suffering from 'manic-depressive psychosis'. Once the researchers were admitted to hospital, no further voices were heard and 'normal' behaviour was pursued. The length of hospitalisation ranged from seven to 52 days, with an average of 19. During this time, the researchers kept extensive notes of drug administration (over 2000 tablets) and interaction between staff and patients (minimal). This writing behaviour appeared in some of the false patients' clinical notes as 'pathological behaviour', but no staff detected the false patients, indicating the strength of medical labelling. In three settings, however, one-third of the real patients recognised the false patients as not being mentally disturbed. This research clearly illustrates the dangers of misdiagnosis and the power of labelling.

Criticisms

The concepts of 'labelling' and 'stigma' have been criticised on the grounds that:

- The judgements attached to labels are subject to change over time, causing variations in the level of stigma.
- The process of labelling implies a passive recipient or victim, underplaying the active individual who has the capacity to counter its effects.

Goffman's (1961) work in a mental institution, in which he identified a distinct culture that had been developed by inmates to enable them to cope with their environment, is an example of the latter. Regardless of these criticisms, the concept of 'labelling' (and its associated 'stigma') does have significant relevance for the study of disability, ageing, and chronic physical and psychiatric illnesses.

Weber (1864–1920)

Max Weber also emphasised potentially powerful individuals but recognised that their existence was constrained by strong social structures such as class, status (education, occupation and lifestyle) and party (the groups in which one had membership).

Weber noted several types of *authority* within the social system of his time. Authority could be:

- *traditional* (based in habit);
- *affectual* (guided by emotion);
- *wertrational* (influenced by humanitarian values); or
- *zweckrational* (positivist, scientific, objective and cause–effect oriented).

Weber viewed these last two types as *rational*, while viewing traditional and affectual authority as *irrational*. Irrationality was linked to magic and alternative healing styles within the health context, but writers such as Ivan Illich (1977) included doctors' charismatic power in this category. Charisma here is seen as the power held by virtue of doctors' healing capacities. Illich criticised this godlike view of doctors. He noted that the medicalisation of illness had taken away people's capacity to believe that they could best cope with major life events such as birth, illness and death. Most people had been conditioned to assume that medical personnel are more expert in these areas.

Weber's experiences as a health service administrator during World War One influenced his view that institutions such as hospitals are best run by proper bureaucratic administration based on principles of rationality. He believed that systematic, measurable, impersonal and objective techniques, together with humanitarian ideals and democratic participation, provide stable management (Weber, 1966). He was particularly concerned at the move to 'efficient' economic, political and social management. He saw this resulting in two likely outcomes:

- Administrators would be reduced to inhuman automatons, promoting minimalist services and mediocre practice.

- Increasing bureaucratisation would affect all aspects of people's lives, and independent action would be constrained.

Criticisms

Weber has been criticised for his rather pessimistic predictions. His apparent lack of awareness of the potential for a clash between the two 'rational' types of authority, 'positivist' versus 'humanitarian', has also been criticised. This clash can be observed currently in hospitals. On one side, bureaucrats (positivists) enforce 'effective' and 'efficient' use of resources, in line with *economic rationalism* policies (the systematic maximisation of profit through bureaucratic means). On the other side, health professionals (humanitarians) battle against cutbacks, emphasising the need for *best care* practices based on humanitarian principles. Contemporary theorist Jürgen Habermas views this clash as one result of capitalism in crisis.

Habermas (1929–)

Jürgen Habermas is particularly interested in 'rationalisation', ideal communication, colonisation of the *lifeworld* by medical expertise and communication between health professionals and patients/clients. His 'lifeworld' is defined as the symbolic arena shared by members of a culture or community through the understandings, convictions and expectations achieved via the intersubjective (consensus among people) recognition of truth, sincerity, appropriateness and comprehensibility (undistorted communication). Habermas' exploration of *rationalisation* provides a focus on social action and emancipation, which sets people free by giving them the knowledge to challenge previous belief systems.

Rationalisation

Habermas' (1976) exploration of 'rationalisation' is based on his assertion that capitalism is in a state of crisis (*recession*). In a recession, *conflict* arises between the owners of capital, who want to make more profit, and the demands of the increasing numbers of people on social welfare. The government's role is to provide a suitable climate for the achievement of capital gain, while maintaining harmony in the wider population through provision of employment and support services. Governments have chosen 'rationalisation' as a means of supporting the capitalists. They have cut back social welfare payments and support services, effectively forcing people into the labour market in search of other sources of income. This abundance of labour in turn gives greater power to employers, resulting in punitive employment practices and greater conformity of behaviour of those who do gain jobs.

It has already been mentioned that one of the service sectors experiencing cutbacks is health. Strong health institutions, information, choices and legal recourse are all needed by the people if they are to create effective resistance to 'rationalisation'. Habermas implies, therefore, that the major challenge for governments lies in an attempt to create a proper *balance* between the needs of the system (which are negotiable) and the needs of people. He sees open (ideal) *communication* between governments and people as a necessary ingredient in achieving such a balance (Habermas, 1984).

Ideal communication

Habermas explores many forms of knowledge in his writings, including 'emancipatory knowledge' and its effects on the process of emancipation. '*Emancipatory knowledge*' (Habermas, 1984) involves reflection and awareness, which empower people to assert themselves and take control of their lives. In an ideal world, communication would involve spontaneous, unlimited discussion among free and equal people (agents).

Placed within the context of health, this ideal communication would result in much more open interaction between health professional and patient/client. The release of controlled knowledge and the resulting open debates would offer prospective patients/clients two options:

- treat themselves; or
- being fully informed and aware of all alternatives, decide to consult a professional.

Hierarchies of power would need to be removed to ensure debates that were status free, incorporating equality, justice and the best possible outcomes for all. One possible interpretation might incorporate an egalitarian round-table discussion involving the patient/client, nurses, doctors, physiotherapists or other appropriate health professionals (including those from alternative health areas), lawyers, social workers and representatives from the patient's/client's family and relevant community support groups. The purpose of this meeting would be to determine the best location and best form of treatment for a particular person's condition. This process of determination would require all participants to develop a critical analysis of the historical discourses (theories and arguments) that influence all aspects of current practice, including the evolution of diagnoses and treatments. Participants would use this knowledge to critically assess current practice in an attempt to provide themselves with the best possible information.

Colonisation of the 'lifeworld' by medical expertise

Habermas is particularly concerned that there are elements of our social structure and culture that deny individual freedom and growth by imposing unnecessary forms of social control. He views medical control as one such element. The development of expert systems such as medicine and law has removed whole areas from the control of the 'lifeworld'. Those who have gained power within these expert systems colonise the 'lifeworld' by replacing 'lifeworld' communication with other discourses (Habermas, 1970). Habermas suggests that this is the case with medical expertise.

One example is the relabelling of certain areas of women's health. 'Normal' events become 'illness' events, requiring medical intervention. Hospitalisation of birthing practices, increases in foetal monitoring, routine ultrasound monitoring and caesarean sections, routine hysterectomies for non-pathological conditions and the introduction of hormone replacement therapy (HRT) are some of the consequences of 'relabelling'.

The shifting of death from a home-based, family-centred event to an institutionalised scientific phenomenon is also an example of the colonisation of the 'lifeworld' by replacing its communication with medical discourses.

Communication between health professional and patient/client

Habermas (1970, 1984) sees three levels of validity claims within 'lifeworld' communication:

- *objective*, which involves treating events as being external to the mind, from a position supposedly free of bias and prejudice;
- *social*, in which events are viewed through the frame of one's cultural beliefs and practices; and
- *subjective*, in which things are viewed through one's own perspective.

Practitioners have allowed issues of power to limit patient access to objective (medical) knowledge. They have also used power-laden communicative techniques to downgrade social and subjective views and restrict patient behaviour.

This distorted communication has been used to facilitate the 'lifeworld' colonisation process, but in doing so it has created four areas of potential *conflict* within the parameters of health professional–patient/client interaction. These are:

- the patient's/client's view of the situation as 'normal' (part of their 'lifeworld'), compared with the health professional's view of it as pathological (medically oriented);
- the individual's 'lifeworld' knowledge versus medical knowledge;
- individual control of the situation versus control by a health professional; and
- limited/restricted communication where patients'/clients' questions are often ignored or labelled 'neurotic' (Graham and Oakley, 1981).

Criticisms

Habermas has been accused of idealism and naivety, particularly in relation to powerful vested interests, such as those of doctors. He has also been accused of overemphasising shared understanding, failing to take into account the fact that all interaction and communication are inherently distorted. Despite this, Habermas' theories of 'rationalisation', 'communication' and 'emancipation' have become key references in the health area.

Summary of Mead, Goffman, Weber and Habermas

Mead, Goffman, Weber and Habermas have been particularly useful in two areas. They have refocused attention on the potential autonomy and power of people, and indicated that processes of interaction may constrain an individual's view of self, especially when others' views and actions involve distorted communication, labelling and stigma.

Mead and Goffman's ideas have been criticised for the limitations of frameworks that view individuals largely in the process of constructing and reconstructing social arrangements. The obvious lack of equity in resources does not fit the assumption that all persons negotiate from a position of equality. Another criticism is that Mead and Goffman have not adequately explored history, constraining social institutions and power.

Weber, and more recently Habermas and Anthony Giddens (1987), have attempted to connect influential structures and active people in a more meaningful way. They have also recognised processes by which 'negotiation' in context, and 'emancipation', may lead to more equal outcomes.

These positions have limited themselves to a focus on individuals and social structures, while postmodern and poststructural approaches critique accepted 'truths', their history, and their current portrayals.

Postmodern/poststructural research

Postmodernism and poststructuralism share a common interest in the *representations* of social reality and the '*deconstruction*' of these representations. They do, however, differ in emphasis. Postmodernism explores issues of meaning within cultural contexts. It rejects modernity and values fragmentation and multiplicity, while poststructuralism limits its focus to linguistic matters, contesting the meanings of language. The process of 'deconstruction' is a method of analysis that pulls the text apart to reveal and critique its assumptions. A new text, with its biases recognised, should emerge.

Postmodernism

Postmodernism, which can be traced back to early this century, is a transitional movement, defined by what follows. It concentrates on culture, history and change within *all disciplines* (particular areas of study). This movement critiques the social foundations of modern thought. Jean Baudrillard and Jean François Lyotard are the two theorists most commonly associated with postmodernism. Other major contributors include Hans George Gadamer, Umberto Eco, Julia Kristeva and Luce Irigary. Important aspects of postmodernism involve reactions against past representations of 'reality', 'truth', time, space, history, scientific objectivity, politico-economic rationality and 'representation' (accepted, usual depictions of particular things). These reactions have resulted in:

- de-emphasising the subject;
- decentring the author (by focusing on the margins); and
- highlighting the text and the reader.

Other traits of postmodernism include:

- the rupture of identity;
- a focus on ambiguity and the proliferation of meanings; and
- an emphasis on many explanatory perspectives, rather than one.

Early postmodern developments can be seen in the discipline of architecture, with its emphasis on incorporating historical influences into present structures and exposing formerly hidden functions. The National Centre of Modern Art and Culture in Paris (Centre Georges Pompidou) is an example. This glass construction's internal spaces resemble those of Renaissance times. It has a magnificent Renaissance stairway featuring a tortured hand and arm on the banister, recalling memories of people being dragged off to the guillotine during the French Revolution. Exposed electric cables and pipes interrupt this historic splendour.

Literature, film and art provide examples of other developments, in particular self-reflexivity, subjectivity, uncertainty, ambiguity and multiplicity of perspectives.

John Fowles' writing technique in *The French Lieutenant's Woman* (1969) illustrates self-reflexivity, disruption and a focus on subjectivity in which the author's voice may appear in his/her own right within the text. Fowles enters the text and addresses the reader with his concerns regarding the story's characters and ending.

Many of Luis Bunuel's films (such as *La Fantome de la Liberté*, 1974) feature uncertainty and ambiguity, particularly when he juxtaposes and re-examines the concepts of freedom and detention, and practices that are socially accepted and those that are not. The reversal of feeding and eliminating processes is a good example of this. Here people sit on toilets around tables for social interaction, politely congratulating each other on their eliminatory capacities. When they want to eat, they retreat to toilet-sized cubicles and feed in private.

Akira Kurosawa (1950) uses a multiplicity of perspectives to illuminate the complexity of the location of 'truth' in the film *Rashomon*. Four witnesses to the same incident describe what they see. Each story is completely different, reflecting, refracting and distorting from different perspectives.

Carol Shields uses a similar but more complex scenario in her book *Mary Swann* (1990). The text is divided into five sections, four of which reveal the contextual environments and subsequent perspectives of four people whose lives have in some way fleetingly come in contact with that of Mary Swann, a long-dead poet. The four perspectives are juxtaposed, then amalgamated when all four people meet at a symposium. The character of the invisible Mary Swann is created from the four perspectives, which have in turn been created from secondary sources, fantasy relationships, non-existent biographical material, and insight gained by one of the people through a brief one-hour meeting with Mary before she died. Mary Swann's life, through the four people's actions in creating their own perspectives of it, becomes interwoven with theirs, and impacts on them in a significant way. In this instance, the reflection, refraction and distortion arising from each perspective impacts on the others when all four are brought face to face.

Baudrillard (1988) represents the more pessimistic end of the postmodern continuum, emphasising diversity, meaninglessness, the death of the subject, the impossibility of 'truth', redefinition and the endlessly dynamic nature of postmodernism.

Application to research

The postmodern researcher would reject *'meta-narratives'*. These are the grand theories that are presented as providing complete answers. She/he would approach a research topic with a particularly critical eye to her/his own biases and the socially constructed 'realities' she/he is about to investigate. Based on the assumption that 'truth' is multifaceted and in a state of constant transformation, a multiplicity of perspectives would be called upon to refract images from different aspects of the topic. Multiple voices would also be heard, including that of the researcher.

Contradictions

Pauline Rosenau (1992, p. 176) has pointed to some inherent contradictions within postmodernism:

- The discrediting of theory building is in itself a theoretical position.
- The reaction against reason, logic and rationality does not prevent postmodernists from utilising these tools for their own analysis, particularly in the form of deconstructive techniques.

She also sees contradictions within poststructuralism.

Poststructuralism

Poststructuralism emerged during the 1960s and 1970s. One aspect of it looks at the *structures and uses of language* by social agents. Theorists Claude Levi Strauss, Roland Barthes, Jacques Lacan and Umberto Eco have had the most influence on this aspect. The *deconstruction of language* and discourse, reflected in the work of Jacques Derrida and Michel Foucault, is another major aspect of poststructuralism. Language is seen as the place where social meanings are defined, constructed and contested.

Ferdinand de Saussure (1983 [1916]) developed early theories regarding language, which he equated with social reality. In de Saussure's theory, language was seen as an abstract system of *signs*. Each sign was made up of a written sound or image (*signifier*) and a concept or meaning (*signified*), which were connected. The word 'spring', for example, might trigger images of fields of daffodils or of mechanical springs, depending on the context. Meanings were created within the language's structure, not by the objects to which the words referred. Meaning was clarified by *differences* in concepts and other symbols. A 'blue' sky, for example, was understood in terms of its difference from a 'grey' sky.

Jacques Derrida (1982) questioned these apparently fixed meanings of signs. He asserted that they were not fixed: each sound or image (signifier) could appear in different *contexts*, providing a range of meanings (signifieds) that could be deconstructed to identify the *diversity of discourses* present, thus deferring any possibility of locating fixed meanings. The word 'homosexual' is a good example. This has shifted contextually from 'deviant' to 'sufferer of a chemical imbalance' to an extension of what is regarded as 'normal'. This discourse of a marginal group could be further located *within* the social structures and processes of particular systems (such as the medical system), *within* a discursive field. (*Discursive fields* consist of the relationships among language, institutions, subjectivity and power.) All dominant discourses were viewed as reflecting particular value structures and powerful interests. Individuals were seen as being shaped by these dominant discourses, which either supported or challenged the status quo.

Criticisms

Rosenau's (1992, p. 176) criticism of poststructuralism is that, like postmodernism, it is contradictory. Its focus on the marginal and the invisible indicates an internal value in an environment that has dispensed with valuing and prioritising (supposedly), while the focus on *intertextuality* (the play of texts upon each other) comes into conflict with the Derridan focus on the isolated text. The inconsistencies of which modernism and structuralism are accused thus appear acceptable within postmodernism and poststructuralism.

Implications and application of postmodernism and poststructuralism

Methodological implications

The methodological implications of postmodernism and poststructuralism are complex. In postmodernism, the researcher/author is decentred. The text, the participants and the reader are centred. Texts are dominated by small designs, personal experience, intuition, a focus on the margins, the display of narratives that have had minimal interpretation, and unique forms of representation. Prediction is no longer valued.

Theory building is unacceptable. Reflexivity, ambiguity and a rigorous and continual questioning of the text, without conclusions, are favoured.

Everything is defined as 'text' in poststructuralism. Intertextuality and the deconstruction of 'texts' are encouraged. The aim of this deconstruction is to reveal powerful discourses, hierarchies, presuppositions, deliberate omissions and polar opposites. Deconstruction and intertextuality are seen to enable *transformation*, which is the process of *becoming* (changing identity) and knowing how to write this as lived experience.

Application to health research

If these orientations were applied to health research, all aspects of the health system would become open for inspection. On the one hand, past 'realities' based in hierarchy, control of knowledge, institutionalised practice, economically rationalised health policy, and hospital-oriented rather than patient-oriented care and diagnostic and treatment regimes, which were all decided without community consultation, would be included in the negotiation of new 'realities'. These new 'realities' would emerge through processes of deconstruction and reconstruction of knowledge and policy; removal of status, power and hierarchy; and the construction of different, more egalitarian discourses. Institutions would be viewed as 'mythologies constituted discursively to serve particular interests of power, and contested by other interests of power' (Fox, 1993, p. 49). Following this, hospitals and health departments would be viewed as reactive and process-driven rather than as social systems with structures and goals. They would be seen as comprising self-referential discourses of 'illness', 'disease' and 'care'. These discourses could be viewed as having become inscribed on the bodies and minds of patients and the general community, to be countered by individual and group desires.

Postmodern or poststructural?

The difficulty in separating postmodernism from poststructuralism (culture and language being inextricably intertwined) is illustrated in the following example of 'poststructuralist' health research by Elizabeth Turnbull (1992). The research in question involved writing the recovery experiences of adult children of alcoholics in Al-Anon (Alcoholics Anonymous) meetings. The study's focus concerned transformation. The text emerged from the researcher's experiences of the intersubjectivity she inhabited (how she was positioned to observe change in both the group and herself) in her desire to write the quality of becoming. The result is a story about stories of becoming (changes in identity). The analysis of such data occurs within the interweaving of the stories presented in the Al-Anon meetings, the researcher's response to these, and the relevant theoretical positions.

Feminist research

Although the term 'feminist research' is often used, it enjoys considerable diversity of interpretation among the many feminisms and different versions of feminist thought (Tong, 1989; Olesen, 1994). Some insist that there are no particular methodological approaches (Reinharz, 1992) or theories that can be separated out as purely feminist, because feminists are diverse in their approaches. Others insist that there is a distinctiveness in the combined ways of seeing, knowing and being in the world of research carried out *on* women *by* feminists (Stanley and Wise, 1990).

Despite these differences, there are some fairly enduring *principles* that have become attached to feminist research. These include:

- a need to centre the social constructedness of gender;
- an acceptance that women are oppressed, although views of their responses to this oppression vary from total powerlessness to active verbal and other forms of interactive negotiation;
- a non-exploitative, hopefully egalitarian and emancipatory relationship between researcher and researched;
- an exposure of the researcher's position, emotions and values, how these affect her view of reality, and how this reality is managed in terms of the analysis and interpretation of the realities of the researched; and
- a presentation of research results that addresses issues of power, honesty and ownership.

Power relations

The focus on power relations, the unravelling of power and the avoidance of exploitative relationships have encouraged an emphasis on egalitarianism, equality, the insider view, friendships with participants (Oakley, 1981), caring (Gilligan, 1982), reciprocity, 'empowerment' and participatory action research. Some researchers have resorted to payment, the sharing of knowledge, or the provision of support beyond the study in an attempt to minimise differences. Others have attempted to develop empathy with participants by misrepresenting their positions (as researchers). Others still have insisted on the insider position as preferable in achieving and appreciating the experiences of those being researched. This involves some form of sameness of life experience, such as being of the same race or sexuality, or sharing the same experiences of oppression. Kirin Narayan (1993, p. 676) suggests that the insider–outsider debate should be abandoned because of the multiple subjectivities within which both researcher and researched move during and beyond the research process.

Feminist researchers also favour other techniques, such as a focus on oral and life histories, which records the experiences of women and presents them with minimal interpretation. The benefit to those researched is not always clear, nor is there any indication of how this gathering of their views will improve their lives or result in emancipatory changes. It may, however, avoid some exploitation.

Another approach is to include the research participants' names as co-researchers and to share any royalties. This can occur only when participant numbers are not large and issues of anonymity are irrelevant.

The decentring of the researcher is a further technique used to adjust power relations, but this approach will affect participants as well as the kind of data gathered. The assumption that removing the researcher from centre stage will reduce the power equation is flawed. It does not allow for the impact of the multiple reflexivities, realities and selves of both researcher and researched in an interactive process where the location of dominance shifts and is in a constant state of change. An exploration of the impact of breast cancer on a group of women (Kasper, 1994) provides a good example of successful decentring. The researcher listened and avoided asking questions. Only issues raised by the women were discussed, thus allowing them to define what the researcher should analyse and interpret.

Empowerment

The outcome of *empowerment* is also problematic, however desirable it may seem in intention. What does 'empowerment' mean? What does 'empowerment' look like? To whom does it mean this or look like that, and why? The term 'empowerment' has condescending overtones similar to those of 'consciousness raising'. Both terms imply that individuals or groups operate at a lower level than the researcher, who takes it upon her/himself to liberate them. Seen in this light, the researcher's position is similar to that of the early missionaries, who were so firmly convinced that their culture and belief systems were part of a higher order along a continuum of belief systems, that they saw it as their duty to impose these on 'the natives'.

The results of an investigation into the 'meaning' of 'empowerment' for 15 women who believed that they had experienced it (Shields, 1995) showed it to be multi-faceted. The experience centred on the development of an internal sense of self (which enabled them to take action) and on the development of interpersonal connectedness (a balance centring more on the self). These women had achieved their definition of 'empowerment' without the aid of researchers.

Anne Opie (1992) asserts that 'empowerment' of individuals can occur through their contribution to the issue under research, through the process of reflection and evaluation of their own experiences, and through the potential of subversion when the researcher's interpretation challenges particular belief systems.

Participatory action research has been another approach taken in an attempt to improve women's life conditions. This approach has been little utilised (Wolf, 1996), possibly because it is the participants who initiate research in the ideal situation. In addition, all planning, interpretation, analysis and writing up (documentation) are shared. The difficulty of achieving consensus may place another hurdle in the way of a project's completion.

Current debates (Wolf, 1996) indicate that the achievement of feminist goals may be fraught with problems. The basic issue of *what knowledge* is being produced *for whom*, highlights the fact that most feminist research is carried out by middle-class female researchers to further their careers. Open and honest sharing of information with persons under research, and attempts at intersubjectivity, may be neither appropriate nor desirable in situations where value systems are dramatically different (Reinharz, 1993).

Friendship is equally problematic. The short term, casual and shallow relationships that characterise field research should perhaps not be elevated to this status. Where true friendships do develop, those under research may use them to prevent a situation in which their sharing of 'secrets' may make them vulnerable to later identification and abuse.

The hierarchical and status differences that exist in the majority of studies where 'researching down' has occurred are very difficult to erase or even minimise. Ultimately, power lies with the researcher, whose final conclusions and interpretations will stand. Opie (1992) points to the restrictive nature of the feminist view, which renders insignificant other experiences or incidents that have the power to challenge or disrupt interpretations. This makes it difficult to avoid taking the views of marginalised groups and interpreting them in such a way that they reinforce a particular ideological interpretation (*colonising*).

Criticisms

In conclusion, the principles involved in carrying out feminist research are perspectives that are not always easily achieved (Reinharz, 1992). These are:

- the equalising of relationships;
- the minimisation of differences; and
- the sharing of power and knowledge in the research process.

It is hard to argue that these orientations are unique to one particular form of research as opposed to other approaches in the qualitative tradition. It must be admitted, however, that feminist researchers have been most active in creatively changing the research boundaries (Fine, 1992; Ellis and Flaherty, 1992).

The theory/concept-generating approach is said to dominate feminist research (Stanley, 1990). Within this approach, it is very difficult to argue that all women are oppressed. This statement can only be justified after the situation and responses of *all* women have been explored, and are then continually revisited. The need for continual revisitation is due to possible changes in results as women's life experiences, or their recollections of experiences, change. A solution to this problem of constant flux has yet to be found.

Summary

This chapter has examined the major approaches to the utilisation of theory in qualitative research, particularly in the context of health. The inclusion of feminist research may spark some debate, since it is not a theory as such. As stated earlier, it is included for its valuable contribution to research approaches and its influence on thought within the health arena.

In summary, then, there are four broad approaches to the utilisation of theoretical perspectives in qualitative research:

- theory/concept-driven;
- theory/concept-generating;
- postmodern/poststructural; and
- feminist.

Theory/concept-driven research is heavily underpinned by one or more theoretical perspectives or concepts, which direct and refine the major questions and design. A critical analysis of the findings and designated perspectives is developed through examining each in light of the other.

Theory/concept-generating research is generally more lightly underpinned by one or more perspectives or concepts that must also be considered when developing new theoretical propositions from the collected data.

Postmodern/poststructural research rejects grand narratives, even though it may incorporate aspects of many of these. It critically examines historical and current contexts, discourses, language and power differentials. It focuses on 'multidimensionality', 'subjectivity' and the processes of 'deconstruction' and 'reconstruction'.

Finally, feminist research highlights the oppression of women. It has come to the forefront in pursuing concepts of 'empowerment' and 'emancipation' in the qualitative research process.

The next chapter concentrates on issues and debates surrounding qualitative research design. Many of these issues have their bases in the theoretical concepts just discussed.

Further readings

Belenky, M., Clinchy, B., Goldberger, N. and Tarule, J. (1986) *Women's Ways of Knowing: The Development of Self, Voice and Mind*. New York: Basic Books.

de Saussure, F. (1983) *Course in General Linguistics*. trans. Roy Harris, C. Bally and A. Sechehaye (eds). London: Duckworth. First published 1916 as *Cours de Linguistique Générale*. Paris: Payot.

Eco, U. (1984) *Semiotics and the Philosophy of Language*. London: Macmillan.

Foucault, M. (1973) *The Birth of the Clinic*. London: Tavistock.

Goffman, A. (1959) *The Presentation of Self in Everyday Life*. New York: Doubleday.

——(1961) *Asylums: Essays on the Social Situations of Mental Patients and other Inmates*. New York: Anchor.

——(1964) *Stigma: Notes on the Management of a Spoiled Identity*. New Jersey: Prentice Hall.

Habermas, J. (1984) *The Theory of Communicative Action*, vol. 1. Boston: Beacon Press.

Lather, P. (1991) *Getting Smart: Feminist Research and Pedagogy with/in the Postmodern*. New York: Routledge.

Marx, K. (1971) *Capital: A Critical Analysis of Capital Production*. London: George Allen & Unwin. First published 1893, 1894.

Mead, G. (1934) *Mind, Self and Society*. Chicago: University of Chicago Press.

Parsons, T. (1978) Health and disease: a sociological and action perspective, in T. Parsons (ed.), *Action Theory and the Human Condition*. London: Macmillan.

Sarup, M. (1993) *An Introductory Guide to Poststructuralism and Postmodernism*. Athens: University of Georgia Press.

Smith, D. (1996) Telling the truth after postmodernism. *Symbolic Interaction*, 19 (3), pp. 171–202.

3 Research design issues

This chapter endeavours to expose some of the current debates about issues of research design. In doing so, it provides brief definitions of key terms that influence research design, and undertakes an exploration of what the terms represent and how researchers view them. In the past, research design was often inextricably linked to terms such as:

- 'objectivity' (separating the researcher emotionally from the data);
- 'validity' (ability to verify data);
- 'reliability' (ability to produce acceptable outcomes);
- 'subjectivity' (researcher's own perspective);
- 'sampling' (searching for a representative group); and
- 'ethics' (the accountability of the researcher).

It is necessary to explore the debates surrounding each term to understand the significance of their role in research design.

Objectivity, validity and reliability

Traditional scientific discourse held the view that *objectivity* was based on the assumption that all knowledge was built on a solid foundation. This foundation consisted of either *human experience* (uniform sense impressions prompted by external physical stimuli) or *human reason* (based on beliefs so well tested that they appeared unlikely to be affected by future challenges). It was presumed that all activity could be explained in terms of *linear causality* (cause and effect along a straight line). It was also presumed that a properly trained researcher could maintain a distant, neutral, professional stance, which is the essence of the objective position. This objective position, together with the careful use of sampling techniques, design procedures and peer review of published material, should ensure that proper standards, 'validity' and 'reliability' of the data were maintained in the search for 'truth'.

Validity in qualitative research lies in the reader being convinced that the researcher has accessed and accurately represented the social world under study. *Reliability* is also assessed by the reader and lies in the capacity of the researcher to present a coherent, complete and meticulously checked exploration of all aspects of the topic under investigation.

The unresolved debate

There has been considerable, largely unresolved, debate about 'objectivity', 'validity' and 'reliability'. Much of the debate has attempted to resolve questions such as:

- Are they achievable?
- Are they desirable?
- What constitutes a 'fact'?
- Can objectivity ensure certainty?
- Can research be value free?
- Whose valuation is dominating?

Contention surrounding these issues can be traced as far back as Thomas Hobbes (1588–1679) (see Hobbes 1991 [1651]), who queried whether a higher order of knowledge beyond human patterns and behaviour actually existed. If it did, was it accessible to researchers? Hobbes' query pinpointed the separation of 'facts' of a scientific nature from the 'values'/'valuations' that made up patterns of social and political interaction.

Karl Popper (1969) held a similar view. He insisted that there was no secure starting point for knowledge, as nothing could be known with such certainty that future revisitations would not result in change. This led to the question, 'If no knowledge is certain, can objective research techniques, based on clear definitions and carefully controlled processes of inductive logic, get any closer to 'truth' than a 'subjective', intuitive view clouded by bias?'

Wilhelm Dilthey (1833–1911), a German philosopher (see Dilthey, 1976), took this argument further by suggesting that it was impossible to account for the observed 'reality' of social interaction without acknowledging that human beings had an innate capacity to understand each other. In other words, both observer and observed were subject to similar influences and prejudices. This made it impossible for any researcher to achieve a level of objectivity comparable with that of an alien investigating a new planet, although the socially constructed aspects of his/her previous environment would necessarily limit such an alien's perceptions.

Karl Mannheim (1954 [1936]) added to the debate by pointing to the multiplicity of perspectives (later referred to as 'biases') that could impact upon a researcher's judgements.

Gunnar Myrdal (1970, p. 43) emphasised that as social scientists we are deceiving ourselves if we naively believe that we are not as human as the people around us, or that we do not tend to aim opportunistically for conclusions that fit prejudices remarkably similar to those of other people in our society. He suggested that value-laden concepts should be clearly defined in terms of their origins (*value premises*). In exposing our biases, we need to recognise that not only our socially constructed perspectives but also our methodological techniques, concepts, theories and models are heavily biased by the dominant discourses of our culture, in particular the culture of the middle-class academic researcher. It can then be argued that most social research is merely a highly sophisticated procedure for documenting one version of 'reality', where researchers' biased and often hidden views may 'lead to a false perception of reality and to faulty conclusions' (1970, p. 47).

Bias versus objectivity

The arguments surrounding bias continue to provide an important area of debate within qualitative research. Critics have insisted that social science research is not only ideological, but also part of the ideology of society's ruling classes. Techniques of 'objectivity' have been viewed as actions aimed at co-opting victims of the present system of domination into serving the powerful and providing rewards for social scientists. Alvin Gouldner (1970) argued that background assumptions, which are conservative and value laden, determine how people interpret what they see. Myrdal (1970) suggested that it is not only our political, religious, ethnic and cultural biases that need to be addressed. Those arising from personal vanity and our intellectual traditions must also be examined. But would an awareness of this, through exposure, be sufficient to overcome the operation of such biases? Even if researchers were able to produce acceptable research, what control would they have over the further bias, misrepresentation, censure and moral criticism that may develop when their reports enter the domain of public discourse?

Jürgen Habermas (1972) has advanced the argument against objectivity by suggesting that mutual understanding and emancipation should replace the presumption that there are indissoluble links between knowledge, methodology and human interest that render objectivity impossible. Most feminist researchers take a similar view, tending to emphasise trust, empathy, non-exploitative relationships and empowerment as key factors in carrying out research. This partnership between researcher and researched is the dominant aspect of feminist research, which aims to achieve emancipatory social action.

Max Weber (1949) took a more pragmatic approach, arguing in favour of objectivity. He asserted that the truth of factual propositions can be established in an objective manner, even though evaluative judgements (valuations) have impacted on the selection of problems and their investigation. Denis Phillips (1990) has echoed a Weberian position by suggesting that objectivity is possible in qualitative research when there is evidence of the researcher's critical responsiveness to the paradigm/s he/she is using, exposure of his/her biases, and review and acceptance by the research community.

The only certainty when discussing 'objectivity' is that for every argument for or against it, there will be a counter argument. And so the debate continues . . .

Rigour

The questioning of the terms 'objectivity', 'validity' and 'reliability' has polarised positions between those who have emphasised the importance of rigorous qualitative research and those who regard 'rigour' as inappropriate. *Rigour* is the researcher's attempt to use as tight a research design as possible. The major concerns within these positions in qualitative research lie in the assessment of:

- the extent to which the researcher has disturbed the setting;
- the potential for selective interpretation and presentation of findings; and
- whether or not all aspects of the phenomenon have been addressed.

Those pursuing a rigorous approach have set up processes of *triangulation* involving *convergence* (the location of the singular truth of a phenomenon) or *completeness* (the achievement of holistic information regarding a phenomenon) (Knafl and Breitmeyer, 1991) or simply *cross-checking* the data (Guba and Lincoln, 1989, pp. 240–241). These definitions depart from the original orientation in surveying, where several readings of exactly the same kind, but from different positions, are taken in order to locate 'truth'.

Patti Lather (1986) has suggested that triangulation should include multiple methods and multiple theoretical schemas, as well as multiple data sources.

Jack Douglas (1976) has insisted that a long stay in the field can improve reliability, allowing for the generation and testing of hypotheses. Douglas pointed to the difficulties of claiming reliable data with a single method and a one-off cine shot of social phenomena, which are known to change over time. He concluded that without a diversity of methods it is almost impossible to trace the multiplicity of influences impacting on an environment or a relationship.

Other techniques said to improve rigour include:

- *face validity*, often termed *member checks* (checking interpretations by presenting them to a focus group of the participants);
- *construct/theoretical validity* (confronting existing theoretical perspectives with the data or the development of new theoretical/conceptual schemas);
- *catalytic validity* (assessing the degree to which the research process re-orients, focuses and energises participants, who transform their realities through gaining sufficient knowledge);
- *self-reflexivity* (documenting the researcher's biases and assumptions, and how her/his position and perspectives have changed throughout the study);
- acknowledging disconfirming evidence and contradictory interpretations; and
- *audit trails* (tracing the conceptual development of the project from raw data through data reduction, analysis and reconstruction).

Triangulation also has come under scrutiny. The gathering of information from different points (methods and sources) may not serve to consolidate a certain position. It may simply provide more information for the researcher to deal with. Even if the results tally, there is no guarantee that the inferences involved will be accurate. The outcome may be two incorrect, but similar, conclusions (Hammersley and Atkinson, 1995, p. 231).

Radical qualification

Researchers antagonistic to 'rigour' assert that the concepts of 'objectivity', 'validity' and 'reliability' are too problematic and should be abandoned or radically qualified. The process of radical qualification addresses such important questions as:

- For whom is the research being conducted?
- What are the social situations of the researcher and the researched?
- Whose knowledge is being articulated in the field, as well as in the written representation?
- Who benefits from this research?
- Has the capacity to act independently (*active agency*) of the researched and the researcher within the structural determinants of the setting been adequately assessed?
- Do the participants understand the aims, theoretical underpinnings and outcomes of the research, and how have they made sense of these in order to gain greater understanding or to facilitate changes in their situations?
- Were the barriers between researcher and researched broken down?
- Was the researcher seriously involved or just a voyeur?
- How have participants' views and the research process modified the researcher's perspective?
- Has the research clarified the underlying power relations impinging on both the experiences of the researcher and the researched, and how have they responded to these within the process of mutual emancipation?
- What is the reader's role?
- What forms of representation are being used (rhetorical, authoritative, self-reflexive, first, second or third person, descriptive or interpretative), and for what purpose?
- Whose voice dominates, and whose voices are not being heard?

Robert Dingwell (1992) is one researcher who insists on 'radical qualification'. He argues that there is a need for investigation and careful explication of the relationship between what is observed, and the larger historical and organisational contexts. Such scrutiny should also be applied to the relationship between the observer, the observed and the setting. This involves the documentation and analysis of several factors in terms of their historical, cultural environment. These factors are:

- the numbers of participants;
- key individuals, their activities, schedules, division-of-labour hierarchies, routines and variations;
- significant events;
- members' perspectives; and
- social rules and patterns of order and disorder.

Those favouring the abandonment of terms like 'validity' and 'reliability' see qualitative research more appropriately located as a *literary art* than a scientific form (Grumet, 1990). 'Validity' is then demonstrated in the product's capacity to illuminate and penetrate, via the persuasiveness of a personal vision (Eisner, 1981, p. 6). Like art, it displays a relationship to, and a perception of, the phenomena rather than displays of a 'thing'.

Those who do not wish to abandon 'rigour' completely, but who are unhappy with the connotations surrounding traditional terminology, have developed new terms and techniques, such as *dependable*, *credible*, *defensible* (Polkinghorne, 1983) or *trustworthy* data (Guba and Lincoln, 1989), or *scientific legitimacy* (Mishler, 1990). These latter can be developed through displays of the text and its representations. Where this is not practicable, transcripts and tapes can be made available for inspection. In general, exposure of the dialectic between theory, the analytic structures of relationships among textual features, and the data, is seen to enhance the research process's acceptability.

Other forms of trustworthiness are viewed as lying somewhere within the coherence between intention and fulfilled meaning (Giorgi, 1988), or in the development and extension of relationships with participants in a process that should enable the transformation of both researcher and researched. 'Validity' then becomes the display of the research and personal development processes undertaken by the researcher, within a context and a discourse (Wolcott, 1990). This involves 'the social construction of a discourse through which the results of a study come to be viewed as sufficiently trustworthy for other investigators to rely upon in their own work' (Mishler, 1990, p. 429).

Reflexive subjectivity and the politics of position

Postmodern/poststructural traditions have replaced 'objectivity', 'validity' and 'generalisability' with 'reflexive subjectivity' and the politics of position. 'Objectivity', 'validity' and 'generalisability' are all presumed to belong to a dubious empiricist discourse, based on scientific evidence (Kellehear, 1993, p. 42).

Patti Lather (1993, pp. 677–687), however, has identified four problems/directions of postmodern/poststructural research that can be interpreted as moves towards validating data:

- 'Validity' as *simulacra* (copies without originals) or *ironic validity* (in which language and its role in constructing meaning are actively critiqued) views all representations and relations as problematic, and no final conclusion is possible. This is derived from Baudrillard.

- *Neo-pragmatic validity* (derived from Lyotard) highlights differences through paradox, discontinuity and complexity. The juxtaposition of values and *face validity* (checking interpretation of data with the participants) replaces the application of major discourses and the researcher's colonising gaze.
- *Rhizomatic validity* (derived from Derrida) involves avoiding facts and details from within hierarchies. This approach favours co-authorship with participants. Structures and networks feature predominantly, and all theoretical and political assumptions undergo rigorous examination.
- *Voluptuous/situated validity* critiques 'male' knowledge and universal 'objective' claims in favour of positional engagement and self-reflexivity. It aims to decentre both researcher and researched by challenging the public/private division of the researcher's life, and by highlighting uncertainty in the creation of a questioning text. The focus of this approach is the emerging discourse of women with its new forms of representation, such as poetry.

These problems present critical clarification of the spaces that researchers are opening and inhabiting. The dangers of allowing these four directions to become rules or routine pathways to acceptably 'valid' data lie in the probability that dynamic movements in qualitative research will become constrained and concretised.

Reflexivity

Reflexivity, at the very least, involves a process of self-awareness that should clarify how one's beliefs have been socially constructed and how these values are impacting on interaction and interpretation in research settings. George Marcus (1994, pp. 568–572) has identified four styles of reflexivity:

- self-critique based on experience and empathy;
- self-critique designed to maintain objectivity;
- reflexivity as location, emphasising diversity and intertextuality; and
- feminist, subjectivist reflexivity, situated in epistemological positioning.

The process of 'reflexivity' is viewed as instrumental in transcending differences of power, culture and class.

Rahel Wasserfall (1993), however, has pointed to the limitations of these approaches when ideological differences are involved. She suggests a stronger version, which involves the active deconstruction of the researcher's authority, aimed at overcoming the potential for exploitation. She also warns that this may only be realistic when shared perspectives exist. When major differences occur between the beliefs of researcher and researched, the researcher's views will tend to dominate. This suggests that 'reflexive subjectivity' is useful for awareness development, but may have limited impact on participants' transformation, empowerment and emancipation. Such 'reflexivity' may, in fact, be seen as self-indulgence rather than an integral part of method (Marcus, 1994).

Generalisability

Generalisability involves the usefulness of one set of findings in explaining other similar situations. The quantitative notion of generalising in a predictive manner is controversial within qualitative research. Diversity of opinion abounds. Some insist that generalisability is impossible, because some researchers deal with individuals, not aggregates. Others undertake large complex studies and often generalise from descriptive statistics. Still others espouse '*projectability*' (Goodman, 1983), or 'naturalistic' or logical generalisation using schema theory (Donmeyer, 1990).

Schema theory originated from Jean Piaget (1971), who saw all knowledge as being filtered through *cognitive structures* that shape what we 'know'. This process is termed *assimilation* and is followed by *accommodation* (the reshaping of cognitive structures to accommodate the novel aspects of what is being perceived). The cognitive structure will become more integrated and more differentiated as a result of these processes. Donmeyer suggests that the reader's natural processes of assimilation, accumulation, integration and differentiation provide a framework for the generalisation of information gained from powerful narrative case studies.

Joseph Maxwell (1992) also makes a claim for the generalisability of qualitative data. He sees this occurring through the development of theory from the data—a theory that can be applied to similar persons in similar situations.

Broadly speaking, all learning involves generalisation (Berliner, 1988). The application of acquired knowledge to new situations through the ability to generalise skills, images and ideas via formal inference, attribute analysis and image matching (Eisner, 1991) is the test of learning.

Subjectivity

One outcome of the rejection of 'objectivity' has been an emphasis on 'subjectivity'. *Subjectivity* has been viewed in many ways. It has been seen as:

- the link between emotions, the physical body and cognitive processes (Ellis and Flaherty, 1992, p. 4);
- individuality and self-awareness, where subjects are dynamic and positioned in relation to particular discourses (Henriques et al., 1984, p. 3); or
- involving joint construction of meaning (Roman and Apple, 1990, p. 38).

'Subjectivity' has been in and out of favour, according to the dominant research design of any given era. It was to be avoided in favour of researcher neutrality, following the 'rigorous' position. More recently, it has been suggested that 'subjectivity' must be addressed as part of the self-reflexive process, and should be linked to political, cultural and historical contexts and the power relations between the researcher and the researched.

Elliott Eisner (1991, p. 52), in an attempt at radical qualification, suggests joining 'objectivity' with 'subjectivity' to form a *transactive account* (looking from both 'objective' and 'subjective' positions). His reasoning is that all that can be known about the world must be mediated by the mind. Therefore, 'objectivity' and 'subjectivity' are inseparably united. The criteria for judging a 'transactive account' then become coherence, consensus and the utility of the research (via peer review).

Denzin (1984b) asserts that *emotional intersubjectivity* is required to gain an understanding of others' meanings. 'Emotional intersubjectivity' is the process by which we enter the worlds of the researched and bring their experiences into our own frames of reference through the process of sharing. True emotional understanding is not the same as sympathy or empathy (projecting how the other feels then identifying with that false projection) (Denzin, 1984b, p. 138); nor is it the same as awareness or visualisation. Instead it involves some physical manifestation that both researcher and researched recognise as real evidence of understanding the other's position, rather than being part of a managed performance.

Despite these views, most methods have emphasised rational order and researcher neutrality until quite recently. 'Subjective' views, particularly those of an emotional nature, have been treated as belonging to a lower order in relation to processes of cognition and analysis. Any form of emotion was separated from cognition, the body and the social context, and was seen as exhibitionist (Ellis and Flaherty, 1992; Small,

1997). 'Subjectivity' has become centrally situated within postmodern ethnography, however, allowing researchers to access and understand the self from the inside. The process involves managing multiple selves and multiple roles. This form of subjective presentation (poetry, drama or narrative) is judged on its capacity to share emotions and provoke responses from readers who have had similar experiences. Sandra Butler and Barbara Rosenblum's (1991) exploration of the experience of medical error leading to living with, and dying of, cancer is an example of this. Their book comprises journal entries and reflections of the experiences of illness and the partnering of a person with cancer. Marianne Paget (1993) uses a similar presentation method. She interweaves her personal experience of breast cancer with her academic writings on mistakes in clinical medicine and a newsletter to her friends.

Postmodern and poststructural positions favour a subjectivity that is dynamic, multifaceted, contradictory, decentred and located within particular discourses that are open to deconstruction and reinterpretation. Poststructuralism allows recognition of the multiple discourses that have deprived the individual of *agency* (independent action) and inscribed the cultural patterns of desire (prioritised powerful discourses). Researcher integrity can be demonstrated through self-reflection, self-monitoring, growth and transformation. Alexander Peshkin (1985) believes that aspects of our personal biographies, together with the contexts in which we find ourselves, influence which one of our subjective selves will perceive the world at any one time. Each documented perspective enhances the multiple subjective perspectives of others in an ongoing, emergent, creative process.

Sampling

Sampling is a process of selecting individual groups or texts for inclusion in a project. The sampling techniques chosen will vary with the question and the demands of the position from which the researcher chooses to conduct qualitative research. This position may change during the research if the researcher decides to change the question or due to emergent data. Further sampling strategies may be utilised until the researcher is convinced that the topic under investigation has been covered.

At the rigorous end of the scale, and perhaps in conjunction with the collection of quantitative data, a large number of people may be sampled using *probability techniques* (where each individual within the total population has an equal chance of appearing in the database). This form of sampling is said to permit generalisation, but only if the issues raised by uncertainty and chaos are discounted. It can be undertaken using the following techniques:

- *simple random* (allocation of random numbers to each unit of the population);
- *systematic* (every *n*th element drawn from a list);
- *stratified random* (random sampling within specified strata, such as age and sex); and
- *cluster* (random sampling from categories, such as all the hospitals in one area, then the random sampling of patients/staff within those hospitals).

Questions can be structured in two ways: closed-ended or open-ended. Those structured in a *closed-ended* manner use yes/no or rating scale responses to provide data, which can be statistically analysed and is claimed to be generalisable. *Open-ended* questions seek data on the *how*, *when* and *where* of a particular situation. (They are discussed in detail in Chapter 4, and in relation to the quantitative–qualitative debate in Chapter 1.) The key question is whether a large random sample will give richer or better information than a small group that has been carefully selected.

Other issues that arise in deciding on a sampling approach are accountability and relationships with participants. Ann Oakley (1990) explored the ethical and moral dilemmas she faced as a feminist when utilising randomised control trial techniques in a study exploring the topic of pregnant women and supportive services. The women were randomised into either a supported group or a non-supported control group. They were surveyed using open-ended and closed-ended questions during and after pregnancy. Oakley concluded that, methodologically speaking, the use of experimental quantitative sampling techniques had some advantages over intuitive approaches. These techniques posed a number of problems for women's research, however, particularly when notions of choice, researcher accountability, equal participation and emancipation for all participants were foregrounded.

Qualitative researchers usually employ *non-probability techniques*. These are not representative. Their purpose is to select information-rich cases. Patton (1990, p. 182) lists over 15 types of non-probability sampling, including:

- *extreme sampling* (using outstanding cases to explore in detail one aspect of a phenomena);
- *homogeneous sampling* (to explore a particular subgroup of people);
- *critical case sampling* (choosing people who will provide the most information on the topic); and

- *opportunistic sampling* (to take account of new situations that arise during the research process).

Patton's list implies that non-probability sampling includes almost any reasonable approach that can be justified. The most commonly used techniques, however, include:

- *Maximum variation/heterogeneous/quota or non-representative 'stratified' sampling* (Trost, 1986): the researcher carefully selects those who will provide the best representation of the research question's definable aspects (often with the help of a matrix).
- *Snowball sampling*: word of mouth and networks are used to locate people who fit certain criteria. This is often the only way to locate an otherwise invisible group.
- *Convenience sampling* is used where the aim is to locate a group of people as quickly as possible in order to maximise convenience and minimise cost (such as sampling among friends or work colleagues). This technique generally yields information-poor cases. It is regarded as the weakest technique, particularly when issues of validity and reliability are of concern.
- *Theoretical sampling* is used in grounded theory and involves sampling for concepts or examples of particular situations in the data.

Maximum variation/heterogeneous/quota or non-representative stratified sampling sounds very complicated, but the following example should simplify its procedures. Suppose that we want to ascertain the dietary habits of teenagers in town X. One possibility would include identifying the age range, living situations and incomes of those teenagers, then using a matrix to represent these definable aspects of the research question. Cells could be allocated (see following table) in order to locate 30 teenagers. Although the potential total is 30, some cell groups may be difficult to fill. Teenagers with a high income living on the street could be one such category. Using the matrix simplifies and clarifies the research process, providing a readily accessible information map.

Traditional sampling techniques are avoided where 'validity' and 'reliability' are regarded as irrelevant non-issues. This is the case within the postmodern/poststructural tradition, where the researcher looks for information-rich cases instead, whose number is unpredictable. The outcome of such a study may vary from the display of one detailed life history to as many as 30 shorter histories, within which the

Potential matrix for the dietary habits of teenagers (15–19 years) in town x.

living situation	With one parent			With 2 parents			Solo (renting)			Pair/group (renting)			Street/squat		
Income	high	med	low	h	m	l	h	m	l	h	m	l	h	m	l
Sex	m.f.	m.f.	m.f.	m.f	m.f	m.f	m.f	m.f	m.f	m.f	m.f	m.f	m.f	m.f	m.f

researcher seeks to display as many aspects as possible of the diverse results produced by the study's questions.

Ethical issues

Currently, the dimensions of research ethics range from basic protection of participants' rights to active endeavours to improve their lives. Accountability and the relationship between researcher and researched is the key issue. At the 'rights' end of the scale, it is generally accepted that it is unethical to harm anyone in the course of carrying out research. Deception regarding the purpose of the research; creating embarrassment, emotional turmoil or other forms of distress; harm brought to people through studying them without their knowledge; violating promises of confidentiality; or falsifying or presenting results out of context, are all deemed to be 'unethical' practices.

Most *ethics committees* require researchers to send a one-page *explanatory letter* to all potential participants in a study. This letter must include the following information:

- the aim of the study;
- the personnel involved; and
- a description of possible outcomes, including:
  — benefits or lack thereof;
  — any potential harm/s that participants may suffer;
  — an offer to answer questions at any time (the phone number of the researcher/supervisor/secretary of the ethics committee is included here);
  — a promise of anonymity and confidentiality, and an indication of how these will be maintained;
  — clarification that the participant is free to leave the study at any time and is not obliged to answer any questions they feel uncomfortable with; and

— an indication that should any of the above change they will be contacted and their further permission sought.

The following is a typical example.

Dear Mr/Ms _____

I am a student in the [degree] at [university]. I am researching . . .

In this study I wish to talk with [you/ . . .] about . . .

I feel that [your/ . . .] perspective of . . . is extremely important in exploring the experiences that people may have had. To date there has not been much research done in this area, and I am keen to add to our knowledge.

I would be most grateful if you could spare the time to assist in this project by granting me an interview touching upon certain aspects of the topic. All information discussed will be treated in the strictest confidentiality, and none of the participants will be individually identifiable in the resulting paper. You are, of course, entirely free to discontinue your participation at any time, or to decline to answer particular questions.

Since I intend to make a tape recording of the interview I also seek your consent, on the attached form, to record the interview, to use the recording in preparing the paper on condition that your name or identity is not revealed, and that the recording will not be made available to any other person.

This study has been approved by . . . Ethics Committee. The Secretary of this committee can be contacted on . . .

If you decide to participate in the project, would you kindly return the signed consent form so that I can contact you to arrange a suitable time for our interview.

Please accept in advance my thanks for your assistance.

Yours sincerely,

_____

In addition, ethics committees tend to comply with the guidelines of the health ethics committees of their particular state or country; the ethics that must be addressed in researching indigenous people; and those guidelines regarding clinical trials. IVF and embryo transplantation, use of foetal tissue, epidemiological research, somatic cell gene therapy and the introduction of DNA and RNA all require that the researcher adheres to specific ethical guidelines.

Covert research

One of the major debates within the ethics of qualitative research has centred on the issue of allowing *covert research*, which is the observation of people without their knowledge or consent. Those who have successfully carried out such studies insist that there are certain areas of society, and certain individuals' actions and behaviours, that are unobservable within the normal ethical range of research activities. Laud Humphreys' (1970) study of casual sex between men in public toilets, Powdermaker's (1966) investigation of the Ku Klux Klan, and the study of a group practising Scientology (Wallis, 1977) are all cases in point. These researchers assert that they would not have been able to obtain access to such settings if they had openly approached individuals or groups. The more sensitive or legally marginal the activity to be observed, the greater will be the impact of the intrusion of a known researcher. Further instances of previous acceptance of covert research include situations where a researcher's life would come under threat if it were known that she/he was collecting data, or when those under research are indulging in nefarious practices. The benefits of gaining knowledge without unduly impacting on the setting clearly outweigh any potential harm to the participants.

Most researchers condemn covert methods, but some (Holman, 1993) have argued that such research must be judged on both the setting and the likely benefits of proceeding with the research. The issue is particularly complex, as the knowledge of being researched may, in itself, have the potential to produce harm. Take, for example, the case of a carer researching the process of death of a person under their care. If the carer is open about this research, it might well cause considerable distress, because the patient may not be aware or may not have accepted that he/she is dying.

One response to this problem is that, if people are likely to be harmed, the research should not be undertaken. Thus, the cyclical nature of the argument continues. The equivocal nature of many ethics committees' positions and their emphasis on 'likely benefits' has opened the door to covert health research. If the researcher can mount a persuasive argument to convince the relevant ethics committees of the usefulness of such research, it will go ahead.

More questions

Other questions/issues that require consideration in coming to terms with ethical dilemmas include:

- Is it always unethical to misrepresent one's identity in order to gain access to a private domain?
- Is it always unethical to misrepresent the character of one's research in order to gain access to information that is difficult to obtain? What about misrepresentation that some perceive as causing no harm, for example, placing bogus advertisements in personal columns to gather and analyse responses (Goode, 1996)?
- Is being a covert outsider better or worse than being a covert insider?
- Is it possible to fully inform potential participants when the aims and direction of the study may well change?
- What constitutes a 'public' or a 'private' domain?
- Can researchers really protect the identity of places and participants?
- Is it realistic that all persons who participate should provide consent? What about casual conversations and those who wander into the study?
- What does 'beneficial knowledge' actually mean, and who decides this?
- How honest should a researcher be when asked for her/his political views by participants holding views she/he privately disagrees with?
- What happens when a participant is unhappy with the interpretation of his/her interview transcript?
- Should the research assistant who contributes substantially to the project be a co-researcher or a hired hand?

Research in specific areas

Apart from the above general questions that are still under debate, there are several specific issues that must be addressed when undertaking research in certain areas. The first of these arises when dealing with patients whose mental capacity is diminished.

Participants with mental incapacity

The issue of consent from people with mental incapacity is very complex. There are few guidelines, but researchers tend to adhere to certain principles. These are:

- Consent/lack of consent to participate can be presumed to be signalled;.
- Where the participant appears uncomfortable or distressed, the research procedure should stop.
- Agencies and carers should be involved to provide advice regarding appropriate participation.
- Consent may also need to be obtained from the legal guardian.

The main issue with vulnerable people (which includes the acutely ill and those who are terminal) is whether participating will engender harm or risk. Sensitivity to individual needs and states of health is required. Research involving children is an area where this is especially important.

Children

In protecting the rights and welfare of children involved in research procedures, it is necessary to:

- determine the acceptability of the risk/benefit relationship of any research study conducted;
- ensure that informed consent from parents/guardians, and where appropriate the child, is obtained in a manner appropriate to the study;
- encourage the performance of necessary and appropriate research; and
- prevent unscientific or unethical research.

Consent to the research should be obtained from the parents/guardians in all but exceptional circumstances (emergencies), and from the child where he/she is of sufficient maturity or intelligence to make this practicable. In this context 'consent' means agreement following a full and clear explanation of the planned research, its objectives and any risks involved.

Risks may be considered in terms of therapeutic and non-therapeutic research. *Therapeutic research* is where the procedure may be of some benefit to the child. In determining whether there is an acceptable relationship between potential benefit and the risk involved, the risk of the proposed research must be weighed against customary therapeutic measures and the natural hazards of the disease or condition.

Non-therapeutic research is where the procedure is of no direct benefit to the child. Here, the risk to the child should be so minimal as to be little more than the risks run in everyday life. Risks of research in this context include the risk of causing physical disturbance, discomfort, anxiety, pain or psychological disturbance to the child or the parents, rather than the risk of serious harm, which would be unacceptable.

Covert dilemmas in the case of child abuse

The mandatory reporting of child abuse is a special case within the overall ethical guidelines as applied to research involving children. It varies from state to state and country to country. In certain countries, a child (under 18 years of age) who is known to be suffering from sexual, physical or emotional abuse or neglect that is placing his/her physical/psychological well-being at risk should be reported. Teachers, doctors, nurses, dentists, psychologists, social workers and any employee/volunteer in a government/non-government agency providing health, welfare, education, childcare or residential services all have a responsibility to report such cases. Those carrying out 'official duties' for these organisations are also often obliged to report. The ethical dilemma arises from the fact that all of these people are, in effect, 'covert' researchers, reporting on individuals' behaviours without the consent of either the individuals or their parents/guardians. Abusers and abused both become unwitting subjects (participants) in this covert research.

Funding dilemmas

Another area of ethical concern is the issue of sponsorship funding. In most cases, research monies are targeted to areas of need, but within these areas funding bodies may attempt to exert pressure regarding questions to be investigated, methodologies to be used, and the interpretation and presentation of findings. Reports unfavourable to the interests of funding bodies may be suppressed or rejected. Campaigns may be undertaken to cast aspersions upon the researcher's professionalism or the data's trustworthiness. Early negotiation of ownership and publication rights of the data, in the researcher's favour, is suggested as a way of avoiding these problems. Any rights to veto publication should be avoided. Smith (1990) has suggested that a continuing dialogue with participants, funding bodies and all other interested parties tends to pre-empt and obviate many of the problems that may arise.

Postmodern and feminist ethics

Postmodern and feminist researchers have moved beyond what they see as the limited focus of institutional ethics committees in regard to consent, confidentiality and harm reduction. They have suggested instead that researchers take demonstrable responsibility for the issues of power, negotiation and transformation within their research designs and interpretations of findings. The following series of questions (adapted from Davis, 1995) is used to indicate important aspects that must be addressed:

Ongoing negotiation:

- What do we (researcher and researched) hope to achieve?
- Who will benefit/lose by this research?
- What changes can be anticipated?
- How will confidentiality and anonymity be maintained?
- How will accountability be addressed—particularly when suffering and injustice are evident?
- How will decision making and knowledge be shared?
- How will the needs and concerns of all participants be addressed?

Reflective critique:

- Were relationships non-hierarchical, respectful, caring and growth oriented?
- Was the verbal and written language used accessible and demystifying?
- What dialogues are evident (researcher–researched, researcher–policy makers), and what have their outcomes been?

If all these questions were to become part of institutional ethics committees' areas of comment and advice, the committees might be able to increase their domain from ethical/non-ethical behaviours to acceptable/not acceptable research designs. This issue needs serious consideration.

Research process

Deciding what to research

The first steps in undertaking a piece of research are to identify the *area* one wishes to explore and to attempt a process of *brainstorming*. Taking a hypothetical example, such as a study of the phenomena 'iceberg' (Gummesson, 1991), brainstorming might involve the following process of critical questioning to clarify where 'truth' or some illuminating perspectives might be sought:

- Shall we locate only the tip of the iceberg and call what can be observed above the waterline the 'truth'?
- What about the nine-tenths that remain submerged?

We could sit in a boat and circle the iceberg to gain particular measurements and certain perspectives. If enthusiasm persists, we could put on wetsuits and diving gear and brave the icy temperatures to explore the underwater mass. From this exercise the size, shape, rate of flow and our individual subjective underwater experiences could be documented. This information could be presented as one reflection of 'truth'/'reality', but . . .

- What about the genesis and the environment of the iceberg—its transition from a particular shape and position to eventual disintegration?
- What about the animals, birds, fish and humans that have passed/spent time on this iceberg?
- How does our perspective change as we move from above, to around, to below the iceberg?
- How about documenting on film the changing patterns of reflected light from day to night and season to season?

Should we go further? How about an analysis of the term 'iceberg'?

- How did it develop and change meaning in the linguistic patterns of various cultures?
- What discourses have developed around this term?
- What political, social and economic views of the iceberg have been perpetrated and perpetuated in texts and linguistic exchanges?
- Who has benefited from particular social constructions or historical shifts?

It is obvious from this example that a range of approaches and a variety of perspectives are available to the researcher in studying a particular phenomenon. It is also obvious that refining the questions and perspectives to be used is an ongoing process.

Literature review

Once the approach has been narrowed and the broad parameters of the study defined, the next step involves undertaking a literature review, the importance of which will vary according to the method used. All potentially relevant literature should be examined. The findings and implications for the researcher's study should then be documented.

Each researcher has her/his own style of coping with the volumes of literature a topic can generate. I prefer a *face sheet* (a piece of paper attached or placed in front of each article/chapter) which contains two pieces of information. The first is a *summary* of the relevant findings, with critical comments on these and the theoretical/conceptual frameworks used by the authors. The second draws out the *implications* for my own work—the questions I need to consider and the issues I will need to address. I then file the article under some major aspect of my topic, to be amalgamated and cross-referenced with others when I am writing up my review.

The literature review has several purposes. It is used:

- to establish knowledge regarding the current state of research in the chosen area;
- to locate the theoretical/conceptual frameworks that have enhanced or limited progress on this topic;
- to identify gaps the researcher can fill with his/her own findings; and finally, from all of these,
- to draw implications that can then be translated into questions the research will explore.

Question design and data collection, data analysis and interpretation, and data display follow the literature review (in that order). These are discussed in depth in the forthcoming chapters.

Summary

This chapter has sought to discuss the major issues affecting research design. The discussion has led to the following conclusions:

The issues of 'objectivity', 'subjectivity', 'validity', 'reliability', 'generalisability', 'sampling' and the ethics and accountability involved in undertaking research are all highly contentious and have aroused heated debate over the past 400 years.

There is also considerable disagreement among researchers regarding the issue of 'rigour'. There are those who emphasise it, with accompanying techniques to support it, and those who are convinced that 'rigour' is inappropriate.

The main aim of qualitative research is to gather rich information. Therefore some forms of probability or non-probability sampling have been usual to access the most appropriate participants. Sampling techniques have tended to be de-emphasised or discarded, however, with the advent of uncertainty, chaos, postmodernism and poststructuralism.

Ethical issues are important in health, particularly with regard to the observation of those on the margins of society, and the interviewing of vulnerable people and children.

The research process involves decisions as to how much of phenomena will be explored. A critical review of literature and theoretical perspectives prior to decisions regarding techniques of data collection, methods or methodologies is an essential part of this process.

Part Two, following, deals with techniques of data collection, the third step in the research process. Chapter 4 begins the section with an exploration of the factors involved in interviewing.

Further readings

General

Daly, J. (1996) *Ethical Intersections: Health Research, Methods and Researcher Responsibility*. Sydney: Allen & Unwin.

Fook, J. (1996) *The Reflective Researcher*. Sydney: Allen & Unwin.

Kirk, J. and Miller, M. (1986) *Reliability and Validity in Qualitative Research*. California: Sage.

Mitchell, R. (1993) *Secrecy and Fieldwork*. Newbury Park: Sage.

Punch, M. (1986) *The Politics of Ethics and Fieldwork*. Beverley Hills: Sage.

Steir, F (ed.) (1991) *Research and Reflexivity*. London: Sage.

Children

Cassell, J. (ed.) (1987) *Children in the Field: Anthropological Experiences*. Philadelphia: Temple University Press.

Cohen, D. and Stern, V. (1983) *Observing and Recording the Behaviour of Young Children*. New York: Teachers College Press, Columbia University.

Hatch, J. (ed.) (1995) *Qualitative Research in Early Childhood Settings*. Wesport: Praeger.

Irwin, D. and Bushnell, M. (1980) *Observational Strategies for Child Study*. New York: Holt, Rinehart and Winston.

Part Two
Techniques of
data collection

Part Two provides a detailed examination of 'interviewing' and 'observation'. These are the two major data-collection techniques that researchers use 'in the field'. A third technique, the 'location of documentation', is not examined until Part Three (Methodological Approaches), due to its links with methodological approaches such as history method and discourse analysis. The terms 'methods' and 'techniques' tend to be used interchangeably within textbooks on qualitative research. I have used the term 'techniques' here to minimise confusion between *methods* (ways of gathering data) and *methodologies* (ways of data gathering that are underpinned by particular philosophical orientations that impact on both data collection and interpretation).

Chapter 4 attempts a broad sweep of the factors involved in interviewing:

- the personal decisions that interviewers must make regarding their own positions;
- the kind of interview to be conducted;
- the processes involved in undertaking an interview; and
- the design of the interview questions.

The 'focus', 'nominal' and 'Delphi' forms of group interviews are also explored.

Chapter 5 examines participant observation from the perspectives of researcher roles, processes and procedures, and data gathering. Observation using photography and other visual imaging is also explored.

When choosing 'techniques' for data collection, the emphasis should be on flexibility and the best approach for the topic. Most studies will incorporate aspects of both 'interviewing' and 'observation'. All interviews involve some formal or informal observation, while many observations include verbal interactions, which may vary from an exchange of comments to a formal interview.

4 Interviewing

This chapter discusses several interview techniques and processes, and the place of interviewing in data collection.

Overview of issues

Interviewing is the most common technique used to gather research information. But how does a researcher decide which technique should dominate in data collection? It is often appropriate to *trial techniques* before making a final choice.

One of my own studies that utilised interviewing as the main form of data collection was based in the conceptual frameworks of agency and socialisation. It comprised a longitudinal examination of 25 primary-care-giver males (Grbich, 1987), and explored aspects of their lives, in particular their experiences of caring for their young children over an eight-year period. These men were interviewed every four months during the first year, then at yearly intervals. Their partners and parents were also interviewed to gain other perspectives on the information that was sought from the men. I chose interviewing, with some observation sessions, as my major approach for this study, but only after I had trialled several other techniques prior to commencing data collection.

Videos were used to record observation sessions of the fathers interacting with their children, but this approach had to be abandoned. The combination of crawling babies, toddlers and video equipment proved dangerous and distracting! Another problem was the need for two video recorders to capture the facial expressions of both father and child. This proved to be a very high-tech, intrusive approach, unsuitable for home interviews. Diary records, which could provide a basis for interviewing, were also trialled, but the average father at home with very young children is a busy person. Only those of a particularly literary bent were comfortable with this form of recording. Participant observation was also abandoned as the main technique because it would have involved virtually becoming a household member. This is not a practical option for the average researcher, and the issue of disturbing the setting had to be carefully considered.

In another study incorporating combined quantitative–qualitative approaches and exploring educational and health concerns, Garrard and Northfield (1987) used interviewing and survey questionnaire techniques to examine issues surrounding the delivery of drug education programs in colleges. A survey questionnaire was sent to the total school population in one state. Responses to a number of closed-ended questions provided data for statistical analysis. Twenty-two schools were further selected as case studies based on responses to some open-ended questions. These schools were chosen for maximum diversity of their positive and negative experiences in producing and delivering drug education programs. Interviews were organised with staff responsible for course implementation. Focus group discussions were held with students who had participated in these courses, and these students, in groups of six, were interviewed regarding their recollections of the program. The technique of 'pile sorting' was used to ascertain the students' level of knowledge. 'Pile sorting' involves sorting a pile of 'things' according to a particular criterion. The students were given 17 picture cards of various legal and illegal drugs and food substances. They were then asked to place the cards in order of:

- 'most' to 'least' dangerous;
- 'drugs' and 'not drugs';
- 'causing problems for the community' and 'causing problems for individual users'; and
- producing 'long term' or 'immediate' problems.

While students carried out the tasks, their accompanying discussions were taped to provide information regarding decision-making processes and levels of knowledge.

Interviewing or . . . ?

The preceding examples indicate that interviewing tends to be chosen as the most appropriate technique when the researcher cannot gain access to information any other way. This may be because the events being investigated have already occurred, or are not readily observable. The aim of conducting interviews is to gain information on the perspectives, understandings and meanings constructed by people regarding the events and experiences of their lives. The information gained is termed *second-order data*, as it is one step removed from the actual occurrence of the situation and is therefore subject to problems of recall.

Interviewing styles vary from something approaching an informal conversation between friends (where issues of equality have been carefully considered) to a formal interrogation. The style depends on the study's purpose and the researcher's position. The notion of a friendly conversation implies an established relationship with some form of reciprocity. Although this may well be achievable in some situations, in others it is an overglorification of the power-laden, awkward interchanges that actually occur.

The process of gaining information through interviews contains an underlying assumption that interviewer and interviewee actually understand one another: that the signs and symbols used are meaningful to both, and that both share the visual images evoked and the interpretations applied. This broad assumption leads us to ask:

- Do the researcher and researched share a common language?
- What about differences of class, status, education, culture and other perspectives?
- What does this mean in terms of data collection and interpretation?

Eliot Mishler (1986) suggested that the interview is a form of discourse shaped by asking and answering questions. This then makes a nonsense of 'standardised' questions and elaborate coding rituals. Instead, the interview becomes a speech event, the discourse of which is jointly constructed by interviewer and interviewee. Analysis must then take into account both this construction and the context of the interview.

Another assumption underpinning the interview process is that a response to a question will bear some relation to the 'truth' of the person's understanding and knowledge of the issue. It is vitally important that due consideration be given to the disturbances caused by the researcher focusing on one aspect of a person's life experience. This focus may produce a number of effects:

- Protective 'fronts' (Douglas, 1976) may be created, of which only the first few layers may be revealed.
- Public rather than private views may be exposed.
- The researched may undertake a reassessment of their experiences, leading to complete reconstruction. This may either favour themselves or be what they think the researcher is seeking.

The researcher's position is also problematic. Should he/she totally accept, without question, information given? Should he/she meticulously interrogate the informant, cross-check accounts and spend many hours attempting to penetrate the fronts provided? Or should he/she accept that the information provided is only one facet of the multiple aspects of 'truth', only a few of which are likely to be exposed in a single study?

The issue of power in the interview process must also be addressed. Feminist interviewers tend to opt for equal participation and/or action research when interviewing vulnerable people or those perceived to be of lesser status. Other researchers generally interview persons from the same class who are not particularly vulnerable, thus avoiding the need to address issues of power and accountability.

Interviewing elite groups

In recent times, a number of researchers have attempted to interview people in high positions, such as judges and surgeons. This elite research poses a number of obstacles, in particular, access, type of interview and type of data. The process of access is usually protracted. Professional associations may be involved, but actual availability is the most difficult aspect. Most elite people do not have time for interviews. They work long or strange hours and have a well-developed distrust of researchers. Qualitative researchers in particular are frowned upon. They are placed on the same level as journalists, with the added disadvantage that processes of interpretation are bound to promote distortion of anything said.

Daly and McDonald's study (1992), involving elite persons with scientific training, demonstrates the problems such people have with qualitative research. The group of cardiologists to be interviewed decided to become co-researchers after a colleague (who was on the research team) approached them. This group expressed considerable doubt regarding qualitative data's lack of 'scientific orientation'. The research team had to agree to collect both qualitative and quantitative data to complete the study. The latter was used to generate key variables, which were graded according to particular criteria. These variables were then entered into a computer to create and validate the *typologies* (classification schemes) gained from the qualitative analysis, and to provide reliable 'objective' data that might be more acceptable to medical journals.

If access to elites is achieved, further delays may occur. The 'questionnaire' may be requested for prior viewing and critique, resulting in the removal or restructuring of a number of key questions. The interview session rarely occurs outside the elite person's workplace, is usually limited to 'twenty or thirty minutes' and tends to be punctuated by phonecalls and the intrusion of 'urgent' matters. In this situation, the collection of thick descriptive data is often abandoned in favour of whatever responses can be extracted. Verbal statements from these people are very carefully worded, presenting a 'public', and usually already publicly available, view. The process of validating the transcript often involves a complete rewrite, with the final product resembling a press release.

Even when access is gained, participation does not necessarily follow. An example of this is a study by Cassell (1988), who was forced to fall back on family contacts in the relevant area due to difficulties in persuading surgeons to become involved. She concluded that success in researching elites depends on having acceptable contacts, suitable personal appearance, charm, intelligence, a thick skin and a demonstrated ability to be non-judgemental during data collection.

Once a researcher has achieved access, he/she should undertake an elaborate preparation of background information, based on the subject's biography and expressed opinions (Denzin, 1989). Denzin also suggests the avoidance of any form of questionnaire. He favours placing one broad issue on the table and using considerable interviewing skills to draw out opinions, together with very careful presentation of the data to preserve anonymity and avoid litigation. One example of successful elite interviewing (Meredith, 1993) involved surgeons, anaesthetists, other health professionals and patients in a study over a ten-week period. The study explored patient participation in decision making and consent to treatment in the case of general surgery. Consultations were taped and observed, providing rich, comprehensive data.

Postmodern interviewing

Postmodern interviewing techniques allow the researcher to take a decentred position, although this has not been accepted as readily in research as it has been in literature. A decentred research position would involve the researcher in the following actions:

- initial negotiation with participants to orient the topic towards their life experiences;
- passive listening rather than active interviewing, so that questions are kept to a minimum and areas may not be investigated if not raised by participants;
- shared analysis and interpretation;

- collaborative ownership of the narratives or appropriate acknowledgement of the participants' contribution; and
- active seeking of multiple perspectives and information gained from a variety of contexts.

Interviewer

The interviewer is of central importance to the process of interviewing, regardless of the position taken. Qualitative research has no pretested tools for data collection behind which the researcher can hide. He/she therefore becomes foregrounded. Researchers using heavily 'theory-driven' research can stand in a slightly more protective shadow than those who use 'theory-generating' approaches. Neither can avoid the assessing gaze of both the participant and the reader, however. It cannot be overemphasised that the quality and substance of the data collected during interviewing depend largely on the quality of the relationship established between interviewer and interviewee. A good interviewer:

- has the capacity to listen intelligently;
- is enthusiastic regarding the topic;
- is interested in what the (expert) interviewee has to contribute;
- can share joy and sadness;
- is compassionate;
- is totally focused at all times; and
- can handle contradictory information and complex situations with sensitivity.

Journalling

As readers of research we need to know how the researcher thinks, acts, interacts with and feels about the participants and her/his project, and how her/his concerns and values affect the data. This information can be found in the *researcher's diary*, which is kept to ensure that researchers approach an acceptable form of honest self-assessment, are critically reflective of their performances or are attempting to demonstrate a process of transformation. Diaries vary from researcher to researcher and can be quite revealing. Branislaw Malinowski's diary, which he kept during 1917 while researching in the Troubriand Islands (Malinowski, 1967), reveals incidents of violence, coercion, lust and extortion, as well as a picture of a lonely and rather fed-up young researcher in an isolated situation.

An extract from one of my own diaries, written during a project to investigate the access of young people with severe intellectual disability to school curricula, work, services and the community (previously mentioned in Chapter 1), reveals some of my frustrations and concerns:

> 23rd August 1989, 4pm Me—relaxed—'Jan' [pseudonym for a teacher in high school] tense. Storeroom [cramped, size of a toilet] too hot. I felt sleepy. Same issues emerging—stress, too much to do, the ever expanding role of the teacher, unsympathetic administration, no training to cope with primary and pre-primary aged intellects, students very diverse. Does 'mixed ability' mean each teacher has to teach at 3 levels in each class—advanced, mid range and slow, providing 3 sets of worksheets—the '3 in one' class? Who benefits from this? Who loses? Observed 'Joe' all day—he has no aide, he wandered aimlessly and alone all day. Kids circled him, teachers ignored him. I spoke to him in WW class, he grunted, put his head under arm and scuttled away sideways. Does integration = physical presence only? c/w Melanie @ X technical school who appeared involved and heavily supported by aide and teachers, or is the major interaction between the aide and the teachers* (check this). I must visit a class where M. has no aide support/when aide is away. I think my enthusiasm for the problems of integration (i.e. my desire for it to work) is blinding me to the real problems of the teachers who are stymied by overwork and administrative responsibilities and can no longer see how it can work. I feel frustrated with their depressed attitudes—suspect most regard people with disabilities as a waste of time and effort in this economic climate. I think I'll pull out of schools for a bit and go back to interviewing parents and observing and interviewing in institutions. (Grbich, research diary for Grbich and Sykes, 1989)

The twin issues of reflection and accountability, involving exposure of personal frameworks, necessitate maintaining diary records throughout the research process. These records may be published separately, interwoven with the final presentation of text or interpreted alongside the main data set.

Presentation of self

It may well be useful to examine the findings regarding matching the researcher with the researched in order to be fully informed about the factors that may influence the establishment and maintenance of good relations with participants. Currently, the strongest indicator is that the quality of rapport established is the most important factor (Bailey, 1987). In some situations, however, issues of dress, sexuality, gender, age, class and race may need consideration.

Dress and sexual preference

Most researchers accept that clothing should be neutral and should aim to bridge the gap between the interviewer and the interviewee. It is generally considered inappropriate to wear jeans when interviewing a senior executive, or to put on a designer outfit for interviewing street youths heavily involved in drug consumption. Where questions relating to different sexual preferences form part of the investigation, the researcher must ask her/himself, 'Am I the person most likely to gain the best data?' For example, gay male researchers interviewing gay males on their sexual habits with regard to the potential spread of the AIDS virus may more closely approach the truth of the matter than researchers of heterosexual inclination.

Gender and age

The issue of gender has also been canvassed. Do men gain better information from other men and women from other women? Is age important? Can/should older male researchers attempt to gain an insight into the lives of teenage girls? Debate over the work of anthropologists Margaret Mead and Derek Freeman (1983) is of particular interest here. Mead, a young, female, white researcher, asserted that Samoan girls told her that they had sexual relations prior to marriage. Freeman, a middle-aged, male, white researcher, asserted that his informants, who were the male elders in a different location in Samoa, told him that this was untrue.

Despite this controversy, it is generally accepted that quality of rapport is a crucial factor. It is usually possible to locate an appropriate role or category to inhabit in order to facilitate data collection. When interviewing youth, you can be a contemporary or parent figure. When interviewing aged participants, you can be an equal or a son or daughter figure. It must be accepted, however, that the richness and accuracy of the data collected may be compromised to some extent by the category inhabited by the researcher.

Class and race

Research into issues of class and race is also inconclusive. Most research is undertaken by middle class researchers on members of their own class (middle class participants). Where research is undertaken on the working class, middle class researchers generally acknowledge that they achieve a fairly cautious response in contrast to the less conservative discussions recorded by working class researchers. This suggests that both inside knowledge and acceptance may be relevant.

Race is somewhat more controversial. One study (Tixier, Vigil and Elassasser, 1976) involved interviewing Chicana women twice: once with an Anglo interviewer and once with a Chicana interviewer. These women were more open about issues of menstruation and sexual habits with the Anglo interviewer, but spoke more freely about issues of discrimination with the Chicana interviewer.

My own experience has been that it is difficult for a person of one culture to access and comprehend the cultural intricacies of other groups. The best data, which include an accurate interpretation of the cultural clues embedded in both verbal and non-verbal interaction, are gathered by researchers of the same culture. Even when interpreters are not needed, there is often no comparison between data gathered and analysed by interviewers from the same culture and data gathered from the same participants by researchers from another culture.

One problem that must be addressed, particularly in cross-cultural interviewing, is interpretation of the same word. Do the words heard by the interviewer and interviewee have the same meaning for both? Does 'yes' really mean 'no'? What about degrees of 'yes' and 'no'? How will these be addressed? This becomes even more problematic when translators are involved, as they may be tempted to rephrase or reinterpret what is being said. It is important to spend sufficient time in a setting to ensure that the language and non-verbal cues are fully understood before interviewing commences. When translators are required, it is preferable to actually conduct the interview through the translator in order to pick up and address discrepancies as they occur. One approach that may help the researcher gather good quality data involves using members of particular ethnic groups to interview other members of the same culture in the presence of the researcher. This approach allows for the immediate translation into English, on tape, of verbal responses. Access to the meanings of non-verbal responses can then be gained in a debriefing session with the translator.

Researcher position

The researcher's position will depend on his/her values, the theoretical underpinnings of the research and the research design. A phenomenological or heuristic approach, for example, requires the researcher getting as close as possible to the essence of others' life experiences, while documenting his/her own path. Memory work research, in the feminist tradition, requires that:

- The researcher is also one of the researched.
- The researcher's experiences form part of the database.
- Consensual analysis is carried out by all participants.

At the other extreme, if a researcher is carrying out a *summative evaluation* of a department or a policy, he/she will use a distant assessment based on predecided criteria. *Formative evaluation*, however, requires equal participation, constant feedback and action leading to change.

Despite the tendency for particular designs to limit action, it is possible for a researcher to move from one position to another within the same study, depending on the data to be collected and flexibility within the research design.

Interview structures

There are three main interview structures: informal, guided and structured.

Informal interviews

Informal interviews occur largely as an adjunct to participant observation. They involve casual conversations in which the questions are spontaneous and based on interaction between researcher and respondent. No recording devices are used. Information that is often relevant to the research question may emerge in this casual, general conversation. This information may then be used as a starting point for more formal, guided or structured interviews, in which participants' responses are tape-recorded. Once the tape recorder is packed away, there is a tendency for respondents to once again indulge in casual conversation, commenting reflectively on what they have just said. This 'off-the-record' data is often closer to the 'truth' than recorded data, allowing the interviewer to see what is behind the interviewee's recorded responses. The researcher should make a mental note of casual and reflective conversations, and write up her/his observations as soon as possible after the interviews.

Guided interviews

Guided interviews comprise a set of broad-ranging questions derived from theory, previous research and *intuition* (notions that the interviewer has in mind from his/her own experience and that require exploration). The structure, phrasing and placement in the interview process of these questions are at the interviewer's discretion, but he/she must make sure that they are presented in language that the interviewees can understand. A guided interview's major purpose is to provide a minimally directive framework that enables both researcher and informant to access and identify key areas.

Ken Dovey and Joe Graffam's (1987) exploration of the experience of disability set out to engage parents, teachers, carers, employers, the wider society and people with disabilities in an investigation that centred on one major question: 'What has the experience of disability been for you?' A number of major factors emerged from the participants' exploration of their life experiences as seen from their own and others' perspectives. Important factors for those with disabilities were building self-esteem and confidence, the impact of the idea of 'normality', and their experiences with medical and other service providers. The impact of a child with a disability, the quality of family life, the need for increased knowledge and support, and the limitations of the integration model (in particular its administrative problems) were all extremely important issues from the families' perspectives. Although only one major question was investigated, this group of 96 people from various areas provided considerable insight into the issues surrounding disability in the late 1980s.

This example of a large guided interview study that utilised only one major question is fairly unique. Most such studies would include several major areas of investigation. The guided interview approach is quite usual in feminist and postmodern research, with the addition that the decentring of the researcher may lead to greater negotiation of the questions to be asked and of the interpretations of responses.

Structured interviews

Structured, *open-ended* interviews tend to be used when it is important to ask the same questions in the same sequence. When there are a large number of participants and/or a team of researchers, and comparability of data is desirable, this will be the best interview technique. *Closed-ended* questions that can be statistically analysed can be included, if probability sampling has occurred and variables can be controlled. If non-probability sampling has occurred, the results will be specific to the group when it is researched in a particular context. Any generalisability claimed will be logical rather than statistical.

For example, Grbich and Sykes (1989) investigated home tasks, access to community services, and educational and work programs for young people with intellectual disability. In this investigation the random sampling of a total population encouraged the inclusion of closed-ended questions such as: 'Please rate your view of the medical services your daughter/son has received as excellent, very good, good, poor, or totally inadequate.' These questions were used to strengthen the information gathered. Ninety-five per cent of parents rated the services as 'poor' or 'totally inadequate'. These responses were followed by the open-ended questions: 'Which services have you experienced?' and 'Why have you rated this service as you have?' These questions allowed an exploration of the parents' experiences and produced detailed, narrative responses that provided quotes for inclusion in the final report.

The example just given highlights the positive aspects of open-ended structured interviews. There is a negative side to this technique, however. The need to administer a questionnaire in a particular way limits the opportunities to explore areas of interest that may emerge. Also, the structured interview technique relies upon two highly dubious assumptions, according to Denzin (1989, p. 104):

- that it is possible to structure and order all questions in a manner that ensures that they have the same meaning for all participants; and
- that the different interactions and levels of rapport developed will not create vast differences in the quality of the collected data.

Selecting and combining interview structure/s

The 'informal', 'guided' and 'structured' interview techniques tend to favour different research purposes. Each has advantages and disadvantages. Informal and guided interviews allow for extensive exploration in a setting that is as close as possible to a conversational ideal. They emphasise the interviewee's expertise, while the structured interview shifts the balance of power and expertise towards the interviewer. Guided and structured interviews can also be displayed as appendices. Any weaknesses perceived in using only one of these three approaches can be overcome by moving from one approach to another. The informal conversation has already been shown to be a normal part of guided and structured interviews.

One possible scenario where interview structures can be combined is during course evaluations. Interviews with each person taking the course might commence with an informal conversation, followed by a recorded, 'guided' exploration of the participant's view of the course. These could be complemented by some 'structured', open-ended (and closed-ended) questions designed to provide specific data. The interview could end with an informal, unrecorded chat, yet ultimately all discussions would be recorded in one form or another. The interviewer should constantly make mental notes, which would be written up immediately after the interview.

It has been suggested that a mix of interview approaches will produce more comprehensive data, but neither the form/s of interview nor the best rapport can bridge the crevasses that appear in the data when the wrong questions are asked. This crucial problem can be minimised by piloting questionnaires and ensuring that communication lines remain open between researchers and participants, not only in relation to interviewing and verifying responses, but also on a longer term basis.

The remainder of this chapter deals with interview processes, of which there are two main types:

- person-to-person; and
- person-to-group.

Person-to-person interviews

Person-to-person interviews can be divided into:

- face-to-face; and
- telephone.

Face-to-face interviews are the most common.

Face-to-face interviews

Face-to-face interviews are usually tape recorded, carried out in the respondent's home or at an alternative setting of her/his choice, and average two hours in length.

Gaining access

One of the most difficult hurdles to overcome in conducting research using face-to-face interviews is gaining access to suitable participants. Access procedures will differ, depending on whether the researcher must go through government departments or can go directly to the individual or community. Gaining access to clients of government departments usually requires a lengthy negotiation process. Schools are a case in point. The research proposal may need to be cleared by the Education Department, then by all regional offices in whose areas the researcher may wish to access schools, then by head teachers and finally by students' parents.

Suppose that the researcher wishes to attempt a random sample of welfare recipients. If the appropriate department clears the research proposal, it may be prepared to include a note from the researcher, or a questionnaire, in one of its mailouts. The problems with this are that there is no follow-up, and the researcher depends on people contacting him/her.

Hospitals have their own ethics committees and are most reluctant to let their patients be accessed, unless they are convinced that the researcher is not out to harm vulnerable and sick people or to harass overburdened staff. Patients' permission to be interviewed must also be gained.

These scenarios suggest that researchers should consider the strategy of setting up management committees with representatives from funding bodies (if appropriate), representatives of departments/institutions providing access, and representatives of departments whose policies may be affected by any recommendations for change resulting from the research. The disadvantage of such committees is that they may attempt to control the research design and results, particularly if they have reason to fear the outcomes. The advantage lies in having a captive, and hopefully committed, audience for the research results and recommendations.

Access to members of the community also can be a slow process. Researchers have used various techniques including:

- approaching people whose addresses have been gained from electoral rolls;
- standing outside supermarkets and conducting a brief preliminary interview to ascertain the appropriateness of the potential participant and his/her willingness to provide a home interview;
- using television/radio/newspapers to advertise the study and inviting interested people to contact the researcher for more information;
- using phone-in switchboard systems for a phone-in day on a particular topic, such as domestic violence, or a contentious medical issue such as immunisation;
- approaching community support groups to gain access to their members;
- leaving notices at appropriate venues to encourage participation; and
- inviting participation by means of random telephone interviews.

The researcher may have to resort to 'snowball' or 'convenience' sampling to locate a research group from within populations that are difficult to access, such as home-based people with particular medical problems.

Developing rapport

The idea of *rapport* rests on the presumption that the interview situation should be designed to minimise differences in status, knowledge or power. This should create a sense of equality that will enable the free flow of communication between interviewer and interviewee.

Once a person has consented to participate in the study, the following processes should facilitate establishment of 'rapport':

- Make a preliminary phonecall to advise the person what her/his participation in the study will involve. Tell them how much of their time will be required: one two-hour interview in their home or at a location of their choice, or regular interviews over a period.
- Clearly explain the rights of participants.
- Clarify issues such as who is funding the research, what it is about, and who will benefit.
- Stress the importance of the person's contribution.
- Address any concerns raised by the person.

The face-to-face interview should be preceded by a non-recorded, settling-down time, where the nature and purpose of the study and the interviewee's rights may need to be recalled. A cup of tea/coffee is usually offered. This is an important way of breaking the ice. As an interviewer, I always use this time to elaborate on how I came to do this piece of research. I explain that I have always wanted to explore this area because of professional interest, or personal experience, or close family/friend's experiences, or some other relevant reason. I find that this enables the interviewee to gain some insight into my motives, and helps in the 'sizing up' process. I feel that it is important for interviewees to know whom they are talking to. If an interviewer approached you to participate in a tobacco company-funded project aimed at exploring people's views on smoking, you might be extremely doubtful of the researcher's capacity to effectively present any antagonistic responses. You might decide, therefore, that involvement in such a study would be a waste of your time. All participants have a right to know the background to, and purpose of, any study, so that they can make informed choices regarding their participation.

Recording

After the process of informing and establishing 'rapport' with the participant/s, recording can begin. An interview (with permission) can be recorded using any reliable tape recorder or dictaphone. The smaller the device the better, but it must be reliable and have good sound reproduction. Top-of-the-range recorders can cost up to $1000, but equally efficient machines retail at about $50–$150. Some re-searchers use the small microcassette recorders (about $60) with accompanying transcribers (about $200). Transcription machines need a foot pedal that will backspace to a user-selected distance. This facilitates checking back. The researcher should experiment with microphones to decide what is best suited to the situation. Flat or lapel mikes are good for group interviews, while inbuilt or upright mikes are best for two-person interviews. Lapel mikes, which cut down background noise and produce audible responses, are needed for recording in outdoor or locational settings, such as noisy coffee bars. Voice-activated recorders are *not* recommended because they do not pick up quiet voices, the beginnings of sentences or the length of pauses. The researcher should always check the tape recorder before commencing the interview. If electricity is needed for home interviews, he/she should carry an extension cord to save rearranging the furniture, and ask permission to plug into the power source. In the event of a refusal, or a power cut, it is vitally important to have some back-up in the form of batteries. Spare batteries are recommended if the researcher plans to use battery power. A small hand towel is also useful, for placing underneath the recorder to protect any highly polished surfaces that scratch easily.

Participant control

One way of ensuring that the participant has some control over the interview process is to place the recorder within the participant's reach so he/she can press the pause button. This button can be highlighted with a coloured dot or an arrow for easy access.

Once the interview is over and the recorder packed away, the more relaxed discussion that occurs may produce information of greater interest and accuracy than has been recorded, including comments that indicate the private view of the situation. On departure, it is essential for the interviewer to inquire whether there is anything that has been discussed that the participant would prefer was not used (however anonymously). Few people raise concerns at this point, enabling the researcher to drive a couple of streets away and record all that has passed, including material relating to the informal discussion and the researcher's observations. These notes are not returned with the interview transcript, although their contents should be mentioned within it, or at the end of it. Some researchers note only spoken communication. Others may include perceptions of non-verbal communication and their observations, particularly if interpretation of these is regarded as being open to negotiation.

The interview should be transcribed within 12 hours of recording, to maximise recall. A copy should be returned to the participant as soon as possible and followed up with a phonecall or a second face-to-face interview. This serves to verify the information, follow up emerging issues, and provide base data on which to build in interviews with other informants.

Data collection ceases when sampling strategies are exhausted, no new information is emerging, and the researcher is convinced that he/she has come as close to the 'truth' of the matter as possible within given time, funding and other constraints.

Although most researchers tape interviews, some prefer to take notes that can be immediately verified. The disadvantages of this lie in the difficulty of maintaining eye contact, and the problem of incomplete data, particularly when quotes or narratives are desirable.

Professional issues

It is possible that, particularly during home visits, interviewees may misinterpret the interviewer's role. They may consider some relationship apart from the interviewer–interviewee one to be appropriate. If this occurs, it is important for the researcher to clarify the professional nature of the home visit, to beat a hasty retreat if necessary, and to consider other alternatives if she/he wishes to continue this person's involvement in the study. The following incident illustrates how difficult situations may be handled.

A male colleague had arranged a mid-morning home interview with a woman participant. She opened the front door wearing a diaphanous negligee and exuding a cloud of French perfume. He recognised the cues and stepped back, apologising profusely for disturbing her at what was obviously an inappropriate time, and saying that he would ring back later to arrange another interview. This served to emphasise the more distant nature of the interviewer–interviewee relationship and allowed both participants the option of saving face. Strategies employed by some researchers to avoid such situations include going out in pairs (one male and one female), or confining female interviewers to female participants and male interviewers to male participants.

The potential for sexual harassment, however, pales before the issue of personal accountability. The interviewer–interviewee relationship is widely recognised as an exploitative one. Researchers often seek information, sometimes very personal information, from vulnerable people. What happens to this information? What should a researcher do when he/she discovers lonely and neglected people, or issues bordering on malpractice but not sufficiently clear as to invite immediate action? Some guidelines may be useful in coping with these concerns:

- Before entering the field, get together with interested colleagues and brainstorm the problems that may be encountered.
- Be fully informed regarding your legal responsibilities to report certain categories of information, and have up-to-date information about the relevant services and support groups available in the area.
- Properly address the responsibilities undertaken, as a professional researcher, when intruding into people's lives.
- Contract with each participant to provide a full/summarised copy of the research findings in accessible language.
- Build this cost into the application for research funding. Simply stating to participants that their views may contribute to future changes from which they may ultimately benefit (however likely this may be) is insufficient recompense for their time and effort.

Telephone interviews

Telephone interviews, like face-to-face interviews, are usually recorded (with the participant's permission). This is done by means of a small cheap ($8) electronic recording device, attached to the body of the phone by a suction cup and plugged into a tape recorder, or by means of an answering machine with a two-way recording capacity. The latter is more effective, but it will cost around $200.

Telephone interviews have the advantage of being impersonal. Some people appear to prefer this form of interaction, even asserting that they reveal more on the phone and feel more comfortable than they would face to face. The disadvantages from the interviewer's perspective are that body language, which is often very revealing, cannot be observed. It is also much easier for the interviewee to terminate an interview by simply hanging up.

Do people reveal more in verbal communication on the phone than they would face to face? No currently available research has assessed this issue. This form of communication may seem more natural to many people than a formal interview situation, however. Given that the researcher may well be less evident, the 'friendly conversation' ideal may be easier to achieve on the phone than with the 'stranger in the lounge room' scenario. Telephone interviews are often used as second or follow-up interviews to face-to-face interviews. In this situation, the interviewee 'knows' to whom he/she is speaking, having already sighted and 'sized up' the interviewer.

Interviewing children and people who are aged or sick or have a disability

Some adjustments to the general interviewing process may be necessary when children or people who are aged or sick or have a disability are being interviewed.

Children

When interviewing very young children, it should be noted that autobiographical memory is not considered to have emerged until the age of four years (Nelson, 1992). Children under four will recount events they have found memorable, but these require a good deal of probing. Establishing 'rapport' is often complicated by the nature of the adult–child relationship. Once children have achieved school age, the sense that 'correct' answers are expected may be another stumbling block in seeking 'truth'. Interviews should be kept to a half-hour maximum for younger children, and an hour for older children. Techniques that seem to help confidence building are:

- getting younger children to draw a situation and explain it;
- playing back their early responses during the interview with enthusiastic and supportive comments regarding their performance; and
- using pile-sorting cards with coloured pictures, which can be sorted and discussed.

When young children are otherwise occupied during interviewing, their conversation tends to flow more readily than when they are interviewed face to face. In such situations, lapel or flat microphones are suggested, as children's activities will tend to take them out of the tape recorder's range. Questions should be tailored to the age and vocabulary levels of children, bearing in mind that there are different levels of comprehension at different ages. Questions should also be flexible. They need to be more concrete for younger children, relating to action rather than feelings. This is because they have often had less experience in articulating feelings. It may be better for same-sex interviewers to conduct interviews on sensitive subjects, particularly when adolescents are concerned.

Age and disability

Particular effort should be made to accommodate special needs when interviewing people with age, intellectual or illness-related disability. There are several ways in which the interviewer can achieve a successful outcome from interviewing people who fall within these categories:

- Print consent and information letters in larger type, as a sensible precaution for the visually impaired and those on medication.
- Shorten interview times for all participants.
- When interviewing respondents with hearing limitations, directly face them and speak clearly (essential).
- Maintain a comfortable, supportive environment for all interviewees, paying special attention to valuing all contributions positively (essential).
- Keep questions clear, short and simple, and rephrase them whenever any confusion is evident.
- Wait longer than usual for responses.
- Demonstrate exceptionally empathetic listening skills, in order to facilitate a calm, relaxed environment.
- When people with severe intellectual disabilities are interviewed, encourage carers to be present, as they can clarify responses that may be less understandable to the interviewer.

Carers

My own experiences of interviewing young children, people with intellectual disability and older women from different ethnic backgrounds suggest that it is advisable to spend some initial time with carers. This enables the interviewer to ascertain any particular aspects or issues that may need negotiation, and to clarify with carers that there are no right or wrong responses. It is also essential to emphasise the value of their support in gaining the *participant's* views rather than *their* views as carers. You may well be seeking these at another time.

Regardless of what type of respondent is being interviewed, an important element in successful research is 'question design'.

Question design

Interview questions tend to fall into one of two categories: 'descriptive' or 'probing'. *Descriptive questions* aim to provide an extensive response based on the interviewee's expert knowledge of a particular area. *Probing questions* are used to elicit further information, or to focus 'descriptive' responses provided by the interviewees. Descriptive questions are always used during the early stages of an interview when the interviewer is starting out with broad questions. These are then narrowed using 'probing' techniques.

Descriptive questioning

A good descriptive question is one that elicits a stream of information about something the interviewee knows well and is interested in, such as his/her life experiences or expertise in a particular field. Good descriptive questions also help the participant relax. An example of this type of question is:

When did you first learn that your child had a disability?

Other descriptive questions are then used to explore further the interviewee's concerns:

How did you feel about/respond to that?

Researchers use another descriptive technique that attempts to present polar positions to discover the interviewee's stance on a controversial issue. This may involve the interviewer divulging information gained from other interviews to indicate that she/he is aware of what is going on in a particular context. The following hypothetical question/statement could be used when interviewing people in an institutional setting where abuse is suspected:

> *I've been talking to other residents and some have told me about the good things you do here: you go to the beach; you go shopping; and you go to football matches. But some residents have told me about other things that go on here: like people getting left in rooms on their own or missing out on dinner; like people who can't walk getting left on toilets for a long time; and like carers getting cross and smacking residents. Would you like to give me your view of this place?*

This is very long in terms of question construction, but it was deemed necessary to have a preliminary exposé of knowledge already gained if confirmation of certain incidents was to occur. The presentation of extremes in this manner also allowed the residents to focus only on the good things about the institution if they were unaware of other aspects, or if they felt uncomfortable or vulnerable in acknowledging these.

Probing questions

Probing questions can take a range of forms. The most common is an interested silence, with appropriate facial expressions, or verbal cues such as *Oh . . . ! Really . . . ? Well . . .!*

Repetition can be used, although this is a technique favoured by counsellors and can become very frustrating to the interviewee if overused, as in the following case:

Interviewer: *Now what led to that situation?*
Interviewee: *Well I . . . and after two years I finished up there.*
Interviewer: *You finished up there?*
Interviewee: *Yes, after two years.*

This last interchange has added nothing to the data. It could well have been replaced by:

So, what happened then . . . ?

or by a more focused question relating to previously offered information. This would have indicated that the interviewer had actually been listening and was genuinely interested in what was being said.

The interviewer must be alert as well as gently critical if he/she is to pick up anomalies in the story and to query them. This can be achieved by putting in a quick résumé question along the lines of:

Now, let me see if I've got this straight—first this . . . then this . . . now how does that bit fit in?

The aim is not to carry out investigative journalism to the interviewer's fullest critical capacity, but to indicate that he/she has noticed a discrepancy while giving the person credit for their knowledge, compared with the interviewer's lack of adequate comprehension. This ensures that the interviewer is a critical friend rather than a credulous recipient of tall stories. Résumé or summary questions are also useful at the end of an interview. Many interviewees do not sequence events in strict time order. Unless these are clarified at some point, the data set can become very jumbled and difficult to handle. The following summary questions illustrate an effective method of avoiding such difficulties:

Right, now the first thing that happened was . . . (pause here for confirmation and further exploration), *then you . . .* (pause again), *and the final outcome was . . .* (again pause).

Hypothetical questions that pose an ideal, or advocate something the interviewer knows will confront the interviewee's value system, can be used to probe opinions and provoke a lively discussion. For example, this question:

> *I wonder if we shouldn't just get the Education Department to reconsider integration and retain children with intellectual disabilities in special school settings?*

sparked considerable debate, regardless of whether it was posed to parents, head teachers in special or regular schools, integration teachers, aides or other students (Grbich and Sykes, 1989).

Responses

If someone does not respond to a question, the interviewer should first check the non-verbal response. If the interviewee looks uncertain, the interviewer should apologise and rephrase the question:

> *I'm sorry, I didn't explain that well. What I meant was . . .*

This is not as simple as it sounds. Before leaping in and rephrasing, the interviewer should always check that the person is not just thinking. Older people and those from different cultures often take quite a long time to think out a response.

An interview with an older indigenous man provides an excellent example. The first question was posed—silence. The interviewer tried to ascertain from the man's facial expression whether or not to rephrase, but the man's face was impassive and he was respectfully avoiding eye contact in keeping with his indigenous tradition. This made it difficult to judge what was going on. Three minutes passed. Just as the interviewer drew breath to present a rephrased question, the interviewee also drew breath and delivered a lengthy and beautifully constructed response, obviously based on extensive deliberation.

Questions to avoid

There are three types of questions that may cause problems for the interviewee and/or the interviewer: two-in-one, closed-ended and 'why' questions.

Two-in-one questions

Two-in-one questions tend to be confusing. Most respondents answer one question and forget about the other. Consider, for example:

> *What did you do after you realised you had been injured, and how did you feel about that?*

This question brought a response to the doing rather than the feeling aspect. This type of question should not be used unless for a particular purpose.

Closed-ended questions

Closed-ended questions, in particular those structured to produce a 'Yes' or 'No' response (*dichotomous questions*), should only be used as a preliminary to further probing. For example, the question:

> *So you undertook to . . . ?*

pre-empts the probable answer: *Yes I did/No I did not.* This type of question on its own does not encourage the interviewee to provide much information. By contrast, consider the question:

> *Does your daughter carry out any home tasks?*

If the answer is 'Yes', this can provide the information needed to further investigate the details of various tasks.

'Why' questions

'Why' questions tend to put people on the spot and suggest that the interviewer does not believe what they have said.

Parent:	. . . and the doctor said she was a Downs and should be institutionalised, as she would only ever be a vegetable.
Interviewer:	*Why did he say that . . .?*
Parent:	*Well, I suppose . . . well I don't really know, um . . . because of the way she looked, though I can't be sure, she was a lovely baby . . .*

'Why' questions presume reasons and relationships of a cause–effect nature and often add little to information already gathered. They can, however, be used selectively in a fine probing situation where the 'truth' seems very elusive. Even in such a situation, it is advisable to use them with caution.

Person-to-group interviews

Person-to-group interviews can be conducted face to face in the form of any of the three main approaches to group interviews:

- focus groups;
- the nominal group process; or
- the Delphi technique.

Focus groups

Focus groups are semi-structured, person-to-group interviews that aim to explore a specific set of issues. They have recently become very popular. The focus group interview involves six to twelve people in a 'focused' interview lasting between one and one and a half hours. This technique emerged from Robert Merton's research in the 1940s, and from the rating of radio programs in the 1950s. Here individuals operating push-button mechanisms were connected to radio stations. These individuals registered positive or negative responses to particular programs by pressing a green or red button respectively. Marketing and advertising then used the idea for trialling products with groups of people to gain responses to packaging. Later, researchers from other fields decided that it was a useful time-saving technique. They could gather information from a range of people within the same timeframe it would usually take to interview just one person.

Focus groups are currently used for:

- collecting background information or identifying issues that will form the basis of hypotheses, more structured questions, evaluations or needs assessments;
- investigating responses to policy changes;
- pretesting advertising and marketing strategies; and
- investigating sensitive issues that are difficult to broach on a one-to-one basis, though whether this technique does produce better data on sensitive issues is still controversial.

Running a focus group is not just a matter of locating some willing people and interviewing them in a group situation. Careful planning and attention to detail are necessary if useful information is to be produced. Several steps must be followed.

Setting up a focus group

Firstly, the interviewer should carefully consider the selection of the group. Ideally, a focus group is the coming together of *key informants* on a particular topic. The researcher should aim, therefore, for each participant to represent a particular position or group. This helps to encourage interaction. It also gives the group facilitator the confidence to call on individuals to give their opinion of their represented area:

> *Now, I wonder if Jane from the single parents' group would like to comment . . . ?*

A heterogeneous group, representing a variety of perspectives on a particular issue, will probably produce the most satisfactory discussion.

A focus group *facilitator* has control over three major aspects of the interview process:

- the location of the interview;
- the physical environment; and
- the composition of the group.

He/she must address these before the group meets.

Location: The location should be close to the participants' working/living places to avoid extensive travelling. Preferably, the group should not meet in the interviewer's/participants' work area, as this will contain inbuilt distractions such as telephones, messages and requests for urgent signatures. If people need to travel from interstate or out of town, then transport and accommodation costs should be provided, as should tea, coffee, a meal if necessary, child minding and a participation fee of around $30 (if this is deemed appropriate or desirable).

Physical environment: The room chosen should be small but not so cramped as to inhibit interaction. It must be large enough to seat the group comfortably in a circle so that they can all see each other, but not too large, as large rooms often echo, enabling shy people to fade into the background. Most people prefer to sit at tables, but from the researcher's point of view tables inhibit the observation of non-verbal body language. It is better, therefore, to remove them. The walls too should be bare. Distracting elements such as lively posters or eye-catching abstract art should be removed.

Group composition: A mixed group is usual with regard to age and friendship, but this depends on the focus group's purpose. A group of similar age, for example, may tend to show a conformity of response, although this will depend on the topic. A group involving several friends may be inhibited by friendship and issues of loyalty.

Gender also has the potential to affect outcomes. Mixed groups are usually preferable, again depending on the topic, but persons who exhibit 'stereotypical' behaviour in mixed groups should be avoided. Women who become passive and inarticulate in the presence of males, and men or women who become dominating and respond at length to every initiative, or constantly interrupt and talk over others, should all be avoided if they can be identified early. Over-recruitment is sensible in case some individuals cannot come at the last minute. It is advisable to recruit two more people than are really needed.

The status of individual group members also must be addressed. Nothing is more likely to result in silence or minimal response than placing senior members of an organisation with junior members. Equality of status certainly produces more lively outcomes. If it is known that certain group members hold strong views that are antagonistic to those of other members, or that certain participants are involved in long term confrontations with each other over various issues, the facilitator must devise a plan to prevent the focus group from becoming a battleground dominated by a few people with entrenched interests.

Procedure

The researcher must be very clear about his/her research question before attempting to organise a focus group. He/she must also be convinced that using a focus group is the best means of providing the information sought. Once convinced that the desired outcomes can be achieved, the researcher should choose a group/sample by matching participants carefully with the research objectives.

The group should meet for a 'warm-up' (a cup of tea or coffee) before sitting down. This gives the facilitator the opportunity to welcome each person individually; to see that all arrangements have been met; and to have a quick chat with participants, to assess who is likely to dominate or who may need encouragement in the group discussion.

Individuals should then be seated strategically. Persons with known or suspected demanding natures should be placed to the facilitator's right or left. This will enable physical contact of the touch-on-the-arm variety, a technique used to indicate that other people also need to contribute. The position opposite the facilitator should not be given to a dominating person, as this will make it too easy for the facilitator's eye to be caught and firmly held, or ignored, while the dominating person takes over. This position should be reserved for a person suspected of being particularly reserved or shy. This will enable the facilitator to attempt to engage the person in eye contact and encourage participation with verbal and non-verbal cues.

Once the focus group has been appropriately seated, the facilitator should introduce the topic then run through the ethical issues of confidentiality, anonymity, the right of each individual to withdraw from the group at any point without penalty, and the right not to respond to any question.

Running a focus group requires not only the skills of a good interviewer, but also considerable social skills. A good focus group interviewer has:

- empathy;
- enthusiasm;
- alertness;
- confidence;
- a good sense of humour;
- honesty regarding the interviewer's own bias;
- the capacity to be non-judgemental;
- clarity of expression;
- a strong but not too directive personality;
- the ability to terminate long-winded contributions without causing offence;
- the ability to encourage reticent participants without producing discomfort; and
- the ability to intervene gently in heated arguments without becoming bloodied in the process.

Interviewing techniques

The facilitator of the focus group should employ the usual interviewing technique of going from the general to the specific in a *funnelling* manner. This process should take less time than in a one-to-one interview, as it is necessary to get to the main discussion questions fairly early in the interview before people get tired or start thinking about leaving. A maximum of between ten and twelve pretested questions is usual for these interviews, allowing for some limited exploration of issues. If this focus group discussion is to be repeated with different groups of people, questions must be posed in the same order and format to enable comparability of responses across the groups, although their actual comparability remains contentious. In addition, and in all cases, it is important to provide questions that investigate the participant's needs and concerns, rather than concentrating solely on questions that reflect the researcher's interests.

Various other techniques can be used to maximise response. The circle technique is the most traditional of these. Each person is asked the same question in turn. The outcome of this process may be ten versions of the first or most dominant response to each question. This technique can be a useful tactic when certain people are tending to take over, as it breaks the pattern of dominance and ensures that everyone contributes to a key question. Another technique is to throw out one exciting or controversial idea and see what happens. All responses can then be carefully probed. A third possibility is to present a scenario of ideas and develop the response. The success of this strategy depends on group response. Some groups become very lively, while others may submerge under the onslaught of too many ideas at one time. Brainstorming issues, encouraging lateral thinking and attempting to develop a range of potential solutions are other techniques worth trying. Presenting analogies, or ideal or hypothetical situations, can distance the real situation and allow discussion to proceed in a less emotive manner. Various techniques of storytelling, presentation of case studies, and displays of film, video, photos or models are other useful ways to start a discussion or regenerate tired groups.

The facilitator can model the type of interaction wanted by the manner of questioning or the discussion style promoted and encouraged. Careful sampling may well be the key to a lively discussion (Morgan, 1995). It may be advisable to have two facilitators if the topic is particularly technical (Krueger, 1994) or when the researcher comes from a different cultural or racial background from the focus group members. In such a case, the researcher may prefer to co-facilitate with a person of the appropriate race. I have found this approach particularly successful when communicating with older women with different racial origins from my own.

Recording

Focus group sessions can be effectively recorded by using either a flat microphone, which can pick up voices from a range of directions, or lapel microphones. A second researcher records the participants' order of speech and non-verbal communication (stick-on name-tags are useful here), together with the first few words of each person's contribution if identification of each speaker is required for documentation. It is almost impossible to work out who is speaking on the tape without this. Speakers can be asked to identify themselves each time they speak, but this rather unnatural way of communicating tends to inhibit the flow of debate.

Verbal and non-verbal interaction can be captured on video. My own experiments with this have been highly successful in regard to both non-verbal observation and participant identification. A video recorder is placed in the room, but at some distance from the group, thereby reducing its capacity for intrusion. A flat microphone is centrally placed to record conversation. The major advantages of this technique are the permanent visual and vocal records, and elimination of the need to transcribe noisy tapes, although quotes and major points still have to be taken off the screen. The use of a video camera also removes the need for an extra researcher.

Feedback

At the conclusion of the focus group session, the facilitator should debrief the group and provide feedback. This may include pamphlets, phone numbers of support groups or any other relevant information. The transcriptions of focus group interviews are rarely sent to participants, as the numbers involved are viewed as providing instant verification and adequate cross-referencing. Some researchers choose to contact individual members and pursue various issues further on a one-to-one basis to achieve a greater depth of knowledge. Any participant who exhibits distress is usually approached at the end of the session and/or contacted by phone a couple of days later to see whether he/she requires any further support.

Data analysis

Analysis of focus group data usually requires categorisation of responses in terms of the questions, using the theoretical frameworks upon which the researcher has chosen to base these. David Morgan (1995) has utilised an adaptation of a grounded theory approach, however, in which emergent themes direct theoretical interpretation.

Examples of focus group studies

Some of the better-documented focus group studies to date include:

- An exploration of the perceived learning needs of nurses caring for persons with HIV disease. The purpose of this study was to gather information to construct a training program (Halloran and Grimes, 1995).
- An investigation of older adults' coping strategies in caring for an older adult family member with Alzheimer's disease (Morgan, 1992).
- The development of appropriate support programs for retired people (Straw and Marks, 1995).
- A search through the content and effect of media messages about AIDS (Kitzinger, 1994). In this study, 52 focus groups were conducted. Each was composed

of a homogeneous group of participants, and tasks involved writing a news bulletin from photos and card sorting (people at risk and the degree of risk).

- An identification of the service needs of women infected with HIV (Seals et al., 1995).
- A study involving the identification of the barriers to breast cancer screening faced by older Hispanic women (Saint-Germain, Bassford and Montano, 1993).

Advantages and disadvantages

There are many advantages in using focus group interview techniques in such studies, but there are also disadvantages. The following lists should provide a balanced view of the pros and cons of using focus group interview techniques.

Researchers found the greatest *advantages* of using focus groups in the above studies to be that:

- They are particularly suitable for groups with a strong oral tradition and low levels of formal education.
- They are time efficient. More people can be questioned in the same amount of time as it takes to interview one person.
- The group provides instant verification of the data because of the inbuilt checks and balances of a variety of viewpoints.
- A skilled facilitator can build on a single response to develop a rich source of data.
- Both the group and the facilitator can benefit when a reciprocal process of information is built into the debriefing section.
- These groups can provide an interesting perspective on the power of group dynamics and the degree of tendency towards consensus on particular topics.

The *disadvantages* are that:

- Only a limited number of questions can be addressed.
- Questions cannot be explored in detail, nor can interesting leads be adequately pursued.
- The facilitator needs special skills.
- Two researchers (or one plus a video recorder that can be set up and left to run on its own) are needed.
- Some people do not interview well in group situations, while others tend to dominate. Rather than ten views being collected, only two to three sets of views may be reflected in the data.

- The 'public' rather than the 'private' views of individuals tend to be documented.

When choosing focus groups as their approach to group interviews, a researcher must consider all of the above advantages and disadvantages, then ask her/himself:

- Am I collecting good qualitative data, or are the data rather mediocre?
- Are data being collected in this manner for reasons of expediency, or to increase participant numbers to appease funding bodies?

The answers to these questions can be found only within each researcher's assessment of her/his situation, her/his performances and the quality of the data collected.

Variations

There are, of course, variations on traditional focus group approaches. One is anonymised focus groups for sensitive issues (White and Thomson, 1995), in which general practitioners were interviewed via a teleconference link up. Another is synergetic focus groups (Russell, 1994), where the participants ran the focus group themselves after the researcher had introduced the phenomenon. This group was homogeneous. The participants were acquaintances or friends, who were sought as participants because the researcher's focus was on combined insights rather than a commonality of perspectives.

These examples illustrate how each researcher chooses what he/she thinks is the most appropriate interview process for a particular study. Those who do not choose to use focus groups may well use the nominal group interviewing process.

Nominal group process

The nominal group form of group interviewing allows for the pooling of the diverse and expert judgements of five to nine people, who deliberate on issues where there is known disagreement regarding the nature of the problem and/or its possible solutions. The process generally takes about 90 minutes. It can be carried out either as a live round-table discussion or by tele- or video-conference. When setting up the nominal group process, the researcher must first identify the experts in a particular area, obtain their agreement to participate, and locate a suitable time for the discussion. The nominal group process is then undertaken, usually in four consecutive stages:

1 Participants write down their responses to a carefully formulated stimulus question, which is presented to them in written form or read aloud over the phone or via computer, television or video;.
2 Each participant then contributes a justification for his/her response.
3 The collected responses, with justifications, are made available to all participants, who discuss them at length in order to provide clarification.
4 Participants rank the ideas on the basis of their own preferences. Finally, the group discusses the ranked results.

This approach of identifying a diversity of expert opinion has been used extensively in business and government, particularly in program planning, where it enables the involvement of a range of community interests. An example of the latter could be an exploration of the issues involved in providing accommodation for frail but independent older people. A spokesperson from a group of older people, an economist and other people with known expertise or opinions could be invited to participate and to express their views.

This use of the nominal group process as a facilitator of community program planning often precedes the Delphi technique.

Delphi technique

The Delphi technique is usually linked to policy development. It has been used to develop future projections and forecasts, and to generate expert opinion on policy matters. During the 1950s, the Rand Corporation decided that face-to-face committee meetings had several limitations:

- There was intense social pressure to join the majority view.
- Strong opinions tended to override weaker voices.
- People generally avoided conflict.
- There were clashes of personality.
- Status problems meant that those further up the hierarchy were heard most often, and there tended to be undue emphasis on consensus or on changing opinions as an outcome.

The corporation concluded that, if genuine diversity of opinion was to be identified, interpersonal interaction would have to be eliminated. So the Delphi technique was developed.

The Delphi is characterised by four aspects:

- anonymity of experts;
- several rounds of questionnaires;
- feedback between rounds; and
- some form of statistically or descriptively analysed group response so that the strength (or otherwise) of consensus can be seen.

The first stage involves a panel's identification of a broad-ranging, open-ended question and the formulation of related issues (often accomplished by the use of a nominal group process), leading to the development of a questionnaire. A process of peer review is used to select participants. Up to 40 identified experts are each invited to nominate three other experts. The total number (160) is then sampled randomly and between 10 and 40 people are invited to participate. If a homogeneous group is desired, the number will be closer to 10; if maximum variation is sought, the group may comprise up to 40 people.

The questionnaire is mailed out to the group by post, email or fax. The responses are collated and analysed, then sent back to the panel. These results are used to develop a second questionnaire that identifies particular areas of disagreement. This questionnaire is then sent to participants, and the group is invited also to rank the responses to each question in the first questionnaire. The process is repeated, and a third questionnaire is developed and sent out together with the responses to the second questionnaire, which again require ranking. In addition, statements are sought for outsider or deviant rankings. The process is repeated until consensus seems imminent. This may take up to ten rounds, although more usually only three are conducted. The final results are analysed, and the median response is taken to represent the group's position. The resultant report indicates areas of consensus, spread of opinion, minority arguments and deviant responses.

Let us take a step back to the nominal group process example involving research into the breadth of issues involved in accommodating frail, independent older people. A Delphi group could take this a step further, and attempt some solutions by including experts from aged care, older people's support groups, health professionals and others relevant to that area. Once the parameters had been identified issues could be ranked, and disagreements and solutions trialled through successive rounds of questionnaires.

In health, the Delphi technique has been used in curriculum and policy planning to generate debate, determine priorities and identify role competencies. Variations to the technique have become evident most recently. It has been used in conjunction with a data set of face-to-face interviews (Bell, 1993) to establish guidelines for generating communication technology curricula. This study used email and Likert scales to rank responses, which were statistically analysed and compared with the results gained from the qualitative interviews.

Further variations to the technique are evident in a study that aimed to reduce the uncertainties surrounding the associated health and environmental risks involved in the application of sewage sludge to farmland (Webler et al., 1991). Consolidation of expert opinion was required in a very short time, so a 'group Delphi' was developed. This panel of 21 experts was assembled in a hall, in the presence of local citizens, for one day. A two-part questionnaire using Likert scaling and open questions was presented to rotating subgroups, to build consensus and define disagreement. Plenary discussions were held between rounds to foster peer review. This variation of the Delphi process proved to be highly successful. Although anonymity has clearly been abandoned in this version, participants and citizens expressed satisfaction with the outcomes.

Advantages and criticisms

The *advantages* of the more traditional versions of this technique are:

- The issue, rather than individual responses, provides the focus.
- Direct communication among group members is avoided.
- Anonymity is preserved.
- Equal participation is ensured.

There has been some debate, however (O'Brien, 1978), as to whether this process actually reduces *socio-psychological* variables (relating to social or psychological issues) and produces superior research results. Other concerns centre on the capacity of 'experts' to develop future, alternative solutions to problems whose current practice they well may have influenced (Johnston, 1970). The issue of anonymity has also been questioned. A number of studies indicated a lack of significant differences between responses from anonymous and identified participants (O'Brien, 1978). Scientific validity has also been problematic when only quantitative data have been collected (Rowe, Wright and Bolger, 1991). The current adaptations, which include qualitative and quantitative data, appear to be providing more acceptable outcomes.

Summary

A particular phenomenon may be explored by utilising a range of research designs and data collection techniques. The three major techniques include interviewing, observation and document collection. This chapter has undertaken an in-depth examination of 'interviewing'. The following statements summarise the major points discussed.

Interviewing is the most commonly used technique of data collection. It requires decisions regarding:

- the presentation of self (as the interviewer);
- the position of the researcher;
- interviewing style;
- the issue of power relations between researcher and researched;
- diary records;
- interview structures;
- question construction;
- the building of 'rapport'; and
- professional and ethical issues.

Interviews are usually person-to-person or person-to-group. Group interviews may be conducted as focus groups, nominal groups or Delphi groups. Each interview technique or process has its own purposes, procedures, advantages and disadvantages. These advantages and disadvantages dictate when, where and how each technique or process will be used. Researchers are constantly adapting techniques and processes in an attempt to gain better quality (more reliable) data.

The next chapter takes an in-depth look at the second major data-collection technique: 'observation'.

Further readings

Diary keeping

Corti, L. (1993) *Using Diaries in Social Research*. Social Research Update, 2. Department of Sociology, University of Surrey.

Ely, M., Anzul, M., Freidman, T., Garner, D. and Steinmetz, A. (1991) *Doing Qualitative Research: Circles within Circles*. London: Falmer Press.

Interviewing

Hertze, R. and Imber, J. (1995) *Studying Elites Using Qualitative Methods*. California: Sage.

Kvale, S. (1996) *Interviews: An Introduction to Qualitative Research*. California: Sage.

Minichiello, V., Aroni, R., Timewell, E. and Alexander, L. (1995) *In-depth Interviewing: Principles, Techniques, Analysis*, 2nd edition. Melbourne: Longman.

Weiss, R. (1994) *Learning from Strangers: The Art and Method of Qualitative Interview Studies*. New York: Free Press.

Focus groups

Krueger, R. (1994) *Focus Groups: A Practical Guide for Applied Research*, 2nd edition. California: Sage.

Templeton, J. (1994) *The Focus Group: A Strategic Guide to Organizing, Conducting and Analyzing the Focus Group Interview*, 2nd edition. Probus.

Nominal and Delphi techniques

Delbecq, A., Vanderven, A. and Gustafson, D. (1986) *Group Techniques for Program Planning*. Wisconsin: Greenbriar.

Interviewing children

Hatch, J. (ed.) (1995) *Qualitative Research in Early Childhood Settings*. Connecticut: Praeger.

5 Observation

This chapter focuses on the issues surrounding observation techniques in research and the procedures associated with undertaking 'participant observation' approaches. There has been a tendency to use the terms 'ethnography' and 'participant observation' interchangeably in recent times. There are differences between the two, however, which need explanation. Although both derive from the discipline of anthropology, 'ethnography' is a *methodology*, while 'participant observation' refers to a *technique*. 'Ethnography' involves the description and explanation of the regularities and variations within a culture, interpreted within a definable framework. 'Participant observation' is one of the major data-gathering techniques within the ethnographic tradition.

Development of participant observation

A classical anthropological investigation involves spending up to a year living in a community, learning the language, gaining an understanding of societal structures and becoming familiar with the customs and behaviours of the group before starting to record data. This initial settling-in period is followed by several years of data collection, analysis and interpretation, using observation and formal and informal interviewing. The investigation culminates in the researcher leaving the location, undertaking further data interpretation, then returning after a few years to see whether the original interpretation stands the test of time.

Earlier this century Margaret Mead (1928, 1963) and Bronislaw Malinowski (1932) adapted and shortened this procedure. They often learned the vernacular rather than the complete language; used interpreters; commenced data collection soon after arrival; selected aspects of a culture, rather than the complete culture, to study; and only occasionally spent more than two years in a location, rarely returning to test their interpretive hypotheses. The term 'participant observation' is said to have arisen from this process of camping in the study setting and recording observations.

This was in opposition to the tendency of some earlier (armchair) anthropologists, who reportedly never visited the study sites but used the information of others who, for one reason or another, had spent time with a particular ethnic group. The historical link between early anthropological studies and colonialism and imperialism must be taken into account in participant observation. The observer–observed relationship is potentially fraught with power relations favouring the dominant aspects of the researcher's cultural niche (Jordan and Yeomans, 1995).

Early participant observers such as Mead and Malinowski presented the aspects of culture they had observed as being representative of the whole, based on their experiences of having 'been there'. They were certainly observers, but apart from spending time in the setting their participation was minimal. Their positions were also heavily located within the tradition of the researcher as 'objective', 'neutral' and 'expert'.

The technique of participant observation has been adopted subsequently by a range of other disciplines, including sociology and psychology. It has undergone further adaptation and diversification due to time limits and funding constraints, as well as shifts in the researcher's position. In sociology, there has been a broad movement towards participant observation studies in the urban environments of the researcher's own culture. This has been mainly due to the Chicago sociologists' (1920s–1950s) emphasis on human behaviour as a product of both values and attitudes, and on society as 'becoming' (in a state of change). Some of the more well-known of these studies include: *Street Corner Society: The Social Structure of an Italian Slum* (Whyte, 1955); *Men Who Manage* (Dalton, 1959); *The Boys in White: Student Culture in a Medical School* (Becker et al., 1961); *Asylums: Essays on the Social Situation of Mental Patients and Other Inmates* (Goffman, 1961); *Hells Angels* (Thompson, 1967); *Tea Room Trade: Impersonal Sex in Public Places* (Humphreys, 1970); *You Owe Yourself a Drunk: An Ethnography of Urban Nomads* (Spradley, 1970); 'Being sane in insane places' (Rosenhan, 1973); *The Nude Beach Study* (Douglas and Rasmussen, with Flanagan, 1977); and *Massage Parlour Prostitution* (Rasmussen, 1989).

These studies demonstrated a distinct shift away from the neutral, uninvolved observer towards more active researcher participation within the study environment. Dalton, for example, was a senior person within the organisations he studied. This position was essential for gaining access to executive decision making. Erving Goffman was employed as a physical education instructor within an asylum. Laud Humphreys acted as a lookout in public toilets. Jack Douglas and his team became nudists. These researchers sought the understandings, individual constructions of meaning, and action and interaction of individuals and groups, rather than external descriptions of a culture.

Current trends

The advent of postmodernism and poststructuralism and the impact of feminist critique have served to shift the 'documenter of culture' some considerable distance away from neutrality and expertise towards high involvement, decentring, and 'dialogical' or 'polyphonic' interpretation. Some recent researchers are becoming a part of, or even becoming, the total phenomenon they are studying. Carol Ronai (1992) studied her own emotional experiences as an erotic dancer, where she totally participated in the situation before withdrawing to take on the position of researcher.

Dialogical interpretation presumes equality and ongoing negotiation between researcher and researched (or researchers as researched) as they communicate within a particular context. This process may be published as a dialogue to demonstrate the hermeneutic circle the researcher has undertaken in gaining understanding of the meanings and actions of the researched. The hermeneutic circle involves the interpretive process of going out, collecting data, bringing it back, interpreting it, and then repeating the cycle after each interpretation. This results in knowledge enhancement of a specific area of the designated study question.

A *polyphonic* presentation is an open-ended, creative dialogue of subcultures through the display of many voices, which may result from the researcher's decentred, postmodern role. A good example of this is *The Mirror Dance* (1983), Susan Krieger's study of an academic lesbian community in the midwest of the United States. The 'I' of the author is never mentioned, and the responses to particular questions are interwoven in a minimally interpreted display.

Peter Ashworth (1995) has argued against the decentring of the researcher in participant observation, on the grounds that the researcher's position is so intricately interwoven with the group in the joint construction of reality that he/she cannot be merely a pathway for an unbiased display of the studied culture. Ashworth advocates the reintroduction of the subject along feminist lines, using intimacy, reciprocity and co-researching as key factors.

Defining participant observation

A general definition of *participant observation* is that it is a technique of unobtrusive, shared or overtly subjective data collection, which involves a researcher spending time in an environment observing behaviour, action and interaction, so that he/she can understand the meanings constructed in that environment and can make sense of everyday life experiences. These understandings are used to generate conceptual/theoretical explanations of what is being observed.

Use in research

Participant observation is best suited to topics where the insider's perspective is sought, and where such data are accessible and can be gained by observation. This technique has been used to study a range of situations in which the details of everyday life and institutional practices are required. Such situations include:

- tribal groups;
- complete institutions—hospitals, schools, prisons and factories;
- partial institutions—a ward, a classroom or a department;
- groups of street youth, Ku Klux Klan or urban alcoholics; and
- individuals—a day in the life of one person; an examination of the subjective, emotional experiences of the researcher within a particular context; or an exploration of the researcher's 'process of becoming' (transformation) as she/he weaves her/his own responses with the stories he/she is hearing (Turnbull, 1992).

Advantages

The advantages of using 'participant observation' are:

- It allows the researchers to get as close as possible to the action as it is actually happening.
- The researchers can be flexible and adapt to, or follow up, events.

Because data are gathered as they are actually being generated, they are sometimes referred to as *first-order data*. Interview data are seen as *second-order data* because they capture the reconstructed accounts of people who are recalling an event. *Third-order data* comprise textual recordings or material culture from the past or present.

Disadvantages

The disadvantages of using participant observation are:

- Researchers need to have a very high skill level in gaining and keeping the confidence of those being studied.
- Only small numbers of people can be effectively observed at any one time.

Larger studies are more appropriate for a team of researchers. In *The Boys in White: Student Culture in a Medical School* (Becker et al., 1961), four researchers undertook observation and interviews over two years. This enabled them to include in their study most of the medical school students and staff, as well as established medical practitioners in the community. Similarly, the three researchers in *The Nude Beach Study* (Douglas and Rasmussen, with Flanagan, 1977) were able to demonstrate the diversity within this particular culture by comparing insider and outsider observations with interviews conducted over four summers.

Researcher roles

Gans (1982) states that there are three possible roles that a researcher can adopt when undertaking participant observation:

- 'total participant';
- 'participant-researcher/researcher-participant'; and
- 'total researcher'.

As a *total participant*, the researcher emotionally becomes the phenomenon or part of the phenomenon. Two examples are an erotic dancer or a hospital patient requiring a particular procedure. The researcher identity emerges only after the event has passed.

When the researcher is a '*participant-researcher/researcher-participant*', some emotional involvement may occur, but he/she has the option of switching quickly from role to role within an environment. People who study environments in which they work or live are in this category. Erving Goffman (1961) took a position as an assistant athletics director for several months in a mental hospital so he could research the culture of this organisation. His position allowed him to move freely between staff and patients, and to observe and gather the opinions of both groups in a situation where only the top management knew his aims.

As a *total researcher* the researcher is emotionally and physically separate. He/she only visits the setting on regular occasions for limited periods. Observation is the sole purpose of the visits. Robert Bogdan and Steve Taylor's (1975) study, in which they observed staff–parent communication in a neonatal intensive-care ward over four months, is an example of this. They visited the ward two to four times a week for periods of one to three hours, maintaining an emotional and physical distance between themselves and the observation setting.

The issue of *visibility* is paramount along the role continuum from 'total participant' to 'total researcher'. The 'total participant' tends to use his/her legitimate involvement in the setting to carry out *covert* research, where some or all others in the setting are unaware that data collection is in progress. The 'total researcher' generally carries out *overt* research, where everyone in the setting is fully informed regarding the purpose of his/her presence.

Another issue that needs consideration is the number of distinct roles being played and the time available to play them. The 'total participant' may be able to scribble the occasional note or maintain a diary, but generally he/she needs distance from the experience's subjective impact in order to achieve a reflective mode. The 'researcher-participant/participant-researcher' usually divides his/her time fairly equally between these roles, while the 'total researcher' may spend only a couple of hours of a day gathering and writing up data.

It is generally accepted that participation involves the researcher in interaction with a group whose values, actions and behaviours she/he may share to the extent that, in developing an emotional commitment to these concerns, she/he should be able to access a secure and unthreatened position (Ashworth, 1995). Where the researcher does not have an empathy with the values and actions of those under observation, she/he is expected to actively minimise any negative perceptions. It is assumed, however, that any strong feelings of acceptance or non-acceptance the researcher may have towards the group will not prevent her/him from reflecting, analysing and theorising in as unbiased a manner as possible.

The level of participation will also vary from *passive* (watching) to *active* (attempting the activities being observed). The issue of distance between total involvement and distant observer will also impact upon the perceptions of the phenomena that researchers are able to develop. This separation of researcher roles is aimed at presenting ideal types so that differences may be exposed, because in reality a researcher may move at will between visibility and invisibility, and empathy and antagonism. He/she may begin as a covert researcher (a hospital patient, for example), then return later in the overt role of a health worker/researcher.

Issues in observation research

A number of general issues peculiar to the design of a participant observation study must be addressed very early in a study.

Location

The first issue relates to the choice of location. Should the researcher observe in a setting where people are strangers and where the researcher has no prior work experience? Or should he/she use past experiences to facilitate entry and acceptance? There are obviously good arguments on both sides.

Entering an *unknown* setting allows the researcher to observe without preconceived ideas, but that very lack of prior knowledge can be costly in terms of time. Extra time must be spent to gain an understanding of the workings and language of the group, and of the meanings that people have constructed.

Entering a *known* setting means that, although insider understanding of the culture is already in place, the researcher's eye may be limited, or completely biased, by his/her past experiences. This may result in a blinkered approach when interpreting events or incidents relating to colleagues, friends or acquaintances.

Group size

The size of the group to be studied is another issue. William Foot Whyte (1984) asserts that a single researcher should not attempt to observe more than 15 people in a study. Others consider five to eight sufficient for an in-depth study, with larger groups being more appropriate for teams of researchers, or where more general information is being gathered. The process of gaining access and entry into a setting should be minutely journalised. Special attention should be paid to negotiation with *gatekeepers* (people with power to facilitate or inhibit access), as this documentation may give an insight into the hierarchies and dynamics of interaction within a setting. In some situations there are no gatekeepers as such, so making the acquaintance of a key person/persons becomes a priority.

Sampling

Sampling is another issue that must be addressed early. Firstly, the site must be selected. This is usually related to access and ease of entry. Secondly, the group must be defined, using the sampling strategies outlined in chapter 4.

The researcher must also decide what forms of *time sampling* to include to maximise the view of the setting. Is it more appropriate to view continuously for several hours, or to use limited observation periods? Viewing continuously will give broad information only, and may be profitable if used early in the study when the researcher is submerging her/himself in the scene. Limited observation periods are more usual, and are generally used in settings that have a lot of continuous activity (distractions). Steve Taylor's (1984) study of a men's ward in an institution for people with intellectual disabilities is an example of this. Taylor used one-hour observation periods, taken over different hours of different days spread over one year. When intense observation is occurring, one hour is about the maximum most researchers can recall accurately.

Apart from the broad scanning of a setting, another approach involves locating an individual or group of people and focusing on their actions and behaviours over a period. Short term time sampling can also be used in some settings where the researcher, instead of observing the environment, individuals, groups or behaviours continuously, observes in blocks of time, such as every two, five or ten minutes for periods of two, five or ten minutes. This approach can produce intense and very detailed information, which is usually recorded on the spot in a 'total observer' situation.

Needless to say, most researchers vary their approach depending on the question, the stage of the study, the location and the events under observation.

Question structure

Questions for participant observation studies tend to be fairly general. They usually relate to the details of daily living, the organisational structures surrounding the dynamics of interaction and activity of a particular group, or the minutiae of experiences undertaken by researcher or researched. The main question the researcher must address is:

> Does the research problem deal with human interaction or experiences that can best be viewed from the observer's perspective in a situation where everyday life activities are to be documented?

The researcher must allow for the fact that both the question and the focus of the study can change as the study progresses, as happens with all other forms of qualitative research.

Validity, reliability, subjectivity and objectivity

The position of the researcher, be it a distant observer or a subjective one, needs to be decided early, although variations and movement between these polarised positions may occur. The issues of 'validity'/credibility and 'reliability'/dependability also arise in participant observation. At the rigorous end of the scale, *multiple methods* (observation, interviewing and document collection) are suggested, along with team research (including a mix of age, sex, race and status) with members from different disciplines. *Multiple data sets* (different team members observing the same situation), involving comparison, discussion, consensus and re-observation, are also favoured.

This was the form of approach favoured by Jack Douglas in *The Nude Beach Study* (1977). He (a middle-aged academic of high status) and his two co-researchers—a young female postgraduate student who was already a practising nudist, and a youngish male academic of low status who, along with Douglas, became a nudist—spent two summers on the beach familiarising themselves with the culture. They termed this a '*depth probe*'. Each day they met to share their observations and record their developing views. These sessions were taped, providing a record of progress and self-reflection regarding their changing perceptions of both the self and others within the setting. When they began data collection, the two male researchers operated overtly, taping interviews on the beach, while the female researcher remained covert, providing an overview and a double check on the others' observations from her insider position. When the beach culture confronted opposition from the residents above, Douglas, as one of the residents, was able to access and document both insider and outsider views from the opposing groups.

In contrast to this study using multiple researchers and data sources, Carol Ronai adopts a postmodern/poststructuralist research stance. Her observation of herself as an erotic dancer calls on the use of personal emotional experience as a legitimate object of research (Ronai, 1992). Issues of 'validity' and 'reliability' or dependability and trustworthiness (Denzin and Lincoln, 1994) are addressed by systematic *self-intro-spection* (the documentation of thoughts and feelings of the self) and *interactive introspection* (regular interaction with two supervisors), to produce an emergent layered account that reflects multiple images.

Reliability/dependability is generally accepted where there is an indication that the studied subjects' views and meanings have been accessed. At the rigorous end of the scale, there is an assumption that people put up *fronts* (Douglas, 1976) to protect themselves or to reconstruct their identities in a more favourable or acceptable manner. Douglas states that these fronts must be peeled away by cross-checking information against other accounts. But just how far does a researcher need to go to locate 'truth'? Traditionally there has always been a concern that, in going deeper and deeper into a setting and into the participants' lives, there is a risk of 'going native'. This happens when involvement becomes so great that the researcher becomes too absorbed or too committed to see clearly. The same research problems then arise as with the insider who has been in a particular location previously. He/she may omit to document certain data or to critically reflect on data gathered, or he/she may fail to check collected data against other accounts. Particular concerns have been expressed regarding the difficulty of clearly portraying and analysing situations where close friendships/collegiality between researcher and researched have been established. How can we know what reciprocal obligations, both conscious and unconscious, may have been involved? Did the relationships continue beyond the study? If not, how did they end?

Generalisability

Bogdan and Taylor (1975) and Kidder and Judd (1986) have asserted that all settings and participants, while unique, are representative of all others. What is found to be true of people in one situation is likely to be true of other people placed in that same situation. William Foote Whyte (1984) sees the link to theory as one way of strengthening and reinforcing any generalisations that can be made.

However, researchers adopting the postmodern/poststructuralist approach to the meaning of 'truth' have abandoned generalisability. These researchers favour uniqueness and a multiplicity of perspectives, which may reflect and refract in many directions. What people say and do are accepted as constructions of 'reality' that do not require cross-checking to locate an ephemeral or transitory 'truth', although the discourses evident in such cases may be traced historically and pulled apart to locate powerful influences. 'Going native' is viewed simply as one of several levels of involvement where the researcher must be aware of the issue of potential bias with regard to collection, analysis and presentation of data. It is assumed that he/she will take appropriate steps to minimise this. Part of this view is that, the closer the researcher gets to identifying the multiple facets of the situation, the closer he/she may be getting to the 'truth' of the matter.

In this view the fine lines between distorted and clear vision, inextricable involvement and some semblance of objectivity, and the frames of reference being used are rarely clarified. The need to access the 'subjective reality' of everyday life of those under observation necessitates abandoning the conventional dichotomy between 'objectivity' and 'subjectivity'. The researcher, however, must demonstrate access to this world (the 'subjective reality' of the researched); all data must be verified; and this process must be fully exposed (documented). He/she must therefore address many design issues before entering the field and collecting data as an observer.

Other issues to be addressed

Other, more general, issues that need to be addressed include:

- *Researcher's position:* Which end of the continuum will be most appropriate for the research question: a distant role, or a close, participatory role?
  - Can the researcher become emotionally involved yet still maintain her/his capacity for analytical scrutiny?
  - If there is a likelihood of considerable emotional involvement, how will this be managed in researching one's own experiences and those of others?
- *Types of documentation:* Should the researcher use self-reflective documentation, dialogues with others outside the setting, or debriefing from a trusted colleague/partner?
- *Relationship with participants:* Will participants be co-collaborators? If not, what forms of access and control will they have over the researcher's interpretations of their lives? Who defines the boundaries of group acceptance?
- *Identity:* Can the researcher immerse him/herself within the group to be studied? If so, what identity will be best presented to achieve this? How will this affect the data gathered?
- *Concessions:* What concessions will the researcher make in order to locate insider views? Will she/he join the skin group of an Aboriginal tribe, for example, and take on the lifetime rights and responsibilities of a group member, including sharing all her/his possessions?
- *Pressure:* In a group situation, how will the researcher handle pressure to join or support different factions, given that siding with one sector may result in limited access to others?
- *Conflicting views:* How will the researcher manage challenging situations when antagonistic views, violence, racism or sexism threaten his/her presence or values? Will the researcher tend to avoid certain people, but spend more time with those with whom he/she has empathy, thus threatening the representativeness of the data?
- *Intervention:* Are there any situations that may potentially arise in a setting that would tempt the researcher to intervene, such as knowing that a certain person/s

in the group may be at risk? How will this affect the data being gathered? Belief in accountability has led some researchers to intervene once their data is in. Howard Becker (1963) led reform on marijuana laws after studying musicians' use of this substance. Laud Humphreys became active in the Gay Rights movement following his 1970 study of impersonal sex in male public toilets. Steve Taylor led television and newspaper reporters through the institution where he had observed care givers abusing clients with intellectual disabilities.

- *Disturbing the setting:* To what extent will the researcher disturb the setting she/he is to document? It is generally accepted that one person is unlikely to have any long term effect on a culture, but this must be checked. The researcher needs to be attuned to any influence she/he may be having. Any influences noted should be actively minimised and taken into account in data analysis and interpretation.
- *Managing ownership of the data:* What has the researcher negotiated in terms of ownership and publishing rights? Should she/he designate power elsewhere to veto publication if the results turn out to be controversial?
- *Method of data collection:* Should data be collected overtly or covertly?

This large number of issues confronting researchers in relation to observation and other data-collection techniques illustrates how carefully any study must be planned. The researcher's choice of data-collection method, in particular, has broad ramifications for the research design.

Data collection

Perhaps the researcher's most difficult decision is whether to use 'overt' or 'covert' data-collection methods. If she/he chooses a covert observation, what degree of secrecy will best suit the study?

Overt data collection

Research studies have shown that the best data are obtained when people are not being constantly alerted to the researcher's purpose. Overt researchers have the advantage of accessing information and taking notes openly without any recourse to deceit. But just *how overt* is 'overt'? Will the researcher identify him/herself to the authorities once only, to every person who strays into the location, or even to each member of the group whenever observation is in progress?

One disadvantage is that other participants may view him/her as a spy and develop many extra layers of protective covering, thus limiting access to the insider view. Another limitation is that people within busy environments may see the (apparently) idle researcher as another pair of hands to be put to work. He/she may be expected to provide some reciprocal service in exchange for access and information. The taking on of extra tasks must be examined in terms of its potential to distract the researcher from the mainstream activity, either locationally or timewise, as opposed to its potential for giving the researcher greater access and insight into areas not otherwise easily entered.

Covert data collection

Covert research has the advantage that the observer is hidden. Thus she/he is able to observe marginal or illegal activities, but there are also several disadvantages:

- The researcher's life may be in danger if her/his cover is blown.
- Observing people without their knowledge is difficult to justify ethically.
- Covert researchers need a legitimate role in the setting, which may result in considerable time being spent in other roles.
- The role taken by the researcher may have boundaries that it is difficult (though essential) to cross.
- There may be a number of obstacles to note taking, cross-checking accounts and gaining feedback.

Russell Bernard (1994) suggests that there are grades of deception. *Passive deception* includes the kinds of observations that a researcher can undertake in public places (public toilets, public hospitals, public streets, public transport), in which he/she is performing a legitimate role. He/she may take the role of a member of the general public, a visitor in a hospital, a tourist or passer-by in the street, or a commuter. *Active deception*, on the other hand, means going further than discreetly observing in an anonymous fashion. It involves manipulating people or intruding into their lives without their prior consent or knowledge of the potential outcomes of such observations. Following this line of argument, Laud Humphreys' (1970) observations in public toilets would be acceptable. His noting of number plates to identify and interview participants in another guise at a later time would not.

Procedure

Once the researcher has addressed all of the issues influencing data collection, and decided whether to operate overtly or covertly, she/he is ready to enter the field and start collecting data.

It is essential to keep an up-to-date *journal* (as was the case with interviewing), documenting details of the study's progress and the issues surrounding data collection. The journal should also include a creative, interpretive critique of emerging themes and their links to theoretical frameworks.

The researcher acts largely as a camera, scanning and recording detail wherever she/he happens to be focusing, while also recording sounds and spoken language from a broader range. If a broad view is required, early observational sessions should be lengthy. If focus and detail are preferred, early sessions should be shorter, building up to a maximum of one hour.

The three most common areas within a setting from which researchers tend to collect observations are:

- the building/setting/environment (space, colour, smell and observer's responses);
- the people (age, sex, ethnicity, dress, status, relationships, grouping and observer's comments); and
- activities, events, behaviour and the dialogue of those under observation.

Recording

In descriptive observation and following the notion that data collection should be unobtrusive, it is preferable that no notes are made on site (unless limited time sampling is in progress). Observational notes should be written up as soon as possible after leaving the scene and before speaking with others about the observation. A meticulous record of the session should be made on audio tape, videotape or computer or in note form. Talking with others about the observation in the time between data collection and recording should be avoided, as it is most likely to lead to reinterpretation and reconstruction of the observed events. Similarly, the longer the researcher puts off recording the session, the more likely she/he is to lose accurate recall.

The recording process starts with a sketch of the setting, using arrows to indicate people's movement and actions. Key words, beginnings and endings of remarks and brief notes about events all help to stimulate recall. The observation should then be written up, leaving a substantial right hand margin for notes, critical comments and identifying emergent themes and/or issues.

Initial written observations should include detailed pictures of all participants in the setting: their structure; leadership and groupings; and who does what with whom, when and where. Later observations, of course, will note only variations in dress, behaviour, attitude and spatial relations. Spatial relations include such things as positions taken, who interacts with whom, and who initiates activities. All verbal language (agreement, disagreement) should be recorded, including topics of conversation and time spent on each. Full double quotation marks should be used for accurately recalled language, and single marks should be used to indicate approximate recall, when the key words and sense are remembered but one or two words may be missing. The third person narrative voice should be used for general recall.

The setting should be described in detail initially, but with less detail in later observations. These should focus more on change and variation and the researcher's response to these. Events, activities and individuals' behaviour should be carefully described to include movement and non-verbal interactions. The observer's comments appear throughout the observation with a signifier (OC). These comments provide a reflective dialogue of events and ethical and methodological dilemmas. They also expose the researcher's position and clarify the situation in terms of other observations, interviews and theoretical perspectives.

The idea behind collecting data is to blend into the scene and participate where possible, in order to establish close relationships with a range of people. The researcher should also ensure that in the initial stages the questions she/he asks clarify the participants' concerns. Researcher concerns should be clarified later. Understanding the language spoken is important. When conducting his study of urban nomads, Spradley (1970) discovered that 'winos' had a complex language of their own, and that he needed to spend considerable time in the setting learning this language and its variations before he could start collecting any meaningful data. This illustrates that it is wise to make no judgements until familiarity with the verbal and non-verbal forms of communication within the environment are known.

When a research team is involved, each observation should be passed around for comparison with other accounts to provide checks against skewing the data towards one group or individual. Cross-referencing can then occur.

Other techniques that can be used to supplement data from observation and interviewing are the documentary texts of photography, film and video.

Photography and other visual imaging

The technique of including photographs, videos and film in a data set derives from anthropology, where visual records are often taken to provide another dimension on life within distant cultures and communities (Bateson and Mead, 1942). In general, two types of images have been identified: 'public' and 'private' (Berger, 1978). *Public images* are those taken in contexts isolated from the viewer's memory and experiences. *Private images* are those which have meaning for the viewer and can be read or 'read through' in context (Schwartz, 1989).

Images tend to be used either as a complete data source within themselves or as an adjunct to other forms of data collection. One example of the use of photos as a *complete* data source is an exploration of images from a mental hospital, in which 800 photos were collected (Dowdall and Golden, 1989). These were sifted for duplication, sorted into 13 different categories and analysed using a layered approach that involved:

- 'appraisal';
- 'inquiry'; and
- 'interpretation'.

Appraisal involved comparing photos with each other and with existing documentation within a category. For example, 50 per cent of the photos of patients showed males, while 41 per cent showed females; yet documentation indicated that female patients had dominated in numbers. The category in this instance was 'patients'. *Inquiry* involved surveying the internal landscapes of the institution to develop themes regarding patients, the work culture and changes over time. *Interpretation* required the close reading of themes and images to produce explanatory concepts.

This technique is ideal when limited sources of other information are available. Visual images are generally viewed as being incomplete as a sole data source, however, because they lack information about the historical context of the situations and actions that are portrayed.

Images can also be used as an *adjunct* to other forms of data collection. Photo albums can be used as a basis for interviewing, in order to create narratives that are crucial to generating a shared understanding of the context, emotions experienced, and events surrounding the persons and incidents portrayed. In some studies, researchers have deliberately taken multiple photos within a setting and used them to engage respondents in an explanation of the culture of a school (Walker, 1993), or in an exploration of history and change in a community (Schwartz, 1989). Walker and Schwartz both presented current images of locations, events and everyday life. These images enabled the respondents to 'look through' them to see other related images, which in turn were clarified and examined.

The use of videotaping as an adjunct data source is illustrated in an exploration of nurse–patient interaction (Bottoroff, 1994). Video equipment (two cameras) was installed in each patient's room one month prior to data collection to familiarise participants with its presence. Monitoring was done from an adjacent room to minimise interference. Each patient and her/his nurses were videoed for a total of 72 hours over several shifts. The advantage of this approach lay in the permanent visual record, which was enhanced by interviews and verified by participants. The presence of two cameras enabled perspectives to be recorded from both sides of the room.

Limitations of visual data

Images are regarded as being inherently ambiguous, despite their obvious uses. The person behind the camera is selective and biased towards information that may serve to illustrate a particular interpretation of a situation. The ideal of an objective record of a frozen moment in time must be abandoned in favour of reconstructed images that can be interpreted in many ways but that, at best, can provide only one of the many possible perspectives. Techniques that have been used to strengthen visual views of reality include:

- obtaining images taken or controlled by the participants themselves, as a means of contrasting the views of researcher and researched;
- working in a team of researchers who collect and contrast the analysis of their data sets; and
- presenting images without commentary or interpretation so that readers can form their own impressions.

One of the major issues arising from the use of images is the extent to which the camera's intrusion has disturbed the setting. To what extent has this led the people under observation to act/pose for the camera, creating performances that bear little resemblance to the everyday life that the researcher was hoping to record? Another issue involves the frames researchers use to interpret these 'one-off', context-bound images that in all probability reflect only one aspect of 'reality'. Researchers must address these issues if they are to successfully interpret their collected data.

Despite these limitations, visual records are particularly useful in providing glimpses of otherwise inaccessible cultures, historical events and everyday life. They also provide the researcher with an extra dimension of data. In the case of video and film, they provide images that can be played and replayed, portraying precise recordings of verbal and non-verbal action and interaction.

These pros and cons of using visual data as a legitimate observation technique highlight once again how carefully the researcher must choose his/her study methods in order to collect 'valid' data.

Summary

Participant observation is the technique that allows the researcher to get closest to events and actions as they are actually happening. This chapter has highlighted the processes and issues that a researcher will need to address—the range of positions (between 'objective' and 'subjective') that the researcher can inhabit; the data-collection techniques from the eye of the researcher to the eye of the recording device; the contentious issue of covert versus overt research; and the degrees of being an 'insider'. The researcher will need to assess how the above factors might impact on the data and the setting under observation.

It is now time to look at the methodological approaches frequently used in health research.

Further readings

Behar, R. (1996) *The Vulnerable Observer: Anthropology that Breaks your Heart.* Boston: Beacon Press.

Jorgensen, D. (1989) *Participant Observation: A Methodology for Human Studies.* California: Sage.

Kellehear, A. (1993) *The Unobtrusive Researcher: A Guide to Methods.* Sydney: Allen & Unwin.

Photography

Chaplin, E. (1994) *Sociology and Visual Representation.* London: Routledge.

Clancy, S. and Dollinger, S. (1993) Identity, self and personality II: glimpses through the autophotographic eye. *Journal of Personality and Social Psychology*, 64, pp. 1064–1071.

Collier, J. and Collier, M. (1986) *Visual Anthropology: Photography as a Research Method.* Alberquerque: University of New Mexico Press.

Hagaman, D. (1996) *How I Learned Not to be a Photojournalist.* Lexington: University of Lexington Press.

Sontag, S. (1979) *On Photography.* Penguin: Harmondsworth.

Wagner, D. (ed.) (1979) *Images of Information: Still Photography in the Social Sciences.* Beverley Hills: Sage.

Ziller, R. (1994) *Photographing the Self.* Newbury Park: Sage.

Part Three
Methodological approaches

Part Three consists of three chapters. It explores a number of methodologies that have been used frequently in health research. The methodologies presented tend to fall within the theory-generating tradition, and many have their own philosophical underpinning and preferred data-collection techniques.

The part begins with an investigation of library-based research methods (Chapter 6). These include a wide variety of personal (private) and impersonal (public) *documentation*, *historical method* (checking the documentation's authenticity) and *discourse analysis* (the study of language and written documentation). Personal documentation consists of such things as diaries, letters and photographs, while impersonal documentation relies on bureaucratic, 'official' records such as births and deaths.

This is followed in Chapter 7 by an exploration of six more approaches, all of which have a theory-generating capacity:

- *Ethnography* allows a focus on a researcher-defined culture.
- *Phenomenology* uses intuitive knowledge to provide a pathway for identifying the essence of the experience of a phenomenon.
- *Grounded theory* focuses on the common symbols that individuals and groups within particular contexts share and interpret.
- *Biography* explores individuals' life stories.
- *Memory work* helps in the development and reinterpretation of life experience in an emancipatory fashion.
- *Case studies* are an approach rather than a methodology, but can be used in a variety of ways to display and consolidate data.

Chapter 8 focuses on *evaluation* and *action research*, exposing the different ways in which health researchers are currently using evaluation, and showing how action research can produce different outcomes depending on whether it is being used to impose, or generate, change.

This part highlights once again that the researcher will choose his/her preferred methodology only after considering the research topic, her/his position, and the orientation that seems most likely to provide the best data.

6 Library-based methods

The three main library-based research methods are documentation, historical method and discourse analysis.

Documentation

Documentation provides a valuable source of data for researchers. The gathering and analysis of personal and impersonal documentation provide a useful source of information for the historical method and, more recently, for discourse analysis.

Personal documentation

Personal documents comprise diaries, fiction, autobiographies or journals, photographs, letters, films, paintings, music, computer imagery, landscapes, tombstone inscriptions, graffiti and any other collectable or observable artefacts that serve to illuminate the lives of the individual/s or group/s under study. Clothing, hairstyles, jewellery and garbage are also forms of material culture. Diaries, letters and photographs provide the most usual sources of documentation of the personal aspects of people's lives.

Diaries

Diaries tend to provide the richest source of subjective information, especially when these have been written as a personal and ongoing record of the writer's emotions and feelings. This rich data source is probably the closest to 'truth' that can be obtained, given the managed public performances that may be produced by general interaction and the interview process. Some diary sources are not so personal or revealing, however. They may contain only a logbook style account of events, omitting individual responses to these.

When assessing diary documentation, it is essential for the researcher to take into account the context of the situation of writing. The researcher must ask:

- Was it solely a record or conversation with the self, or was it directed at a potential readership?
- Was it a fairly public document that could be, and probably was, read by others around the time of writing?
- Does it contain a careful reconstruction of events? If so, why?
- When was it actually written? Daily? Weekly? Does it document the events of that period as they actually happened, or was it written many years later as a memoir of a particular time still clearly recalled, like wartime or birthing experiences?
- Was it an honest portrayal never meant for publication, such as Malinowski's (1967) diary of his research in the Troubriand Islands? His loneliness, unhappiness and despair intermingle with beautiful environmental descriptions and expressions of his frustration with the participants in his study.
- Was the writer a person of position in society, who was involved in some highly contentious political situations, the 'truth' of which she/he wishes to see clarified posthumously in an effort to 'set the record straight'?

These queries highlight the fact that the purpose and context of writing will clearly affect the data produced.

Letters

Letters are another well-used, potentially rich source of information, but must undergo similar questioning to diary entries. The context in which they were written, the writer's position, the reader's position and the writer's relationship with the reader will all impact upon both style and content. The level of intimacy, trust and closeness in age and status may also affect presentation. Consider the letters each of us may have written:

- *Thank-you notes to relatives*, although short and focused, often contain brief references to important life events, such as moving house, relationship breakdown or the loss of a family pet.
- *Lovers' letters* often contain subtexts and innuendo regarding intimacies shared in the past or anticipated in the future. Coded references to these make it difficult for other readers and researchers to unravel their 'true' meaning.

- *Lifelong correspondence between colleagues, friends and rivals* provides the most revealing data on the minutiae of daily life and the impact of political and social change over time.
- *Formal letters* can be an indicator of practices that have not otherwise been accurately documented. Annette Summers' (1996) study of the letters written by community midwives to the Medical Board early this century is an example of this. The time had passed for these women to apply for registration, but their letters reveal that the practice of unregistered and untrained (but very experienced) women serving as independent community midwives continued long after it was supposed to have ceased.

Fiction

Fiction is another form of personal documentation, particularly where storytelling has been used to communicate things that have actually happened but that the author wishes to present in a reconstructed manner. What appears as fiction is really a disguised version of events. This form of documentation requires careful deconstruction and meticulous cross-referencing with other sources to make it credible.

Photographs

Photographs documenting public events or persons, and family photos, provide another rich data source. They are usually stored in archival collections or family albums. Archives of photographs can be accessed from library collections (via computers) but will need to be placed in their temporal and cultural contexts. The advantage of using family photographs as documentation is that family members can usually provide the context, meanings and interrelationships of the individuals and events portrayed. The carefully posed and smiling group photo may well hide tales of violence and passion. The researcher has access to these subtexts only through the partial memories of living family members, many of whom may have limited, biased or carefully reconstructed memories of past events.

Although the accompanying narratives produced by photographs' owners can provide rich detail and clarify meanings, photograph albums can be analysed without this source of information (Walker and Moulton, 1989). These researchers examined more than 40 different photograph albums. The basis of their research was the assumption that each album was constructed on the basis of some implicit narrative, and therefore had the power to communicate this narrative to them. The following steps (adapted from Walker and Moulton, 1989) can be taken in attempting this type of task:

1 Determine the purpose of the album. Is it a record of a family in general or of a specific family event, such as a wedding or holiday? Does it focus on a hobby? Is it autobiographical, presenting a collection of scenes and persons important to the photographer?

2 Determine what form of narrative is present. With reference to family albums, who comprise the family? Who are friends/acquaintances? What relationships are evident, and how are these indicated? Look at body language, the subjects' positions in the photos, and the position of photos in the album.

3 Identify themes. How are people portrayed? What are they doing and how are they doing it? What locations are used? What evidence is there of possessions or status symbols? What changes are evident over time?

It is also possible to take a single photograph and conduct a rich analysis. Denise Farran (1990) took a photograph of Marilyn Monroe, used Erving Goffman's (1976) gender signifiers to analyse the construction of a 'sex goddess', and applied Harold Garfinkel's (1967) documentary method of interpretation to bring Marilyn's biography into the frame. Farran concluded that people tend to read the photograph with reference to their own biographies. They will view it either as a contrived sexual image or as a photograph of a powerful woman who has the capacity to exploit as well as to be exploited.

Ethical issues

The ethical issues surrounding the collection of some forms of personal documentation are complex. Allan Kellehear has examined these, along with film, television programs, graffiti, garbage and cemetery documentation, in his book *The Unobtrusive Observer* (1993). In general, ethics permissions should be sought where appropriate, and confidentiality and anonymity may need to be carefully negotiated.

Impersonal documentation

Impersonal documentation comprises the public records by which cultural patterns can be examined: court records; political debates and decisions; births, marriages, divorces and deaths; unemployment; crime statistics; social surveys; media accounts;

advertisements; cartoons; children's rhymes; and works of fiction, non-fiction and journals.

Examples of impersonal documentation in the health area are: health and other social indicators; rates of disease; hospital records—admissions, discharges, case notes and case histories; and records of workplace accidents, compensation outcomes and rehabilitation. Achanfuo-Yeboah (1995) undertook an examination of indigenous health statistics that revealed inaccurate, incomplete and unreliable records. Differences in definitions made comparability difficult and showed that a combination of quantitative and qualitative data collected by indigenous people themselves would be desirable in the future. Achanfuo-Yeboah concluded that the poor health profiles evident from the data collected were linked to land deprivation, mass poverty and unemployment.

Most published material is publicly available through libraries. Unpublished material tends to be stored in archives or other private locations around the country. The first hurdle for an aspiring researcher is tracking down original sources. This may involve travel. Much archival documentation cannot be photocopied. It must be searched 'in situ'. Small battery-operated tape recorders, laptop computers and pencils (if notes are to be taken) are essential. There are also legal responsibilities involved in reproducing archival documentation. Copyright rules must be checked, as permission is needed to take quotes from specified documents.

Using documentation in research

Documentation can be combined with other approaches. The inclusion of letters in a participant observation study is one example. Spradley (1970) uses the letters of William Tanner, an older man on skid row, in *You Owe Yourself a Drunk*.

The advantages of using documentation as data are that:

- It can provide sources of comparison for field data;.
- It can be analysed by processes of either theory testing or theory generation.
- It can provide insight and an earlier view of subjective experiences that have often been reconstructed or overlaid by 'fronts' by the time they are discussed in the interview process. This is the case when personal diaries are involved.

The problems with collected documentation lie in the information gaps that become evident, and in the more general problems of authenticity, bias, legibility (particularly when the writing and phrasing of previous centuries is involved), and potential errors of coverage, classification, recording and processing (Bulmer, 1984).

Once the researcher has collected data as documentation, she/he will probably choose the historical method to analyse it.

Historical method

The historical method is the approach used in the analysis of much personal and impersonal documentation. After identifying the research questions and locating documentation, the first stage of historical method involves establishing the documentation's authenticity.

Establishing authenticity

Authenticity is established through seeking answers to the following questions:

- Where does the documentation come from?
- Who wrote or produced it, and when?
- If life events are being reported, was the writer/painter/cartoonist actually present (as an eyewitness) at these events, or was it written up later by someone relying on the reports of others (secondary source)?
- Who was the writer in this process?
- Where was he/she located?
- What was his/her purpose?
- What were his/her relationships?
- Why were the documents actually produced? For money? As part of a job?
- Has the documentation been translated from another language? How may this be problematic? Umberto Eco has stated that the translation of his text *A Theory of Semiotics* (1976) into English produced a completely different slant, so much so that he suspected that in retranslating from English back to Italian he would be able to produce quite a different text.
- Do other documents exist that vouch for the documentation forming the focus of the study?
- Has the author produced other documentation? Does it match? How original are the ideas presented?
- In what context was the document produced?

- Was it freely produced for the self, or for others?
- Or was it produced under coercion? If so, what effect may this have had?

The overall idea is to demonstrate that the information is genuine; that it can be corroborated from at least two other sources; and that all relevant data (both primary and secondary) have been assessed and verified. Clearly, this rigorous and critical process of authentication would be inappropriate where some personal documentation is concerned, unless it involves the diaries of famous people who have left other sources of writing that can provide verification.

Interpretation

Once authenticity has been established, the data must be interpreted. Interpretation occurs in one of two ways:

- by establishing and applying a theoretical position or positions through which the data are viewed and compared; or
- by creating ideal types or theoretical categories that provide a structure for analysis.

The use of an *established theory* to explain the details of historical documentation is contentious within the discipline of history (Tosh, 1991). However, some researchers advocate an approach in which the researcher identifies an *ideal type* (Weber, 1915). This is a labelled pattern of social action that has persisted over time and is relevant to the research topic. It provides a basis for comparison with the documentation being interpreted. Miguel Bedolla (1992) used Lain-Entralgo's (1964) ideal type for the structure of doctor–patient relationships. This incorporates cognitive, operative, affective and ethico-religious components. Although this approach can produce stimulating hypotheses, there is a tendency towards a 'one dimensional interpretation which distorts the true complexity of the historical process' (Tosh, 1991, p. 182). The preference is to let the data speak for themselves first. Their diversity and richness can then be explored using a range of perspectives and, where possible, more than one researcher. This should avoid narrow interpretations towards any single researcher's pet theory.

Analytic induction is the approach to theory generation that is most appropriate to historical sources. It involves close examination of one document to produce a low level explanation or generalisation that can then be applied to other documents. This enables the generation of categories and propositions that inform the interpretation of other documentation while continuing to pick up new aspects. The *grounded theory* technique is another approach to theory generation that can be applied to documentation. Within this, theoretical sampling and the constant comparative process can be used to develop generalisations and generate theory. Ken Plummer (1983), however, believes that the *intuitive approach* is most common. Here, generalisations, hunches and concepts emerge, and in most studies there is no clarification as to how the researcher has moved from the data to the construction of explanatory frames.

The communication of findings will vary from the scientific, objective presentation of 'facts', to a creative, subjective approach, informed by documentation. The meticulous documentation of sources is essential in both approaches. The author's biases must also be exposed, particularly if there are any hidden agendas in the interpretive process. Regardless of the approach chosen, credibility is the desirable outcome. Authenticity of the located material must be proven, and the best or most representative of the sources must be available, together with an interpretation that demonstrably fits the collected information.

The argument for theory generation is strong, especially from researchers who have tried using established theoretical positions from which they have attempted to code and quantify data. A study of 56 diarists (28 men and 28 women) who wrote between 1820 and 1870 (Hansen and Macdonald, 1995), explored hypotheses relating to the social dimensions of everyday life through descriptions of visiting practices. Major difficulties arose in defining a 'visit'. Although data regarding visiting abounded, visiting people were often not identified, particularly in times of stress. The distinction between household composition also varied daily, with many additional family members and workers regularly staying overnight. This confusion led to creative refinements of definitions, a heightened awareness of the problems of coding and a challenge to census data, which previously portrayed household composition narrowly. The problems encountered in this example match those experienced by other researchers who favour creative interpretation and triangulation rather than enumeration.

Postmodern approaches

Here there is no assumption of truth—historical stories will always be biased, based on stories of lived experience. These stories are constructed by historians and they reflect and create relations of power. The issue then becomes the constitution of the past in the present through particular cultural and linguistic re-presentations. Texts are viewed as montages, and multiple approaches and perspectives are needed to capture reflections of reality. (See Wolf, 1992 and Bell and Apfel, 1995 for examples.)

Discourse analysis

There are particular problems in defining the meanings of words, due to the many influences affecting the speaker/writer and the listener/reader. Discourse analysis provides a methodological approach to interpreting documentation and the spoken word by examining different ways of interpreting these 'texts'.

The study of language and written documentation was evident up to 2000 years ago (Van Dijk, 1985). It emerged in the 1960s under the term *discourse analysis*. Since then, many disciplines—including anthropology, sociology, philosophy, law, information processing, history and psychology—have used the technique to examine language usage.

Speech (verbal and non-verbal), written documentation, cultural practices and artefacts are viewed as comprising sets of *signifiers* (symbols) that can be read. These readings can take one of two forms:

- an exploration of language structure through form, regularities, meanings and linguistic patterns that can be compared and constructed; or
- contextualised events based in particular cultures that shape, and are shaped by, social context and identifiable power relations.

Those concentrating on language (e.g Bloom et al., 1994) derive their perspectives from de Saussure (1983 [1916]) and the practice of *semiotics*, in which the meanings of a language exist only in relation to each other within a system. Thus meanings do not pre-exist. They come from language, and variations lie within individual usage. Although researchers with skills in linguistic analysis have managed to combine the two approaches of language and language in context (Fairclough, 1993; Silverman, 1987, 1993), most health researchers have focused on the latter social approach, underpinning their analyses with Michel Foucault's views on knowledge and power.

Power relations and discourse

Dependence on Foucault has led to a rather narrow emphasis on issues of power, ideology, dominance, hegemony, inequality, and the production and legitimation of forms of knowledge that have enabled certain individuals, groups or ideas to dominate social processes. According to Foucault (1977a), 'panopticism' can be observed in the hidden and generalised control processes that serve to 'normalise' individual action and behaviour. These processes will be reflected in the researcher's choice of theoretical orientation, which will determine the research focus. Will interpretation involve the search for previously identified constructs of textual exploration in order to explain the discourses and discursive practices that emerge, and will the researcher's own views further limit the interpretive process? The unravelling of language should also involve unravelling the researcher's personal views, processes and agendas, as well as their cultural and contextual origins.

Feminist researchers usually presume the existence of gender-specific power relations favouring men at the expense of women, so that any textual search should reinforce the discourse of gender inequality. Kathy Davis (1988), for example, explored the discourse of 'paternalism' to interpret an encounter between a male general practitioner and an older female patient. Some feminist researchers have also used patriarchal interpretations to trace the discourse changes that served to consolidate the movement of men into the previously female-dominated domain of child birthing (Murphy-Lawless, 1988). Others have used a poststructuralist approach, accepting cultural hegemony but concentrating more on the microprocesses of legitimation and resistance that allow historical practices to be revealed. Julie Hepworth's (1994) work on anorexia nervosa is an example of this approach. Her exploration of written, historical, medical documentation, recent feminist interpretations and interviews with current health professionals, together revealed the medicalisation process of the disorder, its maintenance within this perspective and the enduring discourse of *femininity* (the idea of a female disease experienced as irrational and emotional behaviour).

Discourse analyses treat documents as 'texts', but focus on their theoretical categories rather than viewing them as reflecting aspects and meanings of peoples' lives in the generation or testing of theory. Each 'text' is 'an historically produced discourse embodying the power relations of a certain moment' (Plummer, 1983, p. 131). The 'text' is merely a repository and a reflection of other processes. The experiences of those who produced them, or who are named therein, are not of particular interest except for their clarification of these wider processes of power and their help in exposing discursive practices.

Discourses in health research

Discourses are dynamic dialogues in which meaning is socially and historically produced, reproduced and transformed in interaction. A single discourse, such as medical dominance, consists of *discursive practices*. The discursive practices of a hospital ward, for example, include case notes, treatment modalities, and interaction among health professions and between health professionals and patients. These practices are linked to others, both structural and ideological, within the hospital, which are in turn linked to practices in the wider society. All these discursive practices make up the *order of discourse* in a particular domain (Fairclough, 1992), within which practices and particular discourses can be identified.

A discourse should be examined within the natural setting, where possible, in order to locate the context appropriately. One such exploration in the poststructuralist tradition (Fox, 1994) used interviews and observations in operating theatres to explore power relations between surgeons and anaesthetists. Two discourses emerged from this:

- patient fitness; and
- the disease imperative.

Competition between surgeons and anaesthetists was exposed through their attempts to give one of these rival discourses precedence over the other, using the patient's body as the site of their argument. The battles between the two tended to favour the surgeons, reinforcing an illness orientation that often created problematic outcomes for the patient.

A further example is the exploration of the discourses on diet, cholesterol control and heart disease (Lupton and Chapman, 1995). This study examined media coverage (1991–94) and general public response, in the form of 49 participants in focus groups. The general public's representatives expressed considerable cynicism regarding media and health promotion information on the above topics. Their cynicism was fuelled by conflicting reportage, the discourses of pleasurable indulgence, and the 'work' required to control one's health. This resistance to 'official' views led to the generation of the compromise 'everything in moderation'. This was regarded as the safest approach in light of conflicting advice and the unknown, incalculable factors of 'luck' and 'fate'. The outcomes of this study reflected multiple levels of information processing and highlighted the individual's capacity to adapt and transform events through the medium of language.

Process

The usual processes that occur in the production of a discourse analysis are:

1 selection of appropriate question/s, given the topic area of the identified discourses;
2 sample selection, and triangulation of documentation if necessary; and
3 the uncovering of themes, identification of codes and emergence of recurring patterns.

Several writers have documented the detailed processes of analysing 'texts'. Van Dijk (1985), Fairclough (1989, 1992, 1993), Potter and Weatherall (1987, 1994), Potter (1996), and Gee, Michaels and O'Conner (1992) are worth reading. All agree that the interactive process of reading the 'texts' will influence the researcher's approach and the language conventions used. All social action takes place within socially and historically constituted locations where words, gestures, phrases and other conventions of speech, acting and writing have particular meaning. This means that the history of the power relations within the setting, as well as the participants' and researcher's views, must be carefully dissected.

The following procedures for discourse analysis are adapted from Potter and Weatherall (1994, pp. 49–65) and Fairclough (1989, p. 166):

- Identify the variety that is evident within the information present. This may help clarify competing discourses.
- Where transcriptions are used, be meticulous regarding any known pauses, hesitations or non-verbals. These may support the variety suspected and alert the researcher to other agendas.
- Seek different levels of meaning and alternative views. Check their reliability within the context.
- Question which values or ideologies are being drawn upon.
- Question what power relations have shaped the discourse/s at the situational, institutional, and broader societal and cultural levels. Trace these historically.
- Seek evidence of challenges or resistance to identifiable discourses.
- Question whether these challenges have resulted in further legitimation or transformation of the power relations, and in what situation this has occurred.
- Find out what processes of 'interdiscursivity' have occurred. '*Interdiscursivity*' is the transformation of past into present via heterogeneous discourses (Fairclough, 1993).

The extensive documentation of process and the display of chunks of documentation enhance the reader's view of process and help to verify interpretations.

Three levels of analysis occur in analysing 'texts':

1   a close analytical description of the texts;
2   a more abstract comparison of meanings across the questions posed;
3   a discussion of the social practices reflected in the texts, viewed both historically and in terms of change.

Examples of discourse analysis in health research

One discourse analysis explored working class women's views of their men's perceptions of cervical screening programs (McKie, 1995). It concluded that the medical process had become sexualised (in the men's view). Consequently, women's self-esteem was challenged when undertaking screening with a male doctor. These data, which were collated in women's discussion/focus groups, demonstrated potential resistance to the aims of national screening programs, thus providing valuable information for those involved in health promotion.

Another discourse analysis was derived from interview data on doctors' and nurses' views of healing (Wicks, 1992). Nurses documented clear resistance to the medical model in areas where they have some control, namely wound care, pain relief and care of the dying. This indicated the complexity (and often contradictory nature) of power relations between doctors and nurses.

Analysis of the case notes of two patients (Cheek and Rudge, 1994) revealed yet another form of discourse. Cheek and Rudge discovered that, as the patients came under increasing medical surveillance, their voices became muted in the webs of documentation produced by health professionals.

Advantages and limitations

The examples given above show that discourse analysis has two main advantages:

* its capacity to theorise the relationship between individual subjective views, environments and historical social processes in the identification of discursive practices; and

- its capacity to provide critical insight into the fine details of the interweaving of hegemony, ideology, power and practice in the development, maintenance and negotiation of discourses.

Like all methodologies, however, it also has *limitations*. Feminists argue that the limitations of discourse analysis lie in Foucault's lack of identification of women as a significant, powerless group (Hepworth, 1994), and in the lack of focus on the transformation of gender relations. The very light and general underpinning of the connection between power and knowledge has also been criticised for enabling a researcher to contrast or highlight particular discourses while ignoring others that are perhaps equally important. Other criticisms lie in the assumption that regularities in language use can be seen in particular cultural groups within a given society, whereas in fact there may be no generalisable regularities (McGregor, 1991).

Summary

This chapter has shown that differing library-based methodological approaches to the interpretation of data and 'texts' provide useful choices for researchers. It has highlighted the processes, strengths and weaknesses of personal and impersonal documentation, historical method and discourse analysis, while stressing the importance of the researcher's inquiring mind in achieving reliable research outcomes.

Historical method provides a useful approach for collecting and handling documentation of a personal and impersonal nature. Discourse analysis also utilises historical knowledge to trace back the development of particular discourses in the development of hegemony.

The next chapter describes six more theory-generating approaches to data interpretation. These come under the umbrella of 'field-based methods'.

Further readings

Personal and impersonal documentation

Hill, M. (1993) *Archival Strategies and Techniques*. California: Sage.

Plummer, K. (1983) *Documents of Life: An Introduction to the Problems and Literature of a Humanistic Method*. London: George Allen & Unwin.

Webb, E., Campbell, D., Schwartz, R. and Sechrest, L. (1972) *Unobtrusive Measures: Non-reactive Research in the Social Sciences*. Chicago: Rand McNally.

Photography

Becker, H. (1986) *Doing Things Together*. Illinois: Northwestern University Press.

Harper, D. (1994) On the authority of the image, in N. Denzin and Y. Lincoln (eds), *Handbook of Qualitative Research*. California: Sage.

Hirsch, J. (1981) *Family Photographs: Content, Meaning and Effect*. Oxford: Oxford University Press.

History method

Tosh, J. (1991) *The Pursuit of History: Aims, Methods and New Directions of Modern History*, 2nd edition. London: Longman.

Discourse analysis

Foucault, M. (1981) The order of discourse, in R. Young (ed.), *Untying the Text*. London: Routledge and Kegan Paul.

Potter, J. (1996) *Representing Reality: Discourse, Rhetoric and Social Construction*. California: Sage.

Van Dijk, T. (1985) *Handbook of Discourse Analysis*, 4 vols. London: Academic Press.

7 Field-based methods

Field-based methods involve the researcher entering the field and exploring particular phenomena by using interviews and observation techniques, although textual data may also be collected. The following six approaches are commonly used:

- ethnography;
- phenomenology;
- grounded theory;
- oral biography;
- memory work; and
- case studies.

This chapter examines each approach, describing processes, giving examples, and highlighting advantages and problems.

Ethnography

Ethnography comes from the anthropological tradition and is concerned with the study of culture. *Longitudinal* observations are undertaken within particular contexts. These observations seek the participants' views of reality through interviews and other sources recorded by camera, videotape and audiotape. Anthropology's detailed cultural studies have been replaced within health by more contained versions or mini-ethnographies, characterised by an eclectic use of techniques. Participant observation, for example, has been combined with surveys, non-participant observation, socio-linguistic and Foucauldian discourse analysis, and interviews of a quantitative or qualitative nature. An ethnographic study of risk management among illicit drug injectors (Power et al., 1996) used a multisite approach (inner city, regional town and semi-rural); participant observation techniques; semi-structured, face-to-face survey interviews; and focus groups. The purpose of such research is to obtain and display, in as much detail as possible, the understandings and meanings constructed by people as they undertake daily activities. The focus is on the description of these activities.

Types of ethnographic studies

Ethnographic studies can be divided broadly into three types:

- classical ethnography;
- critical ethnography; and
- postmodern/poststructural ethnography.

Classical ethnography

Classical ethnography is usually underpinned by theories of structural functionalism or interaction. It has been linked with colonialism and late nineteenth-century imperialism. It seeks the frameworks of a culture, and explores the relationships between these structures and the actions, meanings and interactions of individuals and groups. The researcher's position is that of a 'neutral', reflective (dialoguing between the research process and the product) documenter, who is presumed to have minimal impact on the setting. She/he attempts to gain the 'emic' or insider view through rigorous observation over time.

This approach can be criticised, however, in that it provides a time- and context-limited cine shot, dominated by researcher interpretation and separation of the culture from its historical origins.

Critical ethnography

Critical ethnography uses the perspectives of Karl Marx, Louis Althussar, Max Horkheimer and Jürgen Habermas to address the issuing and distribution of power. It is based on the assumptions that:

- False consciousness exists among people regarding the hierarchies of power.
- Society is in a state of crisis and people are dissatisfied.
- Society is inequitably structured and dominated by powerful hegemonic practices that create and maintain the continuance of a particular world view.

The critical questioning brought by the researcher challenges this hegemony and seeks the genesis of its construction through deconstruction, the analysis of discourses, and a close examination of the concepts of social class, race, ethnicity and gender. This explicitly political, ideological view seeks to enhance collective action, improve societies, and foster the emancipation and empowerment of individuals and groups. The researcher's position is one of active involvement in the critical, theoretical analysis of inscribed power. This position has the capacity to transform her/him during the process of working towards emancipatory change with the participants.

Critical ethnographic projects have been criticised for their lack of holistic examination of the broader issues of class, state and the social institutions within the larger culture, and for their focus instead on specific locations, such as hospitals and schools (Wexler, 1987). They have also been criticised for their minimal evidence of empowerment, but there are current moves to alleviate this by amalgamating critical ethnography and action research (Jordan and Yeomans, 1995).

Postmodern/poststructural ethnography

Postmodern/poststructural ethnography has led to a greater emphasis on the language and discourse of power relations within which both researcher and researched have been constructed. It has also led to an examination of ruptures in the discursive practices that feature in daily existence, namely the social practice of power rather than the concept. Other foci include the issues of how discursive practices can homogenise and apply general concepts that are not generalisable; and how a 'solution' to one problem simply means the emergence of other problems in an ongoing manner (Popkewitz, 1995). The ethnographer adopts a decentred position. He/she does not speak for others, but displays their voices, as well as his/her own, in exposing the setting's multiple realities.

Combining types

Movement can be seen within these types of ethnographic studies, obliterating the boundaries. Kincheloe and McLaren's (1994) study of workers provides an excellent example. They adopted a postmodern, critical ethnographic approach that enabled collaborative research with workers who became empowered through exposing the power structures of their employer's organisation. The workers analysed discourses, created new economic models, and explored alternatives to current forms of democratic control. In this situation, the complexity of the social world is recognised and validity is not sought, but reconstruction of the known world is essential. The desired outcome of such a process, which is best undertaken by those oppressed by current systems, is a radical transformation of their worlds.

Procedure

Bronislaw Malinowski (1967) advises that it is preferable to enter the field with 'foreshadowed problems' rather than preconceived ideas that limit one's view. *Foreshadowed problems* consist of an awareness of key problems, issues and debates. The ethnographer should be free to 'muddle about' (Wolcott, 1979) in the field, letting issues emerge rather than attempting to prove or disprove predetermined hypotheses.

All ethnographies require meticulous data collection and display. Some areas of a culture where data are sought include:

- the context;
- shared systems of beliefs and attitudes;
- economic, political and social organisation;
- language, customs and rituals;
- social control; and
- events, behaviour and action.

The collected data should contain quotes, stories, legends, artistic and visual representations, and material culture. The collection of *primary (or first-order) data* is of paramount importance.

The generation of theoretical positions is usual, although this may be less evident in classical and critical ethnographies, where structural and 'critical theory' perspectives may provide strong direction for insight and interpretation. Data collection and preliminary analysis occur simultaneously. This allows each set of data collection to inform the next. Ethnographic data are summarised as they are collected. These summaries interconnect with earlier and later versions. The themes that emerge encompass types of people, jobs, processes, things, relationships, concrete sayings from the database, recurrent issues and researcher interpretation. The qualitative techniques used involve formal and informal interviewing, observation, collecting life histories, and sorting groups of things in order to illuminate the differences among participants' views.

Observation process in classical/critical ethnography

In classical/critical ethnography, the process of observation usually falls into three categories:

- descriptive observation;
- focused observation; and
- seeking selective dimensions of contrast for identified categories.

All three can be used together in a *funnelling* process.

Descriptive observation involves the researcher in an attempt to cover the whole setting in a broad scanning manner.

Focused observation takes place after major domains of data have been identified. It involves closer observation to define stages or kinds/parts of the domain. One domain might be 'doctors', with included terms such as 'general practitioner', 'consultant' or 'surgeon'. More focused observation and interviewing would then be required to develop a *taxonomy* (a classification scheme of kinds of doctors, indicating subsets and hierarchies).

The third kind of observation occurs where *selective dimensions of contrast* are sought for identified categories. The subsection 'general practitioner' might involve different relationships with patients in rural and urban settings, or in private and public settings. James Spradley (1980) claims that the general classical or critical ethnographic process involves a movement from the identification of domains through patterns of behaviour within them, to *componential analysis* (the systematic search for the units of meaning people assign to cultural categories). Steps in this process include:

1 identifying domains;
2 making a taxonomic analysis of these domains and identifying subsets; and then
3 employing processes of descriptive, focused and selective observations in conjunction with formal and informal interviewing, to arrive at a componential analysis.

Informal interviewing

The success of informal interviewing in ethnographic studies depends on physical context and spatial relations (Burgess, 1988, p. 141), because the environment will affect the language used. Drug-dependent street youths may share quite different language and information in a conversation held on 'their patch' from what they would use in a conversation held in a government agency office. Regardless of the setting, the degree of potential interruption is also important, as interruption to private reminiscences may mean that the thread cannot be recaptured. Modes of seating or standing can emphasise the hierarchical/non-hierarchical nature of relationships. The ethnographer's public participation in groups, and her/his presentation as either receptive to others or self-opinionated, will also affect the amount of informal information passed over. An empathetic, supportive researcher is much more likely to obtain 'unofficial' information and receive requests for formal interviews so that people can 'have their say', than a researcher who is clearly seeking to explore preconceived ideas about people's meanings and actions.

Analysis

Analysis is ongoing. It varies from the more traditional fragmentation to produce concepts, analytical themes, typologies and codes, to minimally analysed narrative presentations including the voices of those observed. Other variations include a quasi grounded theory approach, and the interleaving of field notes to incorporate the researcher's voice in a rhetorical manner.

John Van Maanen (1988) has identified three broad types of ethnographic writing:

- *Realist tales* is currently the most used format. It is characterised by the researcher's absence. The third person is used to present meticulous descriptions and the voices (through quotations) of those observed.
- *Confessional tales* is written in the first person. The research story is told with the researcher centred in the form of 'I'.
- *Impressionist tales* uses poetry, drama, fiction and polyphonic presentations.

Writing-up process in classical/critical ethnography

The writing-up of realist (classical/critical) ethnography follows the pattern of pursuing a detailed literature review to identify the outcomes of past research, noting limits, and critiquing the theories that have generated or provided directions previously. This is usually followed by a methodological section (although this may be appended), then by various representations of rich ethnographic description of the observed culture. These involve both communication and interpretation in terms that make sense to a reader from another culture. The final section contains a discussion of the ethnographic findings in terms of previous literature and theoretical models, or theoretical propositions developed by the researcher.

Spradley (1980, pp. 162–167) identified six levels of *abstraction* that can be used in realist ethnographic writing to link the studied culture with the reader's culture. These vary from the universal to the particular:

1 Level one comprises general statements than can provide links between the culture under study and that of the reader, for example: 'In every society . . .'.
2 Level two uses cross-cultural descriptive statements to provide a link between cultures, but also indicates the differences that make the observation of the other culture worthwhile.
3 Level three leads into the culture being studied by giving specific information about the location and general situation.
4 Level four provides general statements about the culture. These give insight into the details of daily activities.
5 Level five uses statements and detailed descriptions of events and activities to delineate the practices within a cultural domain.
6 Level six documents activities or incidents as they occur.

It is essential to present examples of primary data throughout these levels. Clearly, the ethnographer's intended audience will dictate the combination of levels chosen.

Ethnographies of the self or of cultures that have received little documentation will tend to use the lower levels of abstraction. This will enable the reader to see more directly through the researcher's eyes. Some researchers have fully documented and analysed the construction of their own views in an attempt to address the issues of bias and their potentially limited view (as a researcher). This may be done either as 'confessional tales' or as a dialogue with supervisors and/or colleagues. When this is undertaken prior to the study, it can provide a useful benchmark against which to assess personal change, decisions and interpretations. One example of a 'confessional tale' is provided by Magda Lewis and Roger Simon (1986), who, as a postgraduate student and lecturer respectively, wrote up the experiences of running and participating in a graduate seminar on language and power within certain literary texts. The two voices are juxtaposed in dialogue form, providing two distinct stories on which the larger narrative is built.

'Realist' or 'naturalistic ethnography' has been criticised (Roman and Apple, 1990) for its positivist orientation towards 'facts', hypotheses and the objective observer, while the more subjective researcher-centred approaches are often viewed as self-indulgent, with a tendency to self-justification.

Postmodern and poststructural ethnography

Postmodern and poststructural ethnographies focus on the disentangling of texts and competing discursive social practices within the different power structures of both the culture under study and the culture that has impacted upon the researcher. There is an acceptance that pattern, coherence and unity are lacking within both the researched and the setting. Culture is viewed as 'a field of contest': a confrontation of signs and practices along the faultlines of power (Comaroff and Comaroff, 1992, p. 18).

Those taking postmodern or poststructural perspectives criticise classical and critical ethnographic studies on the basis of the following (adapted from McLaren, 1995a, pp. 271–300):

- They do not recognise that the researcher's identity is the effect of, and has been constructed by, various historical discourses in differing contexts in which the researcher has resisted/rejected particular signs and/or experiences of political and social practices.
- They impose the dominant culture that the researcher inhabits and whose views he/she reflects. In exploring other cultures, of which he/she may/may not have membership, he/she will tend to carry the dominant culture's negative voices. A person researching gay culture, for example, may negate or further marginalise members by emphasising differences from the heterosexual 'norm'.
- They assume that the researcher's knowledge gives her/him a superior position in the research process, from which to observe cultures that are constructed as bounded or separate (Clifford and Marcus, 1986, p. 122), rather than as unbounded human variation along a continuum.
- They fail to recognise the invisibility of some data and the absences within texts that are supposed to be representing the totality of the situation under study, instead of privileging this silence and recognising that it allows for the legitimate deconstruction of such textual records.

Issue of representation

There has been concern about the issue of representation (Atkinson, 1992; Hammersley, 1992), because ethnographic data are a product of the researcher's participation in the field. There is no clear way for a reader to discern whether this experience, or reflections of the phenomena, are dominating the recording process.

Theory is another disputed area. Should the phenomena speak for themselves, or should they be interpreted/reinterpreted through particular theoretical frames? Martyn Hammersley (1992) has queried why researchers should find it necessary to impose other frames when all 'facts' or observations are theory laden.

Concern has also been expressed that many of the 'voices' of an ethnographic study are not adequately heard (Schratz, 1993) or presented. Various techniques used to collect less audible voices have included photographs and video recordings. These capture interactions and socialisation processes of a verbal and non-verbal nature. Comparative audiovisuals from recordings taken from similar locations, but in different cultures/countries, are also used. Dona Schwartz (1989) has documented the use of visual ethnography (here photography) in the process of constructing a rural farming community's multiple meanings regarding change and adaptation to change. Margery Wolf (1992) has attempted a demonstration of different voices and their interpretations of a particular event. The story is told three times: as fiction (or as a 'confessional tale' with dialogue aspects); as field notes derived mainly from the Chinese research assistant; and as a journal article. Interpretation and analysis of 'muted' voices are complex, and all participants should be involved in this process (Gagnon, 1992).

Issue of reflexivity

Another concern that has emerged in postmodern ethnography (Wasserfall, 1993) is that reflexivity, which is supposed to help decentre the researcher, and which needs to address power relations and encourage non-exploitative ones, may be insufficient to address major differences in status, power and values. Tamar El-or's (1992) study of a community of ultra-orthodox Jewish women has explored the difficulties in equalising researcher–researched relations in a setting where one is attempting to extract personal information from another. The fact that the researched are the object of the study must impact on both current and future relationships.

The emotions aroused by fieldwork must also be displayed honestly (Small, 1996). They should be interwoven with the data they affect, rather than being documented separately in diaries (Kleinman and Copp, 1993).

Auto-ethnography

The ethnography of personal experiences (*auto-ethnography*) is becoming popular (see Ellis and Bochner, 1992). It is often presented using the impressionist techniques of poetry, narrative, drama and visual representation. The self is overtly and centrally positioned; the subjective experience is located culturally and theoretically, and thick ethnographic description and other techniques of presentation capture its immediacy, combining its emotional, physical and cognitive aspects. The focus on the self came originally from George Mead's (1934) creative 'I', and the 'me' that was a creature of the 'generalised other'. Nowadays the self is seen as 'the sum of an individual's changing internal conversations' (Gagnon, 1992, p. 239), where the barriers between self and other have broken down.

Examples of auto-ethnography include an exploration of a researcher's relationship with her lover as he slowly declines and dies of emphysema (Ellis, 1995a); a short story presentation of a meeting with an old friend who is dying of AIDS (Ellis, 1995b); and the experience of being a long term patient without communicative capacities in an intensive care unit (Robillard, 1994).

Ethnography summary

The preceding discussion and examples illustrate the current, considerable diversity in what can comprise an ethnographic study. This diversity ranges from a formal, structured documentation of a culture, to a critical ethnography that challenges inequality, to postmodern and poststructural approaches. The latter include ethnographies of the self, a critical assessment of the researcher's constructed identity, and the minimally interpreted display of participants' voices through a variety of presentation modes.

Phenomenology

The phenomenological tradition stems from the work of Edmund Husserl (1859–1938), with its emphasis on returning to the 'thing' or *phenomenon*, and attempting to gain interpretation and understanding from within. Husserl saw the individual as the originator of meaning and the central point for social analysis. Jean-Paul Sartre (1960, 1963), Maurice Merleau-Ponty (1943, 1962) and others further developed this view in the existential tradition. Martin Heidegger (1962, 1982) also added to it. The impetus for the development of phenomenological ideas was a concern that the foundations of knowledge should be placed upon *reality* as it could be consciously experienced.

Husserl explored the difference between 'facts' and 'essences' in his books *Ideas I* (1931) and *Ideas II* (1989 [1969]). *Facts* are individual objects existing in time and space, knowledge of which is gained through perceptual intuition. *Essences* are objects that do not necessarily exist in space or time and can be known through essential or imaginative intuition. Although the intuition of essences and individuals is different, the two 'objects' are often linked. The 'essence' of the experience of loneliness can be intuited through human interactions, for example.

According to the phenomenological tradition, humans exist in the world as wakeful *consciousnesses* with little awareness of each other, separated by socialisation and other social constructions. These ways of being can be suspended to enable a refinement of consciousness to occur. Multiple processes of phenomenological *reduction* make it possible to *bracket* or disconnect the world's 'taken-for-granted reality', and to gain a state of pure consciousness or *ego*. This consciousness is viewed as a self-contained, self-sufficient entity, existing apart from and continuing beyond the physical world. The disengaged consciousness can then be directed towards a specific *focus*, leading to a dual process of conscious awareness and reflective consciousness. This reflective consciousness involves the complete *transformation* of conscious experience and intentionality as the object of reflection. The 'self' is not involved in this transformation. The essential structure of the experience under focus will be brought to light through this theory of the 'essence' of pure *transcendental experiences*. Thus phenomenological consciousness becomes the foundation of *reality*.

Experience, intentionality and reflection

It is difficult to pull out specific directives from Husserl's writing, but Macann (1993, pp. 31–36) points to the importance of the transcendental stance in relation to three elements:

- experience;
- intentionality; and
- reflection.

Experience involves the dynamic engagement of the ego, and focuses on positional consciousness and the intentional relation of the object. *Intentionality* encompasses the means by which an established world of objects or established way of seeing is brought into being. It also refers to the way a researcher uses these established objects and ways of seeing to judge and analyse experiences. In an intentionality that is reduced phenomenologically, the ego is engaged with the object and this new relationship becomes the focus of a reflective consciousness. *Reflection* sheds light on the research topic either explicitly or implicitly through this process.

'Reality' is referred back to consciousness and forward to meaning in a two-way process that seeks the ideal meaning. The *'ideal meaning'* of an object remains, even though the physical object may be destroyed. The two 'realities'—the physical object and the ideal meaning—are both necessary to comprehend meaning. In other words, the actual spatial and temporal 'thing', together with the memories, feelings and multivisual pictures associated with that 'thing', comprise the whole. There is also an underlying assumption that an experience's structure may sit on an invisible base of concealed meanings that must also be intuited.

Research process

Michael Crotty (1996) has explored the views of transcendental and existential phenomenologists, as well as those of Heidegger, who contextualises the phenomenon within everyday life activities. Crotty has devised a step-by-step methodological research process from the core of these combined theoretical positions. The five steps involved in this process are:

1   Develop a general question (for example, 'What is the experience of being HIV positive?'), and sample those who have intensely experienced the situation.
2   Implement a process of *phenomenological reduction (bracketing)*. To do this the researcher must:
   — Ask more specific questions about the experience, treating it as removed from her/his own experience (for example, 'What is it?' 'What is it like?').
   — Move back further, and remove all theoretical perspectives, symbols and constructs, as well as her/his own preconceived ideas, experiences and feelings regarding the experience being researched.
   — Prepare to reconfront the phenomenon with a blank sheet, rather like taking the position of an alien from a distant planet.
   — Focus on the experience, and become open and passive.
   — Set reasoning aside.
   — Listen carefully, and allow her/himself to be drawn-in in a sustained and receptive manner.
3   Document a detailed description of the experience, based on answers to the question: 'What does the experience appear to be now?'
4   Examine this description, considering the question: 'Does it arise from my own experiences or from other sources (past knowledge, reading, previous personal

experiences)?' All aspects that can be seen to have come from other sources must be abandoned.

5   Locate the experience's essence, and identify and critique the essence's elements. Ask the question: 'Would the phenomenon still stand without any of these?' Negotiate the essence's elements with those observed. (Adapted from Crotty, 1996, pp. 158–159.)

Descriptions of the experience's essence are gained through intuition and reflection. Didactic interpretation should reveal different perspectives that can be written thematically, through metaphor, or through other theorists' ideas. The researcher must aim to reflect as closely as possible the essence of the experience. If the researcher is certain that the description and interpretation correctly reflect his/her experiences, and that readers can recognise the experience's description as mirroring aspects of their own experience of the same phenomenon (Van Maanen, 1990), then credibility is ensured.

This process is said to avoid the tangents that have developed in the phenomenological tradition, particularly the paths taken by North American researchers and nurses. In these cases, the focus has been the identification and surface description of the respondents' subjective 'lived' experience, rather than the objectifying of the researcher's subjective view through processes of phenomenological reduction, in which the researcher's consciousness engages with that of the object.

Complete reduction is impossible, however, because one must first experience oneself as existing in order to experience other aspects. As individuals, we are inseparably part of the world. The fact and nature of our existence will affect the form taken by our conceptualisations of any essences (Merleau-Ponty, 1962).

Criticisms

Phenomenological approaches have been criticised because it may not be possible to suspend all empirical and metaphysical presuppositions about the world through bracketing (Merleau-Ponty, 1962; Morris, 1991). Access to concealed meanings has also been problematic, as has the tendency for phenomenology to produce only superficial narratives of social phenomena. These narratives are based in language that covers an underworld of hidden or partly hidden discourses of power and self-interest. We must therefore deconstruct these discourses if we are to make further sense of the essence of the structure of experience.

Phenomenology summary

The phenomenological tradition, incorporating the works of Husserl, Sartre, Merleau-Ponty and Heidegger, has generated a specific process whereby the researcher can become open to the structure of the essence of others' experiences of a particular phenomenon. It is essential that researchers take care not to reduce this technique to a process of superficial description of others' subjective experiences.

Grounded theory

Grounded theory is an analytic *inductive* technique (going from observed instances to the development of a law or model of action in a rigorous manner), based in the interpretive tradition, with an emphasis on individual power, choice and construction of meaning (Znaniecki, 1934). It includes a rigorous guide to data collection and analysis in the generation of substantive and formal theory. There is an underlying belief that all researchers are capable of generating theory, and that research should be analysed as work, paying meticulous attention to the organisation and management of the total project, and to careful interaction with participants.

Barney Glaser and Anselm Strauss developed the technique in the 1960s (Glaser and Strauss, 1965, 1967). It emerged in response to a perceived lack of grounding of the then current theoretical perspectives within the empirical world. These perspectives dated back to the late nineteenth century and often appeared irrelevant to the realities of the mid twentieth century.

Grounded theory may well have been influenced by the phenomenological tradition, in particular the Husserlian concept of 'back to the things themselves'. It was definitely influenced by the Chicago School of Sociology (1920s–1950s), with its focus on field methods (observation and interviewing) and on the documentation (from the actor's perspective) of action, interaction and the experience of complex phenomena. The structural, functionalist tradition of the 1940s and 1950s, with its orientation towards 'scientific' quantitative methods, may have been another influence.

Theoretical underpinnings

Grounded theory's theoretical underpinnings can be found within both philosophy and sociology, especially in the writings of John Dewey, George H. Mead and Charles Pierce. All three emphasised change, continuous action and interaction, complex social processes and phenomena, the actor's view, and the researcher's engagement in the research process.

John Dewey (1934, 1937) emphasised the link between common sense and scientific inquiry, as well as the creative interaction and collaborative dialogues between researchers, researched and the settings under investigation. Emotional and intellectual involvement were both expected to play a part in adequately constructing meaning. There is a realisation that the researcher may be affected by the research process, even though the concept of 'transformation' was not broached by Glaser and Strauss.

Charles Pierce (see Hartshorne, Weiss and Bucks, 1958) pointed to the concept of '*abduction*'. This is the crucial role played by the researcher in combining reflection on the phenomena with previous personal or professional knowledge, to create new possibilities.

George H. Mead (1934) provided the social philosophy that Herbert Blumer (1969) later termed '*symbolic interactionism*'. This perspective locates the phenomenon of human experience within the world of social interaction. It focuses on the interconnection between the dual processes of the construction of self within the social processes of society, and the refraction of the social world by the self, in the relationship between society and the individual. '*Meaning*' is constructed through the use of symbols, signs and language, and the self's ability to take the position of others and interpret one's own actions from that position. Language and interaction with significant others enable individuals to undertake a lifelong process of viewing their behaviour from others' positions, as well as in terms of their society's (the generalised other) norms and values. However, individuals and groups can, and do, negotiate and adapt these norms through the two phases of consciousness of the 'I' and the 'me'.

Focus

Using the above theoretical underpinnings, the focus in grounded theory then becomes the day-to-day life of people as it is actually happening—the empirical, social world 'out there'. This world is viewed as comprising many different layers, as well as public and private views. Motivation, action, interaction and the construction of reality can be understood only if the researcher moves into the setting. He/she must get as close as possible to participants in an attempt to make sense of the verbal and non-verbal interaction and interpretations that occur. Grounded theory technique is best used for small scale, everyday life situations where little previous research has occurred and where processes, relationships, meanings and adaptations are the focus.

There has been an ongoing and very public controversy in recent years in regard to two texts: Strauss (1987) and Strauss and Corbin (1990). Barney Glaser initiated this controversy by asserting that these books 'misconceive our [original] conceptions on grounded theory to an extreme degree' (Glaser, 1992, p. 1). He suggests that Strauss has moved from a process involving the discovery of grounded theory to the development of a verificational methodology for undertaking qualitative research.

Process

Strauss and Juliet Corbin regard the following processes as essential, but accept that some modifications may be made to suit the requirements of the different environments being studied. These modifications, however, should not omit any stages of the overall process. Glaser disagrees on a number of aspects of these stages. The conflicting points of view have been interwoven in the description of the process. Although the technique is best suited to fieldwork, other forms of qualitative or quantitative data may be incorporated. These may be survey, experiment or case study data (Glaser, 1978, p. 6).

Locating an area of investigation

The first stage of this process involves locating an area of investigation and deciding whether it is appropriate. By trying to discover 'What constitutes caring for the human spirit in nursing?' (Van Loon, 1995), or how the development of an alternative service organisation 'operated by and for people labelled chronically mentally ill' can affect self-advocacy and political activist strategies (McCoy and Aronoff, 1994), it can be determined that these are areas where little research has been conducted. Close observation of, and interaction with, the setting will therefore be needed to clarify these questions. The most appropriate questions involve an examination of problems and processes.

Barney Glaser (1992, p. 4) points out the two *major questions* that underpin grounded theory:

- What is the chief concern or problem in the substantive area, and what accounts for most of the variation in processing the problem?
- What category, or what property of what category, does this incident indicate?

Dimensionalising

Once a question has been identified, a process of developing categories and *dimensionalising* and *subdimensionalising* occurs (Strauss, 1987). This involves making distinctions and breaking a property down to its dimensions. The category of 'spiritual care' can then be formulated and dimensionalised into 'mind work' and 'body work'. These two dimensions can be broken down further by asking particular questions that relate to structure, function, process, relationships, change and transformation. Some examples of these questions are:

- What is involved?
- Why is this done?
- When are these tasks carried out? By whom?
- What are the outcomes?
- What happens when they are not carried out?
- Is carrying out these forms of work pleasant/unpleasant, uplifting/draining, necessary/unnecessary?

Theoretical sampling

The dimensionalising process leads to the development of hypotheses for testing in the field, directing the researcher to deliberately seek instances of X or Y (*theoretical sampling*). The ongoing process is one of induction (the process of inferring a principle from the observation of particular instances), *deduction* (reasoning from general to particular instances) and verification. The theoretical sampling of events, incidents and populations directs data collection from the earliest stage.

Glaser focuses on the emergent process. He avoids both dimensionalising and constantly critiquing the data because he believes that the insertion of too many preconceived, substantive questions detracts from the data's true nature and produces only 'forced conceptual description' (Glaser, 1992, p. 5). He also disagrees with the emphasis on the development and testing of hypotheses, viewing theoretical sampling as a process of data collection in which codes emerge from raw data. These codes are used to direct further data collection, resulting in code saturation and integration into emerging theory (Glaser, 1992, p. 102).

Literature reviews are also contentious. For Glaser, they should be avoided until the first core variable or category has emerged. Only then should the substantive area relating to that variable or category be reviewed and from there the literature review should be ongoing. For Strauss, a literature review may (or may not) take place when the initial variables/categories emerge and may (or may not) occur after this time.

Theoretical memos

Theoretical memos are a crucial part of the development of theory. These are written whenever a code is identified, and after coding sessions and discussions with other researchers. These memos are kept separate from the empirical database. Early in the project they tend to be brief, comparing empirical indicators, then indicator to concept. The emerging major strategies and their connections with each other then dominate as the study progresses. Memos provide a descriptive record of ideas, insights, hypotheses and code development. The purpose of memoing is:

- to raise the data to a level of conceptualisation;
- to develop the properties of each category that enable it to be defined operationally;
- to present hypotheses about connections between categories and/or their properties;
- to integrate these categories with others to generate theory; and
- to locate emerging theory within existing relevant theoretical positions (Glaser, 1978, p. 84).

Documentation of people and events occurs in the empirical database, while memos are conceptual, analytical and theoretically focused. Periodically, memos are summarised and further memos written.

Coding

Strauss (1987) and Strauss and Corbin (1990) have identified three different types of coding:

- open coding;
- axial coding; and
- selective coding.

Open coding

Open coding is a word-by-word, line-by-line analysis that occurs every time data are collected. This process is designed to fracture the data then group them conceptually, generalising concepts that emerge from it and fit within it. These concepts and their dimensions lead the researcher to more focused data collection. Some rules of thumb for open coding, adapted from Anselm Strauss (1987, pp. 30–32), are:

- Look for *'in vivo' codes* (terms used by those being studied), and attach existing sociological concepts such as power or class;
- Give a provisional name to each code.
- Question all aspects. What are these data about? What is actually happening? What category does this incident indicate?
- Focus on dimensions that seem relevant to words or phrases.
- Locate comparative cases through these dimensions.
- Make sure that the coding has meticulously accounted for all data.

The idea is to allow categories to emerge from the data, rather than impose already constructed ones upon the data.

Barney Glaser (1992) argues that open coding should be either line by line, sentence by sentence, paragraph by paragraph, or document by complete document, depending on the data's type and purpose and the density or thinness of ideas. The focus should be on the constant comparison of incident to incident, not on the fracturing of data. When concepts do emerge, the focus should then be on the comparison of incidents to concepts. Otherwise, labelling and conceptual forcing are the likely outcomes. The application of such preconceived questions as 'What is happening?', 'What is the data about?' and 'What category does this incident indicate?' may be irrelevant to both the process and the problem.

Axial coding

Axial coding involves intensive analysis of one category that has been developed in open coding. It is used to develop connections between this category and its subcategories. The process requires a search through the empirical data, the re-searcher's life knowledge and experience, and her/his theoretical and research literature knowledge, in order to adequately develop an expanded category. Van Loon's (1995) exploration of what constitutes spiritual care in nursing is one example of this. 'Connecting with the patient' emerged as the core category, and axial coding linked the breadth of this category's dimensions, which included the following aspects:

- connecting as a blending of spirits;
- connecting as intersubjective energy flow;
- connecting as caring touch;
- connecting as an assisted passage in the dying process;
- connecting as allowing the spirit to travel on after death; and
- connecting as a liturgy to celebrate the spirit's transcendence (its destination home).

A researcher would tend to move between open and axial coding. Anselm Strauss (1987) provides a large number of meticulous procedures for axial coding that Barney Glaser (1992) views as unnecessary overload. Glaser asserts that the constant comparison of incident to incident, and incident to emerging category, should be sufficient to focus and strengthen substantive codes. These are the conceptual meanings given by generating categories and their properties.

Selective coding

Selective coding (Strauss, 1987) is the process of validating the relationship between a *core category* and other categories. The core category can be identified by its centrality, frequent occurrence, good connections to other categories and implications for more general theory. Once again, Glaser (1992) takes a simpler view. He delimits coding to those variables relating only to the core variable. Further theoretical sampling and data collection then help to focus memos and integrate theory, leading to saturation of the story line. Strauss sees axial and selective coding as parallel developments with open coding, once the latter has been established. Although interactions and interpretations feature in grounded theory, the structural conditions in which these occur can also be documented through theoretical sampling, which links empirical data with memos.

Integration

The final stage of a project using a grounded theory approach is that of *integration*—putting the memo and empirical files together. The empirical data are checked for holes, while the memos are cut and pasted, and sorted into conceptual sets. The operational diagrams that have developed throughout the study are finalised and written up as drafts.

Examples of grounded theory research include an investigation of the strategies emphysema sufferers adopt to help them manage daily living tasks (Fagerhaugh, 1993); the problem of funding for people with chronic renal failure (Suczek, 1993); and negotiating a division of labour among professions in a state mental hospital (Schatzman and Bucher, 1964). Clearly, the process of undertaking a grounded theory approach requires an extensive knowledge of relevant literature and a broad theoretical and conceptual knowledge. The emerging theory would tend to be rather thin without the constant comparative process. Glaser (1978, pp. 9, 11) suggests that the idea is to have broad scholarship that is used to stimulate questions and enhance the development of a range of theoretical footnotes that recognise the derivation of particular concepts. This theoretical sensitivity should encourage the researcher to continually read in a range of fields to prevent being dominated mentally by one specialist discipline. Glaser (1978, p. 139) also suggests that, during the development of final drafts, in-depth reading in the substantive and theoretical areas under study should occur. This should enable the researcher to appropriately locate the emergent substantive theory.

Formal theory

The development of formal theory may take many years after completion of the actual study from which a core category has emerged. The core category 'status passage' (Glaser and Strauss, 1971) moved from substantive to formal theory through a process of theoretical sampling and coding of other status passages, such as single → married; defendant → prisoner; dying → death; and dying → recovery, where → stands for the transition from one status to another. The same coding and memoing processes are applied to documentation. Creative comparisons with other topic areas enrich codes and memos. Formal theory cannot be claimed until one considers all authored works on status that have any attached stage-to-stage connection or transition.

A 'good' grounded theory investigation can be judged by the provision of clear information on sampling, core categories, key events, hypotheses and negative cases, and the relatedness of the propositions that are generated to broader theoretical concepts (Denzin, 1994).

Criticisms

Grounded theory is not without its critics. Criticisms tend to imply that, on the basis of the following statements, it should not be seen as a reliable research technique:

- The nature of grounded theory has never been properly clarified (Brown, 1973, p. 6).
- Grounded theory has close affinities with positivism (Roman, 1992).
- The link between theory and data has never been properly explicated (Hammersley, 1989).
- The researcher is centred in a quasi 'objective' manner (Denzin, 1989).
- It is not possible to 'ignore' existing research and theoretical positions prior to the emergence of categories from the researcher's own data (Blumer, 1978).
- There is an overemphasis on linking to previously discovered theories (Gerson, 1991).
- The process is more suited to concept generation than testable hypotheses (Williams, 1976).
- The various refinements of the process have resulted in a focus on method and prior knowledge rather than on data. The elaboration of theoretical sampling procedures (Strauss and Corbin, 1990) has resulted in five different sampling procedures. These have only managed to produce poorly integrated theoretical explanations (Robrecht, 1995).
- Strauss and Corbin have failed to define clearly the relations between some of the basic concepts, especially categories, properties and dimensions that are sometimes interchangeable (Lonkila, 1995).
- The 'theories' are rarely tested by other researchers (Hammersley, 1989).
- Grounded theory 'departs' from the assumptions of symbolic interactionism. It assumes 'strongly determined' (Glaser and Strauss, 1965, p. 270) relationships among variables, where 'symbolic interactionism emphasises creativity and indeterminism of human action' (Hammersley, 1989, p. 204).

Despite these criticisms, grounded theory has enjoyed a resurgence in the health area over the last decade. Method modification has dominated, with Heideggerian hermeneutics combining with grounded theory (Wilson and Hutchinson, 1991). Judith Wuest (1995) has suggested that grounded theory can be undertaken from a feminist perspective. Leonard Schatzman (1991) presents dimensional analysis as an alternative approach to the current problems experienced in analysing grounded theory data. Links between grounded theory and postmodern and poststructural approaches have also been investigated (Star, 1991). It is clear that the changes undertaken by Strauss (1987) and Strauss and Corbin (1990) have focused more on method. This has been emphasised by Strauss's appointments in nursing faculties and by pressure from nurses for a step-by-step approach.

Barney Glaser (1992), however, sees these changes as a departure from the original method. He believes that they have quite dramatically limited the capacity for theory generation.

Grounded theory summary

Grounded theory is a rigorous technique within the theory-generating approach. It has the potential to enable researchers to develop theoretical propositions, or even theories, of the middle range that may explain the empirical world. In the health area, however, researchers with minimal conceptual/theoretical knowledge have often used this method to produce 'theory' that is little more than a reaffirmation of their own biases. Those hoping to use the grounded theory method would be wise to fully inform themselves of the theoretical sensitivity issue prior to commencement. They must also indicate which version of grounded theory they are attempting.

Oral biography

The purpose of collecting *biographies* is to reveal, from the inside, how people give meaning to their life events and how these events impact upon themselves and others. Biographies gathered in the field (*oral stories*) may comprise one person's total, partial or edited social life experiences, relationships, interpretations and definitions of situations; or those of a group, an organisation, a process or a culture. These stories are usually collected over time, and the actor/s' perspectives are paramount. These data are gathered via conversations and interviews. They are often supported by material or written documentation, and may form the *single focus* of a study or the *partial focus* of a larger study. When presenting the biography, the researcher must be careful not to display overlarge volumes of unedited voices, as this may create problems with regard to ownership. It may also prevent sufficient space being given to the impact on the data of the researcher's position, views and interactions.

A life history may attempt to cover a person's/organisation's total life to date, or only part of that life. Manzo, Blonder and Burns' (1995) exploration of stroke patients' stories about their 'stroke' experiences provides an example of a *partial life biography*. Such stories can be displayed unedited in the interviewee's words, but they are presented more usually in an edited form, with or without researcher comment at the end that links the text to other literature. Theory generation is the most common outcome. The story of transsexual Jane Fry (Bogdan, 1974) is an example of a *full life biography*. One hundred hours of discussion were taped over a three-month period. The final product is predominantly in Jane's words, supported by documentation (letters, photos and diaries), and edited and interpreted theoretically by Robert Bogdan.

Data collection

Life history data are obtained primarily through interviews in an attempt to gain an understanding of the respondents' meanings and explanations of life's events. A grounded theory approach has been used occasionally in the exploration of multiple lives (Denzin, 1989, p. 196). The benefits of this lie in its generation of codes and categories that are pursued across the lives until saturation is obtained. There is an emphasis on *life course analysis* within oral biography (Dex, 1991). This derives from the Chicago School of Sociology, and involves a longitudinal study in which individuals' lives are placed in context and overlapped with the lives of their contemporaries. Quantitative (demographic) and qualitative data are combined to provide a complete picture. The blank spaces separating classes of people are used to clarify their differences.

Several documented approaches (Denzin, 1989, pp. 196–197) for undertaking life histories include:

- grounded theory;
- progressive–regressive;
- oral history;
- critical hermeneutic; and
- literary folkloristic.

The *grounded theory* approach treats each life as an individual case. It applies the life course analysis to explore the person's life events, linking these analytically with theoretical explanations until saturation is achieved. The participant's and other cases' subjective views are often diminished or lost in this process.

In the *progressive–regressive* approach, used by Jean-Paul Sartre (1963), the interviewer starts by documenting the present context, then follows the person into the future via significant events and anticipated outcomes, while at the same time collecting information on past incidents that have contributed to current situations. This view of humans as *'singular universals'* (Sartre, 1960), whereby each is singular but universalised within a context and a culture, requires the individual biography and the social system to be read across each other, critically and simultaneously.

Paul Thompson's (1978) *oral history* approach favours triangulation of data. Three possibilities are suggested (Denzin, 1989, p. 197):

- single life history narratives including documentation and life stories;
- a collection of several life stories based on a common theme; and
- cross-case analysis of oral and textual data where each case represents a totality.

The *critical hermeneutic* approach (Denzin, 1984a) involves two steps:

1   a meticulous grammatical and linguistic interpretation of the text; and
2   a deeper level of meaning, gained by:
    — moving as close as possible to the other person's interpretation of their life; then
    — moving back to gain a more distant view from the position of the researcher's prior and gained understandings; then
    — researcher and researched getting together to assess these multiple interpretations and develop a shared consensus.

The *literary folkloristic* approach (Dolby-Stahl, 1985) insists that the researcher must have a shared biography with the researched, such as experience of the same illness. The researcher links these shared events to the researched's life history, then to larger social meanings, bringing interpretive approaches from feminism, poststructuralism, postmodernism and psychoanalysis to bear on the data.

This literary folklorist approach is also used for autobiography or personal narratives that take the form of thick *ethnographic description*. Personal experiences are then linked to life history, culture and theory. These descriptions are subjective, with interconnections between emotional, cognitive and physical experiences. Multiple voices, poetry and dramatic presentations are all being used in an attempt to recover the immediacy of the experience. Carolyn Ellis and Arthur Bochner's (1992) short play on the experience of undergoing an abortion illustrates this technique. The voices of the woman and her accompanying partner interweave throughout a text in which feeling, expression and interpretation are communicated with much greater impact than could be provided by a third-person account. A dramatic performance of the text can also introduce a whole range of verbal and non-verbal interaction, which has the potential to deliver a powerful impact

Feminist oral historians have used *women's narratives* to expose women's unequal positions in society, and to challenge accepted perceptions of the status quo. Approaches vary from third-person portrayal, using sketches or vignettes constructed from the researcher's views, to storytelling that displays the participants' 'voices'. These latter narratives are accepted unquestioningly as 'true' in terms of being perspectives glimpsed through memory. The researcher's role in such narratives is to locate contexts and develop a shared understanding of how each 'truth' is used in the construction and reconstruction of self.

Authorship

The issue of authorship must be addressed here. When significant portions of one person's life are displayed in his/her voice, *co-authorship* is usually acknowledged, and any royalties from publications are shared. Where more than one life is involved, negotiations are necessary to ensure equity and avoid litigation.

Oral historian's position

The oral historian's position at the intersection of history, biography and the narrative permits exploration of a broad range of topics. Most topics involve either an historical event orientation, or a focus on famous, typical (of a group) or little-known but different people, especially those who inhabit the margins of society. A 'typical' oral history might be that of a particular mother's experiences. It might be the story of a mother who has been the long term, sole care giver of her intellectually disabled adult daughter/son. Her experiences will not be identical to those of others in the same situation, but it is expected that similarities will be evident, and her experiences may serve to illuminate theirs.

Bias

There are two possible sources of bias within the more traditional orientation towards rigorous data: the researcher and the researched. The *researcher's* limitations may include:

- avoiding certain relevant issues;
- coming from a different class, status or culture from the researched, so that he/she may therefore 'see' things differently; or
- presenting him/herself, or interacting, in such a way that the interviewee may omit large chunks of their lives, assuming the researcher 'would not understand or appreciate' these aspects.

A pre-interview (Paterson and Bramadat, 1992) can often help clarify the content to be explored and minimise differences through the development of good rapport.

The *researched* have the potential for bias in their recollection of life events. The researcher must ask:

- To what extent, and why, have certain events been dramatically reconstructed?
- How can the researcher accurately determine the degree of reconstruction?
- Is it important to do so?

Validity or trustworthiness can be checked by comparing the recorded life with supporting documentation, with other similar lives recorded in the same or other studies, and with interview data collected from friends/relatives/colleagues who have known the researched.

Editing

The editing process involves removing material perceived as irrelevant to the major theme/s or aspect/s of the life under exploration. When editing first-person narratives, Bob Blauner (1987) insists that the interviewee's style and language should not be changed, regardless of the problems this may present to readers. He also states that a process of immersion in the data, identification of the story line and associated themes and researcher invisibility are essential if editing is to remain true to the original texts.

Despite theory generation being the norm, some documents (Plummer, 1983) are collected and tested within the frame of a particular theoretical position. They are edited, subjected to a careful thematic analysis and interpreted through the chosen theory/theories. When theory generation *is* used, several positions may illuminate the text/s or emergent concepts and themes in order to generate theoretical propositions.

Limitations

Despite some considerable diversity in approach, there has been some identifiable change, over time, in the conceptualisation of persons whose lives are being recorded. An early view was that 'truth' lay in their self-reflective, subjective accounts, which were distinct from the social world. Later views (Sartre, 1960; Scott, 1991) proposed that individuals being researched were located within a context, and were the products of their experiences and language norms. Vincent Marotta (1996) has suggested that this situation may be complicated further by the researcher's representation of the stories. His/her views and interests may overlay or distort the original. Marotta asserts that an individual (researcher and/or researched) is embedded in social structures that are both 'constraining and enabling', and that this awareness should help 'transcend the dichotomy' currently limiting life history approaches (Marotta, 1996, p. 133).

Oral biography summary

Oral biography approaches are particularly useful for exploring the meanings people attribute to life events. Researcher positions can vary from that of a distant chronicler of narrative to that of reflective self-examination and re-presentation using literary modes. This impact of context, in particular societal structures and socialisation, remain contentious and can be explored further utilising the next approach, memory work.

Memory work

Memory work is one example of *feminist narrative* method. This approach has been developed from the work of Frigga Haug (1987) and her collective, who sought to establish an emancipatory feminist focus within Marxism. They aimed to achieve this by exploring how women's work and gender relations enable them to take an active part in female socialisation processes.

The *memory work* method is embedded in critical theory. It joins the subject and the object into a single focus of the research, and attempts a process of transformation via learning and social action. This technique is appropriate for any topic in which the investigation of the construction of individual social scripts is relevant. The principle behind the method lies in the belief that women are oppressed within a patriarchal system. Therefore, the processes of construction and reconstruction that they undergo in the presentation of self and the clarification of meaning result in considerable adaptation and change. These compromises can only be perceived, and change can only be achieved, by tracing experiences from the past to the present through memory.

Process

Memory work requires the researcher to become part of the researched group (Haug, 1987; Mitchell, 1993) or a facilitator (Kippax et al., 1988). It involves three stages over a period of up to two years, regardless of researcher orientation. These stages are:

1   *Writing stories in the third person:* These stories consist of actions or events that are relevant to the topic, and are triggered by remembered feelings from the researched's earliest memories. As much circumstantial and other detail as possible is encouraged, including anything that may seem trivial and inconsequential. No interpretations or explanations are made at this stage.
2   *Collective analysis of memories:* The women in the group interpret meanings, make linkages and develop a clear account. The memories may be rewritten at this point. Further explanations will be sought from such theoretical sources as Marxism, critical psychology, Foucault and theories of culture and ideology.
3   *Reappraisal:* The researcher carries this out in consultation with the group.

Power equalisation between researcher and researched—and strict ethical guidelines relating to emotional safety, exploitation, privacy and dignity, anonymity, and group control of the process—are said to increase subjective validity in memory work. The purpose of writing in the third person is to distance the writer and to make the private events of women's lives public. These autobiographies should then have the capacity to illustrate how the formation of identity and the production of self within a particular social context have contributed to the reproduction of a particular societal order. It is anticipated that the provision of a bridge between experience and theory will enable the development of new discursive frameworks. This disruption and destabilising of past influences should break their continuity and provide the potential for transforming and liberating the women involved.

Examples in health research

Memory work studies completed to date cover the topics of female sexualisation (Haug, 1987); women's negotiation of heterosexuality (Kippax et al., 1988); menstruation (Davies, 1990; Koutroulis, 1992); the experiences of being indigenous (Grant, 1995); and older women's health experiences (Mitchell, 1993).

This last study provides an excellent example of this form of research in the health area. The group's first session explored the women's thoughts on the important health-related issues in their lives. Six issues were identified, and these formed the basis for the writing sessions, throughout which models of health were developed at different stages as the women's perspectives changed. These changes occurred as the women located and explored experiences, eventually centralising their physical/mental and emotional/social selves as the key to their perceptions of themselves as 'healthy', despite 'unhealthy' medical profiles.

Problems

Although there have only been a few studies undertaken using this technique, some problems have been identified:

- Friendship groups are not always ideal for this research.
- Women who are not educated in theoretical analysis may become subjects and experience minimal transformation (Koutroulis, 1992).
- Some women have difficulty expressing deep or buried emotional issues in words (Haug, 1987).
- The level of the group's education may truncate the process of analysing, leaving the researcher with the task of locating and utilising appropriate theoretical explanations (Mitchell, 1993).
- There is a tendency for the group to indulge in primitive psychotherapeutics in the sharing of memories, which is not productive (Haug, 1987).
- The focus on Marxist frameworks emphasises a particular explanation of individual action as conformity rather than resistance, which may not sit well with individual interpretations. Studies that have emphasised resistance and coping rather than victimisation (Mitchell, 1993), despite the restrictions of a patriarchal culture, tend to have a more positive outcome for participants than those which emphasise women as victims (Haug, 1987).

Memory work summary

Memory work is a new and exciting approach currently undergoing some 'teething problems'. These problems are understandable, given that memory work is still in the process of development and adaptation (Kippax et al., 1988). The emancipatory, feminist focus of this technique has considerable potential, however, in field-based research where there is an emphasis on empowerment.

Case studies

The debate regarding case studies ranges from one end of the scale where everything is regarded as 'a case', to the other end where the value of such terminology is totally rejected. Despite this dissent, a variety of disciplines and subjects (including psychology, sociology, anthropology, health, education, economics and political science) have adopted and adapted case study approaches.

In qualitative research, a *case* is generally a bounded unit with some established identity. This stands as a potentially generalisable representative of certain features of the social world. The *case unit*, or study focus, can be an individual, case group, event, instance in action, theoretical category, total organisation, culture, community or country. The 'case unit' can be defined as an empirical entity that already exists in the world, or the composition of the 'case unit' will emerge through the interaction between ideas and evidence as the study progresses (Ragin and Becker, 1992). Families, hospitals and doctors are further examples of 'case units'. 'Cases' are smaller units, such as groups or individuals within the larger 'case unit'. As in other areas of qualitative research, cases are dynamic. They can change over time, with each being a case of more than one thing.

Thick ethnographic description and theory generation have been dominant in case studies. The focus has been the ethnography of individuals or groups, the socio-biographies of social rules, or the social history of a particular group (Feagin, Orum and Sjoberg, 1991).

Types of case study

Robert Stake (1995) has identified three types of case study:

- *intrinsic* (for better understanding of a particular case);
- *instrumental* (using cases for greater understanding of an issue or theory); and
- *collective* (an enlarged instrumental study using multiple cases).

Pauline Prior (1995) provides an example of a single-case case study in her edited account of interviews with 'Samuel' to expose the impact of 40 years of institutionalised psychiatric treatment. Despite labels of deviance and stigma (Goffman, 1959), 'Samuel' was able to maintain a strong personal sense of identity throughout this time. This study would fit into Stake's *intrinsic* approach, although strong 'instrumental' overtones point to the limitation of segregated categories.

Arona Ragins (1995) undertook an extended case method approach in which she interviewed and observed 25 low-income Afro-Americans attending a sickle cell clinic. This *instrumental* approach extends beyond individual cases and explores the social context, joining micro with macro structures to identify the factors that may be inhibiting self-care.

Multisite or *collective* case study research involves the comparison and contrast of different locations. A hypothetical multicase study could involve an examination of staff stratification and decision making in a hospital. A matrix of cells could be drawn up, representing different levels of staff. Individual cases could be investigated from each cell to detail the broadest range of decision-making possibilities. As the study progresses, '*casing*' (the further development of new cases) may occur. Data are collected in the usual manner via interviews, observation and written documentation. Data are then presented in the form of focused incidents and decisions made around a particular issue. Decision trails are traced, and various decision-making models are established and located within the theoretical literature. A study by Burgess et al. (1994), in which they examined four schools, is a good example of a multisite research project. Each case illustrated a different type of school (with regard to size and location) within the district.

Advantages and disadvantages

Disadvantages of the case study approach are:

* Defining a 'case', whether it is established or developing, involves theoretical choices regarding content and framing. The loose application of the term 'case' has often resulted in these aspects being minimised or avoided.
* The researcher's biases need to be clarified, but these are rarely exposed.
* The bounded nature of cases suggests that, in general, the case study approach favours containment, control and causality (Platt, 1992) rather than the

multifaceted complexity, continual change and ongoing interaction of the postmodern tradition.

Advantages argued for the case study approach are:

- Case studies, however defined and generated, can provide powerful stories to illustrate particular social contexts. This is generally agreed.
- The holistic approach allows for the observation and grounding of a particular phenomenon.
- Continuity and change can be documented.
- The approach permits the generation of theoretical propositions that may be generalisable to other groups (Feagin, Drum and Sjoberg, 1991), either naturalistically (Hammersley, 1992) or analytically (Yin, 1994).

Case studies are thus a somewhat contentious entity. Those who favour them view them as either a complete method or, more usually, a way of organising data collection within a larger study. They can be seen as comprising one or several cases, with multiple cases viewed as enhancing typicality. They can be seen as being theory directed or theory generating, and as oriented towards producing policy recommendations from situationally grounded but limited views of social life. They can also be seen as systems with boundaries, or as a contemporary phenomenon within its real life contexts when the boundaries between phenomenon and context are not clearly evident (Yin, 1984, p. 23).

Case studies summary

Despite the fairly contentious nature of the terminology, case studies, whether imposed or generated, provide a useful way of designing and managing a research focus.

Summary

The six approaches to the location, management and interpretation of data discussed in this chapter indicate some of the choices available to the researcher. To recap, these approaches are:

- ethnography;
- phenomenology;

- grounded theory;
- biography;
- memory work; and
- case studies.

As with discussion of other research methods in this book, any decision made by the researcher as to which method he/she will use is shown to be influenced by the research topic, the researcher's position, and his/her preferred theoretical/conceptual perspectives.

It is now time to explore 'evaluation' and 'action research', the final two research methodologies in this part of the book.

Further readings

Ethnography

Atkinson, P. (1992) *Understanding Ethnographic Texts*. California: Sage.

Hammersley, M. and Atkinson, P. (1995) *Ethnography: Principles in Practice*, 2nd edition. London, New York: Routledge.

Reed-Danahay, D. (ed.) (1997) *Auto-ethnography: Rewriting the self and the social*. Oxford: Berg.

Schwartzman, H. (1993) *Ethnography in Organisations*. California: Sage.

Thomas, J. (1993) *Doing Critical Ethnography*. California: Sage.

Phenomenology

Heidegger, M. (1982) *Basic Problems of Phenomenology*. Translated by A. Holfstadter. Bloomington: Indiana University Press.

Husserl, E. (1931) *Ideas I*. Translated by B. Gibson. London: George Allen & Unwin.

Merleau-Ponty, M. (1962) *The Phenomenology of Perception*. Translated by C. Smith. London: Routledge and Kegan Paul.

van Manen, M. (1990) *Researching Lived Experience: Human Science for an Action Sensitive Pedagogy*. Albany, New York: State University of New York Press.

Grounded theory

Glaser, B. (1978) *Theoretical Sensitivity*. California: Sociology Press.

——(1992) *Basics of Grounded Theory Analysis*. California: Sociology Press.

Glaser, B. and Strauss, A. (1967) *The Discovery of Grounded Theory: Strategies for Qualitative Research*. New York: Aldine.

Strauss, A. (1987) *Qualitative Analysis for Social Scientists*. London: Cambridge University Press.

Strauss, A. and Corbin, J. (1997) *Grounded Theory in Practice*. London: Sage.

Biography

Church, K. (1995) *Forbidden Narratives: Critical Autobiography as Social Science*. New York: Gordon and Breach.

Crawford, J., Kippax, S., Onyx, J., Gault, U. and Benton, P. (1992) *Emotion and Gender: Constructing Meaning from Memory*. London: Sage.

Denzin, N. (1989) *Interpretive Biography*. California: Sage.

Gubrium, J. and Holstein, J. (1997) *The New Language of Qualitative Research*. New York: Oxford University Press.

McMahan, E. and Rogers, K. (1994) *Interactive Oral History Interviewing*. New Jersey: Lawrence Erlbaum and Associates.

Case studies

Feagin, J., Orum, A. and Sjoberg, G. (1991) *A Case for the Case Study*. North Carolina: University of North Carolina Press.

Ragin, C. and Becker, H. (eds) (1992) *What is a Case? Exploring the Foundations of Social Enquiry*. New York: Cambridge University Press.

Yin, R. (1994) *Case Study Research: Design and Methods*, 2nd edition. California: Sage.

8 Action-based methods

The two main action-based methods used in health research are *evaluation* and *action research*. Both seek outcomes beyond data collection, analysis and interpretation, particularly in terms of improvements to organisations, quality of life or health. Originally, both methods had distinctly different orientations, but current changes show considerable overlap. Evaluation is now an intrinsic part of action research, while action research approaches (involving interventions for change) are seen as a desirable outcome of evaluation.

Evaluation

Qualitative *evaluation* has attracted a variety of definitions, varying from an economic rationalist orientation on improving human efficiency and effectiveness (Patton, 1990, p. 11), to an emphasis on the participation and cooperation of all parties (stakeholders) in accumulating sufficient relevant information to precipitate a critical debate (Kemmis, 1994, p. 4).

Theory direction (often using economic and organisational theories and/or the concepts of power and bureaucracy) and theory generation both occur in evaluation. Theory generation, using loose conceptual frameworks and ideals, is more common and is seen in the production of models of action. Ethnographic approaches and focus group techniques are the most commonly used approaches in data collection, while phenomenology and grounded theory are used occasionally.

Other popular orientations include social constructionism and the ecological approach. *Social constructionism* aims for consensus among stakeholders, making particular use of the 'fourth-generation' evaluative approach (Guba and Lincoln, 1989, pp. 79–279), which emphasises sharing and collaboration between the evaluator and those being evaluated. The central elements of the evaluation are constructed from stakeholders' claims and concerns, thus giving them some control over the evaluative process. The *ecological approach* (Tesch, 1990) seeks to determine (from a behavioural perspective) how goals are achieved in particular environments.

Formative and summative evaluation

The two major types of evaluation are:

- 'formative'; and
- 'summative'.

These reflect the orientations noted above.

Formative evaluation involves the researcher working with people to solve issues that they themselves have generated or identified as problems they wish to address. Equal communication and empowerment are emphasised.

Summative evaluation is often theory/concept/model directed, and the researcher may develop criteria in conjunction with the initiating or funding body in order to evaluate a situation. Although discussions and interviews with, and observations of, participants will occur, the researcher usually has ultimate control of the evaluation.

Evaluation processes

The processes of question development and literature review follow the usual patterns. Interviewing and observation provide the bases for data collection. Analysis of documents such as memos, minutes and policies plays an important role. This is undertaken through the processes of content and discourse analysis.

The literature abounds with different evaluation *models*, including:

- *goal-free* evaluation (Scriven, 1972), where the evaluator is not informed about the goals of the program she/he is evaluating, but the focus is instead on collecting data that demonstrate the extent to which outcomes have met expressed needs;
- *response* evaluation (Stake, 1980), and the *fourth-generation* judgemental approach, both of which prioritise stakeholders' concerns and emphasise collaborative involvement; and
- *utilisation-focused* evaluation, which is creative and flexible, and calls on qualitative and quantitative data as appropriate.

These and other models are just variations or refinements of the *standard approach* to evaluation, which involves:

- question/problem identification or the development of a set of criteria/objectives;
- the location of theoretical/conceptual/ideological positions and the choice of data collection techniques; and
- a form of interpretation that provides the best answers to the topic under investigation.

The five areas in *health* evaluation where qualitative data have been particularly effective are:

- needs assessment (evaluation for development);
- evaluation of design, delivery and outcomes of programs, policies and strategies;
- evaluation of organisations (processes and output);
- evaluation of health products; and
- evaluation of individuals.

Again, these are simply ideal types. Overlap is common in practice, as illustrated by the examples below.

Needs assessment

Needs assessments are used to identify the discrepancies between actual and desired situations, and to prioritise concerns to enable the development of appropriate programs. The determination of a region's health priorities (Southern Metropolitan Health Advisory Board, 1996) is an example. Three panels from different parts of the region undertook broad community consultations. They collected quantitative and qualitative data, which included questionnaires, health statistics, demographic and epidemiological information, and information on social and environmental factors. They held public meetings and focus groups, and conducted shopping centre surveys, community phone-ins and surveys of service providers. They located 150 health issues, which were sorted into different levels of priority on the basis of six key principles:

- health advancement;
- equity;
- effectiveness;
- solidarity;
- efficiency; and
- cultural diversity.

Mental health was found to be the major concern, followed by family violence and home-based care and carer support. The close participation of the community in information collection focused on, and stimulated, concern. This led to an increased awareness and a stronger voice in the demand for better services. These research approaches provided the basis of impressive claims for priority funding through their emphasis on community-based, empowering research.

Another example of a needs assessment that was totally evaluative in approach explored whether there was a need to introduce a program of national screening for prostate cancer to reduce deaths (Australian Health Technology Advisory Committee, 1996). An extensive survey of the literature on prostate cancer was undertaken; qualitative data were collated through an analysis of the portrayal of prostate cancer in the print media during 1994–95; and submissions were taken from community and health organisations. Based on the evidence and views available, the report recommended against the screening of men without symptoms on the basis that screening would not necessarily improve health outcomes. Action approaches, in the form of a consumer statement and an education program for individuals and medical practitioners, are to be developed from this report.

A further example of a needs analysis (Smith and Smith, 1995) investigated the gap between the needs of indigenous people and the health services currently available to 146 outstations in the Kimberley region of Western Australia. A steering committee of indigenous people and health department representatives helped manage the project. Extensive consultation occurred on each outstation, where an environmental needs index was used to assess environmental problems. This index provided scores for water access and purity; toilet facilities; washing and housing facilities; and general access (roads, phones/radio communication). Environmental structure was identified as a priority, as were health services for children and the aged. Community-based training of health workers was recommended, and an outreach health service was considered necessary to facilitate the other recommendations. As with many other health evaluations instigated by government authorities, the dominant perspective was the delivery of white biomedically influenced services. This perspective fails to take account of indigenous definitions of health and well-being (Anderson, 1996). Nor does it really involve indigenous stakeholders in a partnership for ongoing change in which both sets of views are valued and accommodated. The recommendations in this study simply allow for a 'quick fix' solution, in the form of the imposition of one type of service without adjustment or adaptation.

Evaluation of programs, policies and strategies: design, delivery and outcomes

These evaluations are often formative, involving researchers working closely with participants at all stages.

Design

The descriptive, exploratory nature of qualitative data is particularly suited to the evaluation of processes, as sensitive cultural issues can be investigated, unanticipated outcomes can be explored, obstacles delved into, and solutions developed and trialled in an ongoing manner. In the following evaluation, the barriers to participation in mammography screening for Chinese Singaporean women were explored (Straughan and Seow, 1995). Four focus groups involving 24 women from varied backgrounds were used. The questions sought perceptions on who was thought likely to get breast cancer, how cancer could be prevented and the reasons why women do/do not attend mammography screening. The results were interpreted through value expectancy models relating to decision making. The barriers to breast screening were found to lie in:

- fatalistic attitudes towards death and cancer;
- misinformation regarding mammography; and
- perceived costs (physical, psychological, financial and time).

Motivators included:

- faith in the efficacy of early detection; and
- influences of social networks.

These results will help to inform the design of programs to promote mammography screening in Singapore.

A similar two-stage investigation into the diet of pregnant teenagers was undertaken in New Jersey to inform program design. Identification of the barriers to providing ongoing dietary guidance to pregnant teenagers was sought (Janas and Hymans, 1997). A focus group of ten health professionals was held to discover why teenagers were not utilising the existing community services that provided dietary information. Explanations included:

- difficulties of access;
- lack of health insurance; and
- lack of knowledge regarding available services.

It was concluded from this that the people best placed to deliver nutrition programs to teenagers were school nurses. This finding led the researchers to administer a questionnaire survey to 253 school nurses, who clarified the barriers they perceived in the implementation of such a program. These included:

- administrative problems;
- attitudes; and
- resources (especially time).

Despite these issues, 45 per cent of those surveyed indicated an interest in running brief sessions.

The collation of this preliminary information, gained in an investigative manner, is crucial in preventing scarce resources being committed to the development and implementation of a program that may be doomed to failure.

Delivery

A complex and multifaceted example of design and delivery evaluations can be seen in the assessment of a New Zealand campaign to reduce intoxication in licensed premises (Wyllie, 1997). The focus was on providing support for managers of licensed premises to act responsibly in dispensing liquor. Four years of intervention and evaluation were undertaken, including:

- A mass media campaign was conducted, to clarify and encourage manager responsibility.
- A public awareness survey (random telephone interviews of 657 people) was held, to measure public awareness of managers' legal responsibilities in serving intoxicated people. Results showed an awareness level of 27 per cent.
- Stakeholder response to this was assessed (one year later). Stakeholders, all of whom identified that dealing with intoxication on licensed premises was an ongoing problem, included:
  — members of the national committee managing the interventions;
  — indigenous community workers;
  — health promotion workers;
  — liquor-licensing inspectors; and
  — managers of licensed premises.

The campaign was run using the following steps:

1 Media advertisements were pretested with drinkers and managers, then adapted to be more age inclusive and multicultural.
2 An advertising campaign was conducted, after which public response was monitored through a telephone survey of 1000 people. This survey showed an increase in awareness from 27 per cent to 69 per cent.
3 Ninety managers were interviewed (audiotaped) by telephone to gauge their awareness of responsibility. This was found to be high.
4 a second, shorter round of advertising took place four months after the first.
5 Another public survey (1000 telephone interviews) took place. This showed some decrease in awareness.
6 A stakeholder study reviewed (with managers) the directions of the overall focus on host responsibility.
7 A final public survey (after 17 months of no advertising) indicated a fall in awareness to 50 per cent (among 18–49 year olds).

These results suggested that a combination of factors—public campaigns with follow-up monitoring (also including drink driving), compulsory breath testing, closer monitoring of licensed premises and fear of sanctions—interwove to increase the awareness of licensees and the general public.

The long term interventions and constant monitoring of strategies appeared to be useful in facilitating attitude change. The use of qualitative exploration permitted a dynamic approach that could quickly respond to consumer and stakeholder concerns.

Outcomes

The summative evaluation of a total program usually confines itself to outcomes. The feasibility of a proactive model for worksite smoking cessation (Thompson et al., 1995) is one example. All employees who were smokers were targeted over an 18-month period. An Employee Advisory Board was set up, with smoking and non-smoking representatives from all parts of the industry. A survey of all employees was undertaken to identify smokers and develop a database; 29 per cent of workers refused to be part of this database. Interventions and assessments were undertaken in the following categories:

- health fairs;
- holiday health promotions;

- quit programs; and
- three levels of encouragement to stop smoking:
  — telephone advice;
  — mailed self-help materials; and
  — group help.

The overall program was considered a success, as 16 per cent of identified smokers gave up smoking.

Obstacles to the implementation and the long term effects of such programs are not always easily located using evaluative approaches that tend to work at the superficial level of indicators for outcomes. An in-depth exploration of context, culture, and the social meanings of smoking might have provided a more solid base on which to interpret these results.

Evaluation of organisations (processes and output)

Evaluations of organisations largely determine the effectiveness of institutional, departmental or centre operations, and their genesis is usually resource management driven. One example is an evaluation of a women's healthline (Women's Health Statewide, 1996) five years after its commencement. This organisation provided health information and counselling for women by nurses. The organisation, in conjunction with researchers, undertook an evaluation in order to determine its value to the community and to attract ongoing funding. An independent researcher, who utilised the phone contacts left by past clients when they originally sought information, administered survey questionnaires to 200 of these people. In addition, all calls taken over a four-week period were coded, and their orientations were summarised by the health workers. This provided five years of data. The positive responses received enabled the evaluators to make two recommendations:

- that the organisation should continue with a full time coordinator, rather than a part time one; and
- that sufficient resources be provided for the maintenance and development of the different levels of information being sought by clients (especially by lesbians and women from non-English-speaking backgrounds), as well as for adequate publicity of the service.

Another example of organisational analysis was undertaken by a consortium of academics and corporations with expertise in risk management (CERF, 1997). The brief in this analysis was to evaluate the United States' Department of Energy's current management of installations where nuclear weapons research had resulted in radioactive chemical and mixed waste contamination of soil and water. This evaluation was prompted by public and scholarly concerns regarding worker and tribal safety, and environmental pollution. Six sites were qualitatively investigated to explore issues more closely than previous sporadic, ill-matched quantitative investigations, and to make judgements. The researchers used a panel of nine national experts to review 1600 documents relating to the sites and risk management, and collected information from public workshops. Results indicated that:

- Long term storage of nuclear waste required immediate attention.
- Environmental remediation was needed, but would have to consider the presence of endangered species.
- Risks to the public depended on proximity to the sites.
- Implementation of administrative controls were critical to worker health and safety.
- Many current risks were due to past waste management decisions.
- Incidences of Department of Energy agendas overriding installation contamination priorities were noted.

The researchers recommended that the Department of Energy continue to manage the risks in these installations, taking the above issues into account. Many of these issues related to the limited knowledge and narrow management perspectives of past eras.

The utilisation of both qualitative and quantitative approaches in the above studies fits the current orientation towards the inclusion of multiple perspectives (Hepworth, 1997) to gain as complete a view as possible of the area under evaluation.

Evaluation of health products

New medical products are usually subjected to rigorous laboratory testing (Harvey and Murray, 1995) in either their country of origin or the country into which they are imported, in order to meet that country's standards. After entry into the market, consumer magazines may also compare different versions of the same health product to test their claims of effectiveness. There are a number of health products, however, that do not go through any rigorous testing procedures. These lie within the health food and alternative medicine industries.

A government committee in Australia (Parliament of Victoria Social Development Committee, 1986) conducted an exploratory evaluation of these industries. Surveys of practitioners, manufacturers, retailers and the general public were undertaken. Group discussions, interviews, public hearings, analysis of training courses and site inspections were also carried out. Interpretation of these data led to many recommendations, with particular reference to the content of training courses for alternative health practitioners; the need for proper accreditation; and the need for standards in labelling, advertising and monitoring of alternative therapy programs. The committee expressed considerable concern about the unregulated spread of the health food and alternative medicine industries.

Evaluation of individuals

The assessment of individuals is a very sensitive area, given the biases and hidden agendas that often underpin calls for evaluation. There is no escape from the questions: 'Who is evaluating what?' and 'For what purpose?' Performance indicators can be used unfairly to enforce a performance 'norm' that advantages one group while disadvantaging the remainder. Clinical case investigations and peer reviews are techniques that often provide the detailed information required to target individuals for redundancy. Quality assurance is one aspect of individual evaluation that has the dual purpose of reducing negligence claims against hospitals and health professions, while promoting professional accountability.

Evaluation of individual attitudes can also provide useful information prior to the development of a health promotion program. Researchers in Scotland (Allbutt, Amos and Cunningham-Burley, 1995) attempted to identify the social image of smoking among young people. Focus groups were undertaken with 234 people aged between 11 and 20 years of age. Cigarette smoking was found to be predominantly a social and group activity, about which both positive and negative views were expressed. It was also seen as a weight loss technique. Ambivalence and contradiction were evident when smokers could be seen to hold negative views of the smell, the smoky atmosphere, family members who smoked, and the health and addiction risks, while holding positive views of image, mood alteration, weight control and the passing of time. These findings indicated that addressing young people's meanings and ambivalence within their social contexts might increase the success of a non-smoking program.

Post-structural evaluation research

Postmodern methods rarely emerge within the ordered and focused world of evaluation. Aspects of poststructuralism, however, can be seen quite often in the deconstructive techniques used in analysing the discourses that are evident in many years of policy statements, memos, minutes and case notes. The webs of documentation that interweave throughout medical case notes (Cheek and Rudge, 1994) enhance the power/knowledge axes of certain health professionals, while muting the voices of patients, their partners and their families. Analysis of this documentation reveals a complex, structured rite that facilitates the discourse of medical dominance.

Action research

In general, *action research* involves a process of enquiry, intervention and evaluation, and is most appropriate when improved practices and problem solving are core concerns. It has been applied in organisations and community groups.

Action research arose during the early 1900s from the work of J. L. Moreno, a physician who used group participation and co-researchers when undertaking community research with prostitutes in Vienna (McTaggart, 1994). In the 1940s Kurt Lewin, a social psychologist, further developed this approach. He described the action research method as 'rational social management' (Lewin, 1946, pp. 205–206), where combined knowledge generation regarding particular social systems could lead to change. His approach involved a repeated cycle of planning, action and evaluation. This allowed each step to be assessed; then this assessment would determine the next step.

Action research has undergone a fairly dramatic shift since Lewin's time, with regard to the researcher's position. It has shifted from the 'researcher as expert' to the current emphases on collaborative or participatory action research. The 'researcher as expert' searched for information about an issue for those at high management levels, devised action/s or experiments to be tested within a location, collected information from respondents, and analysed this and produced a report The collaborative or participatory action research position involves those at lower levels of the hierarchy defining the issues to be addressed and instigating, implementing and assessing action for change in a co-researcher manner.

These two approaches illustrate the polar opposites of a *continuum*. There has been some fairly considerable movement within and between these two, but four orientations have been identified in the health area (adapted from Hart and Bond, 1995, pp. 39–44). These are:

- *experimental*, where the emphasis is on scientific experimentation, and the researcher devises, conducts and evaluates interventions with the aim of enhancing administrative control;
- *organisational*, where change is brought about by working for or with managers, though some negotiation with lower level workers may occur;
- *professionalising*, where the researcher works in collaboration with practitioners who wish to improve their practice; and
- *empowering*, where a co-researcher situation includes both health users and practitioners, with the aim of understanding the complexity of the issue in order to develop negotiated change.

The prime foci are clearly social groups, problems and change. There is variation in the positions taken both by the researcher and by those on whom the outcomes of the research will impact. Just as the positions of researcher and researched vary across the continuum of action research, so too do the procedures used.

Directed action research

At the more experimental end of the continuum, the focus is on the following aspects:

- identifying the issue of concern and the orientations of the stakeholders—their positions, views, levels of power and control over areas that may be subject to change;
- seeking out information about the issue from all parties;
- developing guidelines with the participating group (management, in this instance) to clarify their needs, wants and expectations regarding outcomes and lines of communication; and
- developing, trialling and assessing an intervention, reporting to the group and deciding on further action.

This shows that the researcher's position is central, and that he/she moves between the group who initiated the research and the implementation and assessment of changes with people at lower levels of the organisational hierarchy. The researcher acts as a go-between and a change agent for controlling groups. He/she may, however, have some influence on the interpretation and instigation of change through the introduction of other scientific/theoretical models of practice.

An example of organisational action research (Bond, 1996) was initiated by the manager/researcher of a home for older people. A volunteer sociology graduate cum social worker developed case studies after collecting data from case notes and observations of drug storage and rounds. The results of this exercise were shared with the staff of this and two other facilities. Five areas of concern emerged (abridged from Hart and Bond, 1995, p. 174):

- lack of diagnostic information;
- lack of evaluation of a person's condition before issuing repeat scripts;
- scope for errors between surgery and home;
- compounding of errors when no accurate records were kept; and
- clinical confidentiality acting as a barrier to responsible staff action.

Strategies were implemented to improve these areas. The top-down nature of this project meant that it experienced resistance and indifference from some staff, although it enabled the inclusion of a number of professional development initiatives for staff, and the implementation of new monitoring systems.

Another example of a form of organisational, needs-driven action research was an investigation into service provision for young people with severe to profound intellectual disabilities (Grbich and Sykes, 1989). The project was initiated and funded by a group comprising community representatives and senior policy personnel in a government disability unit. This management group met with the researchers at different times and had input into the methodology. It also received verbal presentations of work in progress and of the final written report. The major areas of concern identified initially by the group were:

- how the integration of young people with severe to profound intellectual disabilities was proceeding with regard to access to 'normal' schooling and to employment in the community; and
- whether females were more or less advantaged than males in this situation.

Random sampling of a total population led to the collection of 80 case studies within which these issues could be explored. Extensive interviews and observations found that minimal access had been achieved; that females were less advantaged than males; and that service provision to parent care givers in this situation needed considerable review. The group then used the resultant report to facilitate changes in service provision. Several years later, when these had been achieved and implemented, the researchers were asked to conduct an evaluation of them. This evaluation could then be used to promote further changes.

The researchers in this situation were little more than hired hands operating within prescribed limits on rigid time lines. They did, however, attempt to empower the participant families by ensuring that the final report was in accessible language, and that each family received a copy. They also spent considerable time 'negotiating' the results with policy personnel in relevant government departments. This study serves to demonstrate that, although a project may be defined by a 'management' type group, researchers still have some leeway to facilitate participation and empowerment through providing access to knowledge for those affected by, and those implementing, policy changes.

A more focused example of directed action research with the potential for empowerment can be seen in an attempt to improve the quality of life of chronically ill older Canadians (McWilliam et al., 1997). This research involved a health professional undertaking active intervention with a recently discharged person in order to effect perspective transformation. (*Perspective transformation* involves an individualised, reflective dialogue leading to a change in expectations, beliefs and values that will result in positive improvements in quality of life). Thirteen chronically ill persons over the age of 65 years were matched with a health professional. Interviews were taped and interpreted. Five stages were noted in the process:

1   building trust and meaning;
2   connecting;
3   caring;
4   mutual knowing; and
5   mutual creating.

Ways of seeing, doing and being were reformed. One woman started writing stories and letters that gained publication and helped her to connect with the outside world, thus enhancing her control over a bed-bound life. The heightening of individual conscious awareness of health rather than illness provides one form of empowerment that nurses can enhance in this situation.

Participatory action research

At the emancipation/empowerment end of the scale (Carr and Kemmis, 1986), in line with the ideas of Jürgen Habermas (1984), action research is seen as more than just problem solving. It is a quest to understand and improve the world by changing it. It comprises collective, self-reflective inquiry that participants undertake in social situations, so that they can understand and improve upon the practices in which they participate. The reflective process is seen as being oriented to action, historically influenced, embedded in social relationships, and culturally and politically influenced. It is a creative exercise in constructing and transforming ideology and practice in social life. Critical theory often provides the underpinning, participation is emphasised and people work towards improving their own situations or practices. The inquiry, action and evaluation cycle of action research, controlled by the researcher, becomes group planning, acting, observing and reflecting. This involves the participant in becoming a co-researcher in a self-critical community, with an emphasis on emancipation through praxis. The ripple effect of changes instigated by these groups may ultimately affect a broader field.

The procedure for emancipatory research involves establishing a group that is anxious to improve an aspect or aspects of health practice. Some time is spent in identifying the history of current practice and the discourses that have developed over time. The implementation of changes, including changes in language and terminology, is critically monitored. Satisfactory outcomes are publicised widely to facilitate the ripple effect. The emphasis on shared and critical reflection ensures that a variety of perspectives are taken into account. It also provides a broader base for further reconstructions and revisions of action.

Action is monitored by the same techniques used in any other forms of quantitative or qualitative research that place an emphasis on anecdotal records (descriptive, longitudinal accounts of relevant situations); document analysis (memos, minutes of meetings, organisational publications, workplans, letters, contents of noticeboards, diaries, surveys, logbooks, visual documents); and questionnaires, surveys and interviews (Carr and Kemmis, 1986).

Procedure

In more detail, the stages of participatory action research involve the following steps:

1 locating a group of people who share a concern and are prepared to work towards its resolution;
2 identifying current organisational aspects and practices that impact on this concern, and exploring their history;

3 defining the concern and identiftying all relevant aspects, such as power relations and resources;
4 designing and implementing a process for investigating all aspects of the concern;
5 developing and implementing changes to alleviate/transform this concern; and
6 evaluating the outcomes, developing further changes, and implementing and assessing these.

Examples

One example of particpatory action research was undertaken by a group of health workers who decided to become co-researchers and explore the sources of stress that they experienced at work (Traylen, 1989). They identified these as coming from 'hidden agendas' emanating from depression, drug taking and suspected child abuse in the families they visited. They observed and recorded their own and others' behaviour, practised confronting the 'hidden agendas' and tried out new behaviour strategies. As a group they then consolidated, developed and periodically reviewed these strategies.

Another example of participatory action research was a study undertaken by Peter Reason (1988). The aim was to explore the practice of holistic medicine with a group of medical practitioners. This group decided the criteria for involvement. The project involved a two-day workshop for planning (reflection), six weeks of application in the surgery (action), and finally a four-day workshop (evaluation). The two-day workshop involved brainstorming experiences, listening to guest lecturers, and developing a holistic care model, together with strategies for implementation. Various procedures of 'validity' were pursued, in particular:

- research cycling (cycles of research involving experience and reflection);
- checking on collaborative issues; and
- countertransference (exploration of underlying tensions) within both the self and others.

The central issues in the move to holistic care were clearly power (particularly medical power) and the autonomy of patients. Other important strategies included:

- skill sharing with patients;
- changing the consulting environment;
- developing personal relationships; and
- role playing (changing positions with the patient).

Empowerment and emancipation

The terms 'empowerment' and 'emancipation' present different stages along a continuum of the desirable outcomes of participatory action research. *Empowerment* (the imparting of power) is the most usual outcome and one that does not necessarily equate with, or lead to, *emancipation* (the setting free from previous controls).

The term 'empowerment' has always been contentious in application. In the *speaker-centred approach* (Patai, 1988, p. 10), where there is minimal researcher intervention, participant definition of topics and free discussions are paramount. This process is viewed as empowering in itself, but it also raises several questions:

- Whose knowledge base is being augmented?
- Who is actually benefiting, and to what degree?
- How can this be clearly ascertained?

These questions can be addressed further by the argument that empowerment occurs in an open-ended interview through highlighting and confirming the participant's expertise in a therapeutic process. In addition, the incorporation of marginal and silenced voices can create a subversive text that questions previously accepted patterns of obligation (Opie, 1992).

The concept of 'empowerment' implies that those being researched are vulnerable or lacking in power. Thus the first issue that must be addressed is 'the establishment of criteria that can distinguish [the] claims of moral superiority which we [as researchers] exercise as outsiders' (McLaren, 1995a, p. 289). The underlying assumption that researchers are already in a superior, 'empowered' position is arguable, especially when feminist researchers are considered. The desire of these people to research *for* and *with* women, to bring about change, cannot obliterate the fact that many feminist researchers are vulnerable members of male-dominated universities. As such, these researchers are struggling to empower themselves at the same time as they are trying to empower other equally marginalised groups of women.

The concept of 'moral superiority' becomes even more problematic when those under research are from different cultures. Although equal participation may be established, it seems reasonable to assume that the researcher's well-established and confidently articulated frameworks (usually reflecting those of the dominant culture) may influence the exchange process in sharing different ways of seeing. There is abundant evidence (Whyte, 1991; Wolf, 1996) that, although participatory action research in third-world countries can result in short or even medium term change, it has not yet succeeded in achieving the greater political and economic impact on the social system that would allow emancipation to occur.

Ideal or reality?

The ideal and the reality of genuine empowerment in participatory action research appear somewhat distant. The emphasis on the interactive nature of participation in the planning and design of projects hides the fact that genuinely equal participation may be rare. Partial participation may in fact be the norm. An example of this is William Foote Whyte's (1991) use of key informants who liaised with the community and collected data for the researcher. The researcher controls data analysis and report writing in many studies. It is difficult, therefore, to find studies where a community group, particularly one of lower socio-economic status than the researcher, has initiated contact with a researcher in order to facilitate change. The reverse is more usual. The basic dilemma here is the conflict between the researcher as an academic who hopes to publish data, and the researcher as a member of an action group.

Another approach involves helping participants to lose their 'false consciousness' and gain a state of questioning previous beliefs and behaviours. This enables researcher and participants to join together in action for change (Lather, 1988). The potential problem with this lies in the academic persona, which again may tend to dominate and direct, rather than elicit, facilitate and co-research in a negotiated manner.

The emphasis on empowerment as one goal may also reduce the possibility of effective evaluation of the project (Reinharz, 1992). If the emancipatory focus is researcher determined, it may also restrict the development of researcher views and action, thus limiting the empowerment process (Opie, 1992). Empowerment that is limited in focus is also an issue. The emphasis in community care has traditionally been on the client/consumer (Stevenson and Parsloe, 1993), but if staff/carers are not empowered also, the longevity and effectiveness of consumer empowerment may be restricted.

Achieving empowerment

Given these limitations, how may empowerment be defined and how may it be achieved? One approach involves evidence of the researched gaining new insights and understandings of their social world. These gains can be demonstrated by applying knowledge to create new possibilities for action (Elden and Levin, 1991, p. 131). Paulo Freire (1972, p. 136) has asserted that both researcher and researched are empowered through the exchange of different frames of reference; the forming of a new, shared frame; and the naming of this world (new frame) in order to transform it.

Several issues must be addressed if we are to turn the concept of empowerment into an adequately theorised and useable entity (rather than a token slogan), and to demonstrate that empowerment has actually occurred. These issues are that:

- The focus of empowerment needs to be identified.
- The power structures currently inhibiting empowerment need to be located and named.
- The processes by which the effects of these power structures are overcome must be documented.
- The outcomes, in particular the long term outcomes, need to be investigated.

Postmodern action research

Postmodern action research is a recent development that de-emphasises the search for truth in the examination of a fixed and easily 'knowable' social reality. Instead, the focus becomes:

- the way this knowledge has been produced;
- who/which group has exerted power; and
- who/which group has benefited.

This requires:

- developing an historical overview of the genesis and implementation of taken-for-granted beliefs and practices;
- identifying frameworks of meaning within organisations; and
- rejecting order and rationality in favour of flexibility, contradiction and the multiple intersection of texts.

Language and the discourses that have developed over time must be deconstructed to identify inherent power structures and to clarify the hierarchies of authority, so that these can be restructured and transformed.

Ernest Stringer (1996, pp. 25–38) places postmodern action research within community research, based on a model of looking, thinking and acting. He has emphasised four working principles to guide potential researchers in this area:

- equal, harmonious, cooperative and accepting relationships with co-researchers;
- appropriate communication, which requires listening attentively and sharing knowledge in a genuinely open and sincere manner;
- effective participation of workers, which requires significant and active involvement and support; and
- inclusion, which not only necessitates cooperation with all relevant groups and individuals, but also addresses all relevant social, economic, political and cultural issues.

The desired outcomes of such a process involve transformation of the researched setting, relationships and communication strategies. The continuing procedures of evaluation and monitoring mean that the process is ongoing, and that defined outcomes will be difficult to assess at any one point in time. Stringer (1996, p. 137) asserts, however, that focused evaluations for funding authorities will still be possible. This approach avoids the criticism that action research is atheoretical and tends to manipulate people (Mies, 1990), but it is unclear whether it will result in empowerment, emancipation or the use and creation of a multiplicity of perspectives.

Criticisms of action research

Action research has been criticised (Carr, 1994) on the basis of its positivist tendencies to focus on 'action' rather than to take into account the social dimensions that will impact on such action, and its tendency to pay lip service to the process of self-reflection.

Another major criticism of action research has been the separation of theory from practice (O'Conner, 1993; Carr, 1994; Hart and Bond, 1995). There is always a temptation to isolate a situation and look for an immediate solution to fit the needs of one sector of stakeholders (those in a powerful position), rather than to spend a fairly prolonged initial phase inquiring into the genesis, discourses and theoretical modes that have constructed that situation.

Also, once consensus as to the solution or best outcome has been achieved, there is rarely any extensive discussion as to where this outcome fits within current theoretical positions. Nor is there much evidence of indulgence in dialogical, reflective processes of philosophical critique.

Summary

The preceding exploration and discussion of action-based research methods has presented various approaches within evaluation and action research, and provided detailed examples of case studies as a means of clarification. The major points to arise from this examination can be summarised as follows.

Evaluation research can be used for a variety of purposes and approaches. The researcher can take the role of a distant 'expert' conducting assessments for various authorities, usually within the agenda of economic rationalism and using predecided criteria; or she/he can work with a group in a co-researcher situation.

In health, the major areas of investigation using evaluation research have been needs assessment, program evaluation, evaluation of organisations, evaluation of health products and evaluation of individuals.

Theory/model generation is the most usual outcome of evaluation research, but deconstruction and discourse analysis are also used to investigate various relevant forms of documentation.

Three forms of *action research* can be identified, even though they tend to overlap. These are: *directed action research, participatory action research* and *postmodern action research.*

Directed action research is a top-down approach that includes experimentation and interventions where researcher control dominates the process.

Participatory action research is a co-researcher approach where joint identification, action, reflection and further action dominate a process that highlights concepts of empowerment and emancipation. The terms 'empowerment' and 'emancipation' are contentious both in definition and application. They require careful interpretation and assessment if they are to be more than meaningless slogans.

Postmodern action-based community research focuses on genuine equality, communication, participation and inclusion in an attempt to restructure and transform settings and relationships.

The next chapter examines the major issues concerning interpretation and explores the processes of data analysis.

Further readings

Evaluation research

Owen, J. (1993) *Program Evaluation: Forms and Approaches.* Sydney: Allen & Unwin.

Patton, M. (1987) *How to use Qualitative Methods in Evaluation.* California: Sage.

Wadsworth, Y. (1991) *Everyday Evaluation on the Run.* Melbourne: Action Research Issues Association.

Action research

McNiff, J. (1995) *Action Research for Professional Development: Concise Advice for New Action Researchers*. Dorset: Hyde Publications.

Noffke, S. (1997) Professional, personal and political: dimensions of action research, in M. Apple (ed.), *Review of Research in Education*, 22, pp. 305–343. Washington: American Educational Research Association.

Reason, P. (1994) Three approaches to participatory inquiry, in N. Denzin and Y. Lincoln (eds), *Handbook of Qualitative Research*. California: Sage.

Part Four
Interpretation, analysis and presentation of data

Part Four consists of three chapters that explore the major issues involved in interpreting, analysing and presenting the data that has been collected.

Chapter 9 examines the major issues in interpretation:

- framing the data;
- the interpretive focus; and
- the role of the reader.

This is followed by a detailed exploration of the processes involved in the four major types of data analysis:

- the *enumerative* mode, which deals with documentation that is approached through procedures of content analysis;
- the *investigative* mode, which is concerned with the analysis of language;
- the *iterative* mode, which is most commonly used for data that has been collected from the field by interview or observation; and
- the *subjective* mode, which involves the researcher in some form of active participation in the studied setting or phenomenon, leading to the analysis of his/her own responses, or in minimal analysis that allows the participants' voices to emerge.

Chapter 10 provides an overview of many of the qualitative computing packages currently available, a critical assessment of what these may be doing to data, and comments from program users.

Chapter 11 looks at ways of presenting qualitative data using visual displays, quotes, vignettes, anecdotes, pastiche, layering and alternative modes such as poetry, drama and dialogue.

9 Interpretation and analysis

This chapter attempts to present the basic issues involved in interpretation, and to display four major modes of data analysis.

Interpretation

The process of interpretation is complex. It involves three potentially contentious areas:

- the frames applied by the researcher;
- the researcher's interpretive focus; and
- the reader's position in relation to the collected data.

Frames applied by the researcher

The concepts of *frames* and *framing* come from Erving Goffman's frame analysis, in which frames are 'the principles of organisation which govern social events and the actor's subjective involvement in them' (Goffman, 1974, p. 10). The focus here is on units, and the links between face-to-face presentation of self and breaching barriers among people during communication. Another definitional source is Gregory Bateson's (1973) metatextual framing of textual situations to make them comprehensible.

In general, the term 'framing' emphasises an active interaction with the text (MacLachlan and Reid, 1994) in an interpretive manner. The act of framing places a frame around a set of data and lifts it out. In everyday life, the frame used will tend to be drawn from the researcher's own life experiences. Agatha Christie's Miss Marple, for example, spends considerable detecting time comparing the situations to which she is exposed with her knowledge of previous events and personalities from her home town of St Mary Mead. Researchers have access not only to their own previous experiences, but also to the experiences of other researchers in similar areas, and these frames are often applied to the setting under observation. Another source of framing comes from the theoretical positions directing or informing the research.

Recognition of the frames that dominate the researcher's interpretation of texts is clearly important, as is an awareness that the act of imposing a frame upon an event may well disturb or distort existing forms. A gynaecological examination, for example, falls under the general frame of a medical encounter. This separates the event from other related frames, such as sexual encounters or attempted abortions. Placing other frames upon this encounter (such as doctor–patient relationships, paternalism, distorted communication, or medical dominance versus lay knowledge) must inevitably unsettle the existing frame, particularly in relation to context and boundaries, as the 'readings' of the frame change.

The importance of context has always been a key aspect in situating events and meanings. However, there is an implicit presumption that context is a static entity that can be located, with its boundaries identified and meaningful connections made. This is antagonistic to the accepted view that context is socially produced (Culler, 1988). It is also subject to a teeming mass of contradictions in the processes of individual and group creation, maintenance, resistance and transformation, as well as the added reactions to, and qualified adaptations of, the frames introduced by the researcher.

Further complexities

Erving Goffman (1974) pointed to further complexities inherent in framing. Some of these are:

- the story within a story, or *frame within a frame*, may be obscured by the outer frame. For example, if an individual is involved in a rescue operation, this frame of perception may be so strong that he/she does not notice, or chooses to ignore, the fact that he/she also is injured. His/her task orientation may be so focused that he/she feels no pain until the task is complete.
- Participants may *fabricate frames* to deliberately mislead researchers or create more favourable reconstructions of events. For example, acts of violence may be reframed as retribution, momentary madness or the lashing out of an individual who is tormented beyond belief.
- *Out-of-frame activities* may be of greater importance than those which have been framed. For example, in an interview with the manager of a health care program, the criteria for running the program may be clarified, but its actual day-to-day running may be completely different.

- *Breaking frames* to present another frame may occur. Both researcher and participant may leave frames to attend to other matters. For example, the frame of the engrossed interviewer–interviewee may be broken by the intrusion of dogs or children fighting, unexpected guests or other unanticipated events.

Types of frames

Some of the types of frames that may delimit as well as enhance aspects of the researcher's view include:

- *language* frames, in which different speech patterns, word usage, tone and accompanying body language may be separated out or combined in some revealing way;
- *cultural* frames, which provide artificial boundaries that segregate and marginalise representatives of particular cultures, delegating them as 'other';
- *specialist* disciplines with particular and highly guarded theoretical frameworks that are less accessible to those without appropriate qualifications and insider knowledge; and
- *gender* frames, in which a particular world view, such as feminism, prevents other interpretive possibilities from emerging.

Researcher's interpretive focus

The researcher's interpretive focus is generally defined by the researcher's intentions. Is she/he seeking to demonstrate the homogeneous nature of her/his data? Or is she/he seeking to reveal the contradictions, uncertainties, unexplainable gaps and disruptions that are evident in the data? Is the text to be viewed as a highly respected entity that contains meaning? Is this meaning one that the researcher will only minimally analyse or edit to enhance reader appreciation? Or will the text be viewed as a superficial and carefully constructed document, requiring intensive deconstruction to reveal created meanings and underpinning discourses of knowledge that have been distorted for purposes of power?

Those favouring minimal interpretation, or none at all, argue that analysis reduces the text to a shadow world of 'meanings' (Sontag, 1966). If interpretation is not undertaken, meaning's dynamic nature can be pinpointed and displayed in a cineflash approach. This will not reveal historical changes, traces of which remain in the words used. A collection of recurrent themes can be examined for their similarities or differences where interpretation is undertaken, but this approach favours centring the researcher's position in the process of conscious reflection and reflexivity, leading back to framing—an approach rejected by poststructuralists as favouring specialisation of particular knowledge bases.

Others (Bloom, 1976) have argued further that there are no texts. There are only relationships between texts, and attempts at any analysis should involve creative misreadings (Eco, 1993) as the researcher engages in a strong and imaginative struggle with the text. Nabokov's *Lolita* (1965 [1958]) is creatively misread in Eco's (1993) short story *Granita*. Eco parodies (or deconstructs by reversing roles) *Lolita* by having an adolescent boy ardently pursue an octogenarian woman, instead of a middle-aged man lusting after a pre-pubescent girl.

Analysis by deconstruction celebrates contradiction, although an awareness of what this may involve for the text has led authors such as Derrida (1972) to write already deconstructed texts. *Glas* is one of these. It comprises texts within a text. Here the first sentence of the text—'What, after all, of the remain(s), today, for us, here, now, of a Hegel?' (Derrida, 1986 [1974], p. 1)—is deconstructed through the presentation of a pastiche of information. Each sound, word and meaning is teased out, and interrelated information is explored and juxtaposed. For example, the name 'Hegel' leads to a sound comparison with 'eagle', which represents various visual images. 'Remains' is interpreted through views of this word's meanings in relation to humans and the texts left by Hegel.

Poststructuralists such as de Man (1979) favour rhetorical deconstruction, which explores the values that underpin the structure and production of meaning in the process of deciding between literal and figurative meanings.

Reader's position

The role of the reader has been explored at some length in literary interpretation. Again, there is a diversity of opinion. Holland (1980) asserts that there is no division between the reader and the text. Each reader's free and interactive response is unique. Interaction occurs on the basis of:

- *defence*—what the reader allows in from outside;
- *expectation*—the reader's wishes;
- *fantasy*—the reader's inside contribution; and
- *transformation*—meaning beyond time (Holland, 1980, pp. 359–370).

'Subjectivity' is paramount in Holland's view. There is a constant interchange between the reader's life experiences and knowledge base, and the information revealed in the text.

Another view (Iser, 1980) is that reading is a dynamic interchange, but is activated by blanks and negations within the text. These break the continuum and force the reader to hunt for hidden meanings, or to create images to fill the gaps. The text is seen as a separate entity from the reader, and the response pattern resembles shock tactics rather than the close and continuous engagement expounded by Holland.

Umberto Eco (1979) sees the reader's interaction with the text as being limited by whether the text is 'open' or 'closed'. Although each text utilises codes to promote a shared understanding between author and reader, various semantic techniques can be used to create either an 'open' or 'closed' text. An *open* text relies on semantic techniques that ensure the widest possible interpretation at all chosen levels. A *closed* text relies on different semantic techniques that ensure acceptance of content without wider interpretation from ideological or intertextual knowledge.

The three aspects of interpretation just discussed—framing, the researcher's interpretive focus, and the meanings taken or developed by the reader—are all part of the interpretive process, and must be taken into account in the analytical process.

Data analysis

There are many types of analytical procedures within qualitative research. Certain approaches have well-articulated (although considerably debated) processes attached to them, such as grounded theory, phenomenology, and content and discourse analysis. Other approaches vary depending on whether an 'objective' (distant researcher) position is involved, or whether the researcher's submergence in the data or his/her subjective view is required.

Broadly speaking, four *ideal modes* of analytical procedures can be generated:

- *Enumerative*, dealing largely with documentation: The recurrence of particular aspects is recorded, and the researcher inhabits a distant position. Content analysis of documents and some material culture best fit this mode. A characteristic of this approach is that data are collected as a complete entity prior to analysis.
- *Investigative*: The researcher collects documentation, but undertakes a form of analysis that searches beneath the superficial words or other forms of evidence to uncover the history, power struggles, myths and language uses that have impacted

on current practice, rather than enumerating predefined categories as in content analysis. Discourse and semiotic analysis fit into this mode, as does the historical method.

- *Iterative:* The researcher collects data from the field by interviews or observations, reflects upon it and notes emerging themes, which are used to inform further forays into the field. Methodologies within this mode include grounded theory, phenomenology, ethnography, oral histories, case studies, and action and evaluative research. Diary records facilitate the development of the researcher's subjective, reflexive views. Parallel analysis of diary field data may occur.
- *Subjective:* The researcher either becomes highly involved in the lives of those under research (as in heuristic phenomenology and memory work), or targets him/herself as the research focus (as in some feminist or other narratives and postmodern approaches). The researcher's subjective experiences are inseparable from the analysis; texts are often minimally assessed, created and/or utilised for transformation; and both the researcher's and participants' voices are usually heard.

These four modes have been identified on the basis of:

- the researcher's position in regard to data collection;
- the types of data collected—existing documentation in contrast to researcher-generated data from live participants; and
- the different interpretive approaches.

Clearly there is overlap. Oral histories may well fall within the feminist narrative tradition as well as the iterative mode. They may also appear as subjective ethnographies. The dynamic nature of qualitative research means that boundaries must inevitably be artificial and that new creative combinations will continue to emerge. This will be illustrated in the following detailed discussion of each mode and its analytical procedures.

Enumerative mode

Quasi-statistical content analysis

Although content analysis does occur in a qualitative form, the enumerative approach has tended to dominate. This approach has been characterised by the production of 'objective' accounts of the content of verbal, visual or written texts; the prior development of codes and categories; and the measurement of units of analysis.

Measurement tends to be based on the frequency of occurrence of particular units—spatial aspects (the amount of space being allocated to the unit measured), the strength of statements (using measurement scales), and appearance (size, shape, colour, race). This approach is used to assess the content of speeches, letters, policy documents and television programs, among others. Considerable documentation may be involved, and sampling strategies can be used. Issues of 'validity', 'reliability' and 'generalisability', as defined within quantitative approaches, are also important factors. Other researchers should be able to replicate results, and the measures used should enhance 'analytic validity'.

The approach will vary depending on whether written or visual (television, video, film) data are involved. In general, the following steps should be taken (adapted from Fields, 1988, pp. 183–193):

1   Gather documentation needs and, if necessary, sample the documentation using probability sampling techniques;.
2   Unitise the content by specifying the units to be analysed (words, themes, characters, sentences, total script, visual images, theoretical concepts).
3   In visual analysis, transcribe the script where necessary. Include spoken language, vocal inflection, facial expressions, body language and scene composition.
4   Apply predecided codes and categories that are mutually exclusive. Modify, test and revise.
5   Explore the content, and note dominant codes.
6   Describe the patterns detected and interpret the interplay of themes in terms of the general hypothesis being explored. Use frequencies, percentages, significance and any other relevant forms of statistics, such as multivariate analysis (Weber, 1985), to present the results.
7   Check 'validity' (using face validity) and 'reliability' (using interrater reliability).

Various *computer packages*, such as Gofer, ZyIndex and Textpack, can facilitate the process of content analysis. These programs take scanned-in documentation and can facilitate:

- string and Boolean searches;
- comparisons of vocabulary;
- cross-referencing;
- dictionary construction;
- retrieval of text units and specific enumeration;

- word frequencies (how many times a particular word actually occurs in a document);
- ordered word frequency lists (ranking the occurrence of all words in a document); and
- retrieving key words in context (which places the key word centrally and indicates the eight to ten words that occur on either side to clarify the context in which it appeared).

The advantage of the key-word-in-context function is that, although it is useful to know how often a designated word occurs, particularly in political documentation, meanings do differ, and it is advisable to examine each word within its original context.

Barbara Downe-Wamboldt (1992) conducted a content analysis of hospice volunteers' self-reported records of interactions with patients. The volunteers' roles were categorised into: listening and responding; giving and receiving information; socialising; providing spiritual comfort; and referring. These five categories proved to be sufficiently mutually exclusive to facilitate statistical analysis.

Content analysis using enumerative approaches has been criticised on the bases of:

- the usual problems within quantitative research regarding 'validity', 'reliability' and 'generalisation' (Manning and Callum-Swan, 1994);
- its tendency to atomise by breaking the data into decontextualised units;
- the problem that connection does not equal causation (Kellehear, 1993); and
- being seen as contrary to the goals of qualitative research (Morgan, 1993).

Despite this, content analysis is often used as an adjunct to qualitative data where patterned precision and comparisons between sets of data are an advantage.

Qualitative content analysis

Qualitative content analysis (Crabtree and Miller, 1992; Morgan, 1993) is also enumerative. It involves the general procedures of document collection, including the development of codes (although in this case codes are derived from careful readings of the data); the application of these codes; and an emphasis on the 'why' and 'how' aspects of contextual interpretation, rather than a focus on numerical strengths.

Several forms of qualitative content analysis have been identified (Crabtree and Miller, 1992). Two of these are:

- ethnographic; and
- qualitative positivism/transcendental realism.

Ethnographic content analysis (Altheide, 1987) raises to an explicit level the implicit 'counting' that often occurs in qualitative research. This approach, which involves a combination of the reflexive analysis of documents (Plummer, 1983) and numerical narrative data, has been used by David Altheide in the study of television news broadcasts and films. Analysis of documentation is through a quasi-grounded theory approach utilising categories and variables in a constant comparative process. This comparison occurs between emerging data and the contextual perspectives that news groups use to select and present news. Five considerations direct these perspectives:

- accessibility of the events (and the capacity to obtain visuals for television);
- visual quality (the clarity of depiction of events);
- drama and action (the graphics, visual and aural portrayals);
- encapsulation and thematic unity (the comparison of the events portrayed, to be summarised and linked to other newscasts); and
- audience relevance (the estimated interest for a mass audience).

In Altheide's study, knowledge of the perspectives used by newsgroups served to inform sampling and data analysis. He collected both numeric and narrative data in the categories of: network; presenter; length of report; origin; sources; and individuals interviewed or presented (their appearance, speech and what was filmed). He eventually achieved saturation by going backwards and forwards through the data in a reflective manner, constantly comparing the emergent themes with other perspectives. Altheide stated that the purpose of ethnographic content analysis is to 'document and understand communication of meaning as well as to verify theoretical relationships' (Altheide, 1987, p. 68).

Transcendental realism is an approach put forward by Miles and Huberman (1984, 1994a, 1994b). This position views social phenomena as existing in both the mind and the objective world, with lawful (stable) relationships between the two. The focus is on sequences and regularities. A researcher pursuing the perspectives of transcendental realism would tend to operate with multiple case studies (Miles and Huberman, 1994b). A conceptual framework comprising interlinking variables (from which hypotheses with causal implications have been derived) is placed over the first case, then reapplied to the other cases to develop a cross-case analysis. Causality is sought in the processess underlying a temporal event. The researcher asks, for example: 'What are the conditions under which this event occurs?' There is an underlying assumption in this process that fully predesigned instrumentation will enhance internal validity and generalisability to other cases and settings, and will improve the manageability of the data collection (Miles and Huberman, 1994b, p. 441). Matrices are used for data display and to show the variables impacting firstly in one case, then across comparative cases. The enumerative aspect is utilised 'to see "what's there"— and to keep oneself honest' (Miles and Huberman, 1994b, p. 432).

Investigative mode

At one end of the scale, documentation is fairly superficially interpreted, usually within the contextual information that is readily available. At the other end, a rigorous poststructural analysis will seek out, and attempt to expose, the myths, contradictions and power structures that have been involved in the social construction of documentation. The methodologies within this mode include:

- historical analysis;
- discourse analysis; and
- semiotic analysis.

Only semiotic analysis will be detailed here, as the first two have been addressed in earlier chapters of this book.

Semiotic analysis

Semiotic analysis is the study of *signs*. It analyses:

- how these convey or generate meaning;
- how they are used;
- what hidden meanings are present; and
- how the reader contributes to this process.

There is much diversity in carrying out this mode of analysis. Some researchers view signs as direct representations of meanings within contexts. Others seek to deconstruct signs, codes and discourses to clarify past influences.

Theorists Ferdinand de Saussure and Charles Pierce are regarded as the initial contributors to semiotics. Ferdinand de Saussure (1983 [1916]) viewed the communicative process as comprising two key entities: a *signifier* (sign-vehicle, comprising words or other signs) and a *signified* (meaning), both of which are meaningful to the persons involved in communicating. He was interested in the relationship (*value*) between the signifier (as a physical form) and the signified (its related mental concept), whereby it determines meaning through connections with other signifiers. For example, the image of a cat is constructed by its sound image, its visual contrast (shape and colour) with other animals, and its position in the text. The image evoked by 'sleeping cats' is much different from that evoked by 'fighting cats'.

Charles Pierce, on the other hand (see Hartshorne, Weiss and Bucks, 1958), focused on three entities:

- a sign;
- its object; and
- its interpretant.

In this instance, the sign stands for something that in turn creates another sign in the mind of the interpretant, and so on in a continuing process.

Semiotics focuses on analysis of the *language system* (speech/writing), but it can be used to view *other systems* (material culture). It does not include sign or body language. The theoretical orientation used provides variation in the levels of semiotic analysis. These range from a structural approach that clarifies the contextual meaning of signs, to a poststructural approach, with its emphasis on complexity and deconstruction. The medical system, for example, comprises various subsystems of signification (Barthes, 1977). There are collections of written material—books, journal articles, case notes and patient information—all comprising particular sign patterns and conforming to the rules of the discipline or hospital. There are collections of visual documentation—photos, films, X-rays and videos of particular conditions and processes. There are patterns of verbal interaction—doctor to doctor, doctor to consultant, doctor to nurse, nurse to patient, other health professionals to patients, and so on. All of these can be analysed both structurally and poststructurally.

Structuralist semiotic analysis

A structuralist semiotic analysis would examine the signs and *codes* (systems of signs agreed to by members of a culture as conveying meaning [Fiske, 1990]) to locate the deep structures that underlie cultural communication systems. This would be done in an attempt to understand how people make sense of the world: the meanings, the relationships between codes, spatial and temporal aspects, visual organisation, and presentation and *metonymy* (the transposition of qualities from one plane of reality to another [Fiske, 1990, pp. 95–98]). An example of metonymy is the substitution of 'crown' for 'Queen'. Here, the name of an easily recognisable attribute (crown) acts as an associated substitute for the name of a thing (Queen).

The identification of *binary oppositions* is essential in uncovering the processes by which categories that exist in nature are used to explain more abstract, culture-specific concepts, such as male/female. This is a biological dimension, but is reflected in the cultural aspects of gender relations embedded in power.

A structuralist semiotic analysis (see Corfield, 1991; Sudnow, 1972 for examples) would include the following processes:

1   Locate all relevant signs, codes and systems.
2   Identify culture, value and meaning through spatial and temporal comparisons. The researcher should ask:
    — How often do signs appear?
    — In what form?
    — In what contexts?
    — What are the apparent meanings?
    — How do they relate to other signs and codes?
    — What conventions/metaphors and metonyms are being used?
    — Are elaborated or restricted language codes evident?
3   Identify binary oppositions (the conceptual categories that separate out the text, such as getting well/ill).
4   Utilise structuralist theories, or concepts interpreted in a structuralist manner (such as power, class, gender or socialisation), to interpret the texts.

Poststructuralist semiotic analysis

A poststructuralist semiotic analysis would view signs, codes and systems as relating to a more complex reality, where many associated images may be evoked. Some signs will have the capacity to generate and transform new structures through being connected, yet sufficiently independent, to enable structural transformation from within at some future time (Kristeva, 1970). This potential for constant evolution has links with Charles Pierce's ideas.

Poststructuralism's focus is the exposure of hidden signs through *deconstruction and clarification* of the perspectives and power bases that underpin the text. In the medical system, for example, the hospital setting could be explored for the power and hierarchical complexities that underlie language and other interactions. In exploring the maintenance of order in such a setting, the poststructuralist analyst would ask: 'What communication has become distorted?' 'What knowledge has been controlled?' 'What definitions of "sickness" or "wellness" have been constructed?' 'Who is powerful/powerless?' 'When and how does this change?'

A framework for facilitating poststructural semiotic analyses is presented below (adapted from Kellehear, 1993, p. 48):

1   Assemble all relevant material, including information on cultural and physical contexts. Include any interview or observational data where these provide useful clarification.

2   Identify oppositional elements (powerful/powerless; sick/well; normal/abnormal; male/female) to clarify which element has been privileged. Reverse these, and critically apply general meanings to the context to deconstruct the text.

3   Compare stories, accounts and versions *intertextually* (across and against each other), to enrich and contrast the layers of meaning. Identify distortions, irrationality and uncertainty, and locate gaps. Actively seek out marginal views and frames within frames.

4   Ask questions:
    — Whose views on discourse patterns dominate? Why?
    — What image of reality is being portrayed? Why?
    — Who benefits? Who loses?
    — Whose voices are less audible? Whose voices are soundless?

5   Utilise appropriate poststructural theoretical perspectives to explain your findings.

Problems with semiotic analyses

The problems with semiotic analyses lie in the limitations of structuralist approaches in coping with change and autonomous individual and group action, and in the poststructural tendency to reduce the text to meaninglessness through overinterpretation (Eco, 1992). The focus on units of signs and codes means that the rich ethnographic description in which these are embedded tends to become diluted, and the broader holistic view is lost. Semiotic analysis's inability to cope with the subjective and emotive aspects of communication (Manning, 1987) means also that it bypasses the diversity of meanings experienced by both the author and a multitude of readers. Roland Barthes (1972), Peter Manning (1987) and Umberto Eco (1992) have pointed to the added complication of reduced cultural formalisation in everyday life (values and rituals), and the increasing commercial formalism (via computers) of monetary and other transactions, which make shifting meanings difficult to pinpoint at any given time.

Other problems lie in the attempt to assess a specific interpretant's perspective on meaning, given that each interpretant understands each sign differently. Umberto Eco (1976) has suggested that the process of interpreting one sign via another sign, which is validated by yet another sign, implies that no real world exists. There are only sequences of self-referential signs. Allan Kellehear (1993) has pointed to the highly abstract, rather dubious, individual analyses that involve tracing the sources and meanings of the layers of meaning involved in poststructural approaches. Finally, the creation of a semiotic analysis involves the production of yet another text, which will in turn also require analysis and interpretation by readers, ad infinitum.

Iterative mode

Iteration, an interpretive/interactive field-based approach, can comprise several levels of analysis, depending on the requirements of the method used. Grounded theory has a three-stage coding process that is specific to this approach. Similarly, phenomenology has a set of unique processes relating to data collection and analysis, and so is not covered here. Despite the different processes of these two methods, their general approach to data analysis fits the iterative mode.

At its simplest level, iteration involves going out into the field, collecting information by observing or interviewing, transcribing this information, reflecting upon it and subjecting it to an initial analysis to determine 'what is going on', then using the information gained to guide the next venture into the field. The levels of analysis that may be undertaken are:

- ongoing preliminary analysis;
- thematic analysis; and
- coding.

Ongoing preliminary analysis

Once the literature has been reviewed, the theoretical concepts/theories that may direct or help to generate theory have been identified, the study has been designed, and issues of access and ethics have been dealt with, the researcher is in a position to collect the first set of data. When interview sessions are undertaken, the researcher will need to transcribe them as soon as practicable. Observation sessions need to be written up within 12 hours of the observation to maximise recall. Interview transcripts are usually formatted with a sizeable margin. This allows the researcher to write in self-assessment comments, particularly highlighting misunderstandings, lack of clarification and unnecessary interruptions to the interviewee's flow of speech. The researcher will also need to make notes about missing information and issues to be addressed either in the follow-up interview with this person, or with all interviewees. Recurrent emerging issues are of particular interest, whether or not they fit into previous research or the theoretical perspectives that have been identified as potentially relevant.

The main aim of preliminary analysis is to critique the data as it comes in, to identify gaps in information, and to start utilising various concepts and frames to see whether they shed further light on the issues being identified in relation to the research topic. In observational field notes, this running commentary tends to be built in through the 'observer's comments function' [OC . . .]. The method I use to complete the preliminary analysis is to take a clean sheet of paper (*face sheet*) and staple it to the front of the transcript with the following information:

- Interviewee's name (usually coded for anonymity):
- Time, place, number and duration of interview:
- Things to do:
    Issues requiring verification:
    Further issues to be pursued:
- Emerging themes/concepts/issues:

A *summary of themes* is attempted every three to five interviews or observations. This will occur every three if the data are complex, covering a broad range of aspects of the topic; every five if the area is focused and a fairly cohesive picture is emerging; or more if the data are being gathered in sets. In the example below, emerging concepts are highlighted and data from three sessions have been accumulated for closer scrutiny:

Disability Study: Views of parents and teachers (summary of three interviews) One of the central issues emerging so far is *how different people view the integration of special school students into regular schools* (1/2–2 days per week). *Parents (X, Y & Z) all favour this,* seeing it as a glimmer of hope, an indication of 'improvement', a move across the great divide from 'special' to 'regular', with the accompanying connotations of normality. All are very anxious their son/daughter should remain in the integration program despite 'fitting' on regular school days (X); isolation and loneliness (Y) when his mate was withdrawn from the program. X seems to be settling down—likes the pop music in practical classes and sings along, the girls think he is 'cute' and ask him to sing songs, Y is ignored (non-verbal, almost blind) and Z has full aide support and a home room to retreat to (for special students), one where regular students come in to play cards (with students with disabilities) on wet days. Z seems calm and settled but aide (?) is preventing any interaction with other (regular) students. *The environment and form/s, or lack of, support are obviously going to influence the students' experiences. Teachers in special settings fear integration,* seeing it as leading to a loss of students with the potential for job loss—they feel that if the students are starting to move to regular settings, they should too, as their expertise would be invaluable to *regular teachers. The latter view integration as ideologically sound practice but pointless unless there is full aide support,* so they don't have to adjust their curriculum (and none do, so far) or have to worry about the presence of X, Y & Z. X & Y's teachers express concerns regarding what X & Y are gaining from the experience, viewing it as negative and stressful for them (and also for themselves?). *It seems clear that High Schools are more academically oriented and more resistant to any disturbance caused by integrating students whereas Technical School (trade oriented) teachers express less hostility and are more oriented to 'giving it a go'.* (Grbich, Data Summary, March 1988, for Grbich and Sykes, 1989).

These procedures of preliminary analysis continue to inform data collection until all the data are in and the researcher is convinced that she/he has gained as broad a picture of the topic as can be realistically achieved.

Thematic analysis

Once the data are in it is suggested that they be left for a couple of weeks, then read (Bogdan and Taylor, 1975). All the data are read (including the researcher's journal), taking care to read against the text in a critical manner by constantly asking: 'Why? How? What if?' This may generate a realisation of holes in the database that require further investigation. Once the researcher is convinced the picture is complete, she/he should get a colleague or friend to discuss what they see as the emerging themes or issues, and to note where they see gaps in the data.

Tentative *themes* should be evident from the researcher's preliminary analysis and this outsider's perspective. The researcher should then:

1 Contextualise each theme, and place it within a *file*. Contexts can be sentences, paragraphs, long speeches or whatever unit is most relevant.
2 Examine each file for theme *typologies* (classification schemes), such as specific language or responses relating to a theme, or specific behaviour patterns relating to particular topics.
3 Examine each typology and attempt to generate *propositions*.
4 Lay these proportions across all other identified themes and typologies to see whether there are *more complex aspects and associations* that need to be incorporated.

North, Davis and Powell's (1995) typology of adaptive repertoires, relating to long term benzodiazepine users, is one example of this. It was developed to demonstrate this medication's symbolic meaning based on the users' relationship with the drug. Users viewed the medication along a spectrum ranging from 'acquaintance', 'companion' or 'workmate', to 'Keeper' or 'Master'. The perceived relationship matched the degree of drug dependency.

Once the researcher is convinced that there is nothing more to be found in the data, she/he should *amalgamate or subdivide* the themes, typologies, propositions and concepts that have been identified, and the final interpretation and writing up stages can begin. The results gained are now combined in a more focused manner at an abstract level by placing them within previous research, and using the identified theoretical interpretations in a theory-testing or theory-generating orientation. Issues of data display then become important.

Coding

Coding usually occurs when the database is large; when theory testing/direction is being undertaken, so that categories and codes can be broadly generated at an early stage; or when qualitative computing packages are to be used. In the generation of codes, preliminary and thematic analyses are usually undertaken first to develop a broad range of themes, typologies, propositions and concepts. Other potential coding categories lie in the setting and in various processes, events and activities, strategies and relationships. The data are checked against these codes to see whether they '*fit*'. If the match is poor, the codes are adjusted. The developed codes are then used to *frame* the remaining data, while the researcher continues to check carefully for examples of negative cases or data that do not 'fit'. He/she must ensure that these are not ignored. The coding process should account for all data in such a way that data are not forced into predetermined frames, but these *frames emerge from the data*. The number of codes will vary, depending on the size of the database. Codes should ultimately be grouped in some way that facilitates writing up. The researcher needs to refine codes and check the content of each coding frame for subcategories or issues that do not 'fit'. The researcher should critically evaluate the data to ascertain his/her effect on the collected data; to ascertain also the range of data sources and the types of responses (directed/spontaneous); and to ensure that his/her own beliefs, values and prejudices have been adequately exposed. It is necessary once again to develop a more abstract interpretation to explain the results.

Subjective mode

In subjective analysis, the researcher has moved light years from the distant role taken in other modes. He/she is now in a position of high involvement, active participation in the actual research, or where the self has been used as the total focus. Those taking a centred position of high involvement have depended upon the concept of 'reflexivity' to actively construct their experiences in the field (Van Maanen, 1988). '*Reflexivity*' varies in definition from an apolitical 'awareness' to 'radical consciousness' of the self (Callaway, 1992, p. 33). At the awareness end of the scale, the researcher continually checks his/her biases in the interpretive process. The concept of radical consciousness presumes the deconstruction of power differences (gender, race, status, culture and attitude) between researcher and researched in the field (Wasserfall, 1993, p. 24), as well as those boundaries between the researcher and the reader.

Power differences

The problem with the emphasis on power differences can be located in the underlying assumption that the researcher has greater power and that she/he has both the capacity and the desire to empower others. Researchers often do not share the researched's belief systems, or they become less and less empathetic as they delve deeper during the research process (see Wasserfall, 1993). The power dimension is usually the other way around in elite research, or the researcher may be as much in need of liberating as those she/he is investigating, particularly when the research issue reflects personal traumatic or emotional experiences. Techniques suggested to reduce the researcher's authority are:

- co-researching, as in memory work;
- acting as an advocate to facilitate change (where power differences are evident); and
- passing on knowledge.

The latter is in itself seen as having the capacity to empower others, despite the contentious nature of the concept of empowerment.

Editing

The awareness of fieldwork's political dimensions has led to an increasing emphasis on *voice* and the editing process. The main aim of editing (where it occurs at all) is to minimise repetition, maintain context and pass on directly to the reader aspects of the researched's lives, told in their own words. The issues that need addressing in this process are:

- Should the language used be displayed phonetically where it is in dialect or heavily accented? Or
- Should it be rewritten in standard English?

It is generally accepted that language as it is spoken should be displayed phonetically. Where meanings are unclear, however, it is appropriate to insert [in square brackets] a word or two of clarification. Constant repetition of words such as 'eh' and 'you know' can also be partially edited (Blauner, 1987). Sufficient of these words should be kept to give the original flavour of speech, but not so many that the reader loses the sense of the unique style of what is being communicated. One situation where editing may well be appropriate is in the transcription of interviews with people from other cultures. The idea here would be to present a clear sense of their communications rather than a meticulous documentation of their less-than-perfect English, as this latter approach could be seen as belittling them or making them appear 'stupid'.

Author's voice

When others' lives or actions form the research focus, the author's voice has a range of possibilities. It may be *submerged or hidden*, as in The Mirror Dance by Susan Krieger (1985), or it may be present as a source of *running commentary*. Between these two extremes, it may appear in some sections of the text as being *separate* from the researched's voices. It may:

- introduce each narrative;
- provide third-person summaries;
- weave in and out of the text as another entity;
- engage the narratives in ongoing and rhetorical conversations; or
- be displayed in questions prefacing each response.

Krieger (1985) has clarified the difficulties she experienced in the process of 'separating out' the self and decentring her position as researcher. She analysed her responses to all the interviewees, both prior to and during the interviews. This process enabled her to come to terms with her own responses and to distance them, while using these insights to facilitate a more sensitive interpretation of the data.

In auto-ethnographies, the self is both the subject of the study and the narrator. The self is connected to others within the contexts of culture and societal structures in an overlapping and interconnecting fashion. Stories are presented in a creative manner utilising fiction, drama or poetry, and the aim is to engage and involve the reader in the writer's experiences. The focus of the subjective view is emotion: the physical and the cognitive within contexts.

Carolyn Ellis and Michael Flaherty (1992) have identified four developing areas in openly subjective research:

- the interpretation of existing texts (books, films, letters, diaries);
- the writing of texts in different ways (dramatic, poetic or fictional representations and the personal narratives derived from auto-ethnography);
- the subjective experiences of time, place and activity; and
- the transformation of identity through traumatic life events (illness, natural/unnatural disasters) or travel and other mind-changing events.

In these instances, the author's voice is the researched's voice, appealing to the readers to relate their own experiences to those presented.

Summary

This exploration of the various modes of interpretation and data analysis in qualitative research has highlighted the complex nature of each. It has also stressed the necessity for interpretation and analysis of data as a means of achieving 'valid' research outcomes at any given time. Issues arising from the diverse approaches that can be adopted both within and across modes have been presented and examined.

The major issues affecting *interpretation* are:

- the frames applied by the researcher;
- the researcher's interpretive focus; and
- the reader's position.

It has also shown that there is considerable overlap among the four ideal modes of qualitative *data analysis*, which are:

- the enumerative mode;
- the investigative mode;
- the iterative mode; and
- the subjective mode.

Having explored these ideal modes of 'human-only' qualitative data analysis, it is now time to look at computer-assisted data analysis as a research tool.

Further readings

Framing

Culler, J. (1988) *Framing the Sign*. London: Basil Blackwell.
Eco, U. (1979) *The Role of the Reader*. Bloomington: Indiana University Press.

Data analysis

Coffey, A. and Atkinson, P. (1996) *Making Sense of Qualitative Data*. California: Sage.
Miles, M. and Huberman, A. (1994a) *Qualitative Data Analysis: An Expanded Sourcebook*, 2nd edition. California: Sage.

Semiotics

de Saussure, F. (1983) *Course in General Linguistics*. Roy Harris, C. Bally and A. Sechehaye (eds). London: Duckworth. Paris: Payot.

Eco, U. (1976) *A Theory of Semiotics*. Basingstoke: Macmillan.

Subjectivity

Ellis, C. (1995) *Final Negotiations: A Story of Love, Loss and Chronic Illness*. Philadelphia: Temple University Press.
Krieger, S. (1991) *Social Science of the Self: Personal Essays on an Art Form*. New Brunswick: Rutgers.
Merton, R. (1988) Some thoughts on the concept of sociological autobiography, in M. Riley (ed.), *Sociological Lives: Social Change and the Life Course*, 2, pp. 17–21. California: Sage.
O'Kelly, J. and Callaway, H. (eds) (1992) *Anthropology and Autobiography*. London: Routledge.
Paget, M. (1993) *A Complex Sorrow: Reflections on Cancer and on an Abbreviated Life*. M. De Vault (ed.). Philadelphia: Temple University Press.

10 Computer-assisted analysis

The most important point to be made initially is that computers are only aids for the management of qualitative data. They cannot analyse it. The process of interpretative analysis rests with the researcher.

Software types

Historically speaking, the development of computer software for the management of qualitative data has involved two distinct stages over the last 25 years:

- systematisation; and
- theory generation.

There is also a third type of program, which carries out content analysis *quantitatively*.

The concept of *systematic data* as 'desirable' came to the fore during the 1970s and 1980s. It was generated by the push for rigour in qualitative data. The major goal of the earlier programs was to provide storage and retrieval of data, and to construct subviews of the data through assigning codes and categories. During the 1980s, there was considerable discussion regarding these programs' capacities, and the methodological and theoretical implications of using computer programs in qualitative research (Fielding and Lee, 1991). Many of these concerns remain today, and are documented in the second part of this chapter. The debate focusing on capacity concluded that, although currently available software was useful for handling data, it could not address the issues of 'reliability', 'validity' and 'generalisability', which some researchers and theorists regarded as the 'problems' of qualitative research. In addition, these programs could not facilitate the combination of quantitative and qualitative data; nor could they promote theory generation.

The debates of the 1980s prompted the development of more complex programs. Programs with a capacity to *generate theory* became available from the mid 1980s.

Using a grounded theory approach, the researcher could move between data (stored in one file) and references to books and articles and memos (stored in another file), and make connections between the two. End-on connections with SPSS packages also enabled the incorporation of quantitative data.

Operation

Both types of packages (code and retrieve and theory generation) are usually menu driven, and based in an abstract model of qualitative research that comprises 'segmentation', 'categorisation', 'comparison', and 'relinking'. They have a theoretical focus on 'theory generation', rather than 'theory testing' or phenomenology. These programs have been developed for data such as field notes, interview transcriptions, observations, narratives, diary records, documents and questionnaire responses. Texts are typed or scanned into a word processor and converted to ASCII (apart from Hyper RESEARCH™). The text is then segmented into words, full lines or other segmented units, and codes are attached. In some programs text segments' boundaries may overlap; and in most programs, multiple codes can be attached and the coding system can be adjusted continually.

Coding and retrieval packages require the marking of text segments and development of codes (usually off-screen), as there is considered to be a 300 per cent error rate reading on-screen. This means that preliminary, thematic and coding analysis will generally have occurred, by hand, prior to any data manipulation using a qualitative computer program. The off-screen coded passages are then entered into the program, filed and stored. They can be retrieved from their appropriate code files and displayed. Programs differ in their capacity to overlap and 'nest' codes (subcodes). They also differ with regard to the numbers of codes that can be applied to each segment (word/sentence/line/paragraph, as defined by the researcher). Other differences lie within procedures for entering codes. Some have one-step procedures (marking text boundaries and entering codes on screen), while others have two-step procedures (marking text boundaries, printing out, coding off-screen, then entering text numbers and code names into the computer). The provision of a graphic user interface (PC or Macintosh) also varies, as does ease of searching and the way results are printed.

Theory-generating programs comprise two file systems and are usually based within the methodology of grounded theory. Again, coding usually occurs prior to data entry, and searches for co-occurrence of codes are undertaken using the Boolean operators 'and', 'or' and 'not'. The researcher explores relationships between coded categories in one file and can also seek conceptual or theoretical explanations for coded data in the other file. Codes focus on the kinds of reactions such as 'expectations about . . .', to facilitate the development of conceptual categories. Data are interrogated for co-occurrence of linkages; hypothesis testing can occur; and theoretical concepts can be generated.

Programs that carry out *content analysis* quantitatively search for strings of characters, word frequency, and key words in and out of context. Some have the capacity to generate cultural grammars.

Packages

An extensive, but not exhaustive, list of available 'code and retrieve', 'theory-generating' and 'content analysis' program packages is displayed in the table below. Most packages come with detailed manuals attached. Again, the terminology has limitations because, effectively, all programs involve coding and retrieving data and some of the 'code and retrieve' packages (notably Enthograph) have developed sophisticated 'memo' capacities that border on theory generation.

The table is followed by a brief description of each package and its distribution agents, after which a discussion of the issues involved in qualitative computing is presented.

Qualitative computing packages

Code and retrieve	Theory building	Content analysis
Ethno (PC)	AQUAD (PC)	
The Ethnograph (PC)		
FolioVIEWS (Mac, PC)		
FuzzyStat (PC)	ATLAS/ti (PC)	
GATOR (PC)		
HyperFocus (Mac)	HyperRESEARCH™ (Mac, PC)	
HyperQual (Mac)		
KWALITAN (PC)	Hypersoft (Mac)	Textpack (Mac, PC)
Martin (PC)		
MAX International and WINMAX (PC)	NUD*IST (Mac, PC)	WordCruncher (PC)
QUALPRO (PC)		
Sonar (Mac)	Qualog (PC)	ZyIndex (PC)
SQL Text Retrieval (Mac, PC)		
Textbase Alpha (PC)		

Code and retrieve packages

Ethno (PC)

This package creates graphic representations of relationships among entities. The process involves defining a framework, then creating and modifying a structure. It is useful for grouping data into logical hierarchies of groups and subgroups.

Distributor: National Collegiate Software Clearing House
                Duke University Press
                6697 College Station, Durham, NC27708, USA
                Tel. (919) 684 6837

The Ethnograph version 4 and version 5 (PC)

This is probably the most widely used of the code and retrieve packages, and it has a large storage capacity. Version 4 can accommodate 6400 files and can attach memos of up to one page (or 2000 characters) to text units. These memos can be independently coded and retrieved. String searches (40 character strings) can be undertaken. Proximity searches for the co-occurrences of code A and code B can occur when they either overlap or occur within 10 lines of each other. Frequency counts can also be undertaken. As in all computer-assisted analysis, data are typed into any word-processing package that can generate standard ASCII files (numerical tags, such as a = 26, A = 27), lines are numbered, and the researcher codes a printout with half the page blank. Up to 12 codes can be attached to each researcher-defined segment, and segments can nest and overlap up to 7 levels. One-step, two-step and on-screen coding are available. Quasi-Boolean searches of up to 6 code words with 'and' and 'not' can occur, and each data file can be prefaced by a face sheet that identifies up to 40 variables for each file. Each piece of data can be retrieved, with identifying markers for speakers and contextual comments and memos. A text editor provides Ethnograph formatting for ASCII files, and can be used independently by another person while the researcher is working with Ethnograph. Code frequencies can be computed and matrices created to compare coding in several files. Limitations lie in being forced to code every line. Version 5 is due for release in late 1998.

version 4:   John Seidel
                Qualis Research Associates
                PO Box 2070, Amherst, MA01004, USA

and

Qualitative Research Management
73–425 Hilltop Road, Desert Hot Springs, CA92241, USA
Tel. (619) 329 7026, Fax (619) 329 0223
Email: Hallock.Hoffman@mcimail.com

version 5: Scolari, Sage Publications
6 Bonhill Street, London EC2A 4PU, UK
Tel. (171) 330 1222, Fax (171) 374 8741
Email: scolari@sagepub.co.uk
and
2455 Teller Road, Thousand Oaks, CA91320, USA
Tel. (805) 499 1325, Fax (805) 499 0871
Email: info@scolari.com

FolioVIEWS version 3.0 (Mac, PC Windows)

This is capable of fast search and retrieve functions, coding, hypertexting, memoing and annotating. It can import directly from word-processing packages such as Word Perfect 6 and Word (but not version 6). It is user friendly with an excellent search capacity, and data can also be directly entered. Footnotes, annotations and endnotes are placed in pop-up notes. Multiple usage is possible, and each user can develop a customised shadow file.

Distributor: Folio Corporation
5072 North 300, West Provo, UT84604, USA

FuzzyStat version 3.1 (Mac)

This program attempts to calculate degrees of membership, where an object has characteristics that may partially fit into other categories. An object may be 'reddish' or 'orangey' at the same time, for example, or the category of 'suicide as rejection' may be coded on an ordinal scale of five points with:

four occurrences	definitely	*in the category*
three occurrences	generally	in the category
two occurrences	sort of	in the category
one occurrence	slightly	in the category
no occurrence	not	*in the category*

These categories are non-metric (minimum to maximum), and no distribution assumptions are involved. FuzzyStat reads a two-way matrix by treating the columns as if they are fuzzy sets instead of variables, and the data as if they represent degrees of membership in those fuzzy sets. Likert scales can be transferred into fuzzy set data. FuzzyStat is user friendly and comes with a tutorial and a user's manual.

Distributor: Dr Michael Smithson
Psychology Department, Australian National University
Canberra, ACT 0200, Australia

GATOR (PC)

The Generalised Automated Text Organisation and Retrieval System (GATOR) compares favourably with the Ethnograph (B. Walker, 1993) with regard to most functions. It also matches approximations rather than exact key words, and undertakes Boolean searches with 'and', 'or', and 'not'. It cannot, however, display overlapping codes through a co-occurrence function. It only displays the coded segment, and has the capacity to embed to 7 rather than 10 levels. It also has master files (key words and associated text) that allow several researchers to work on the same text, and provides audit trails of decisions made.

Distributor: Richard Giordiano
Centre for the Social Sciences, Columbia University
Room 814, 420 West 118th Street
New York, NY10027, USA

HyperFocus (Mac)

This is used to handle focus group or other group interview data. It has a graphical user interface (windows) capacity, one-step coding and uses the *hypercard* system (a set of electronic cards in a stack). This program enables the development of a model through data, description and theoretical notes, as the notes and text are kept separate. The hypercard system tends to be rather slow in operation.

Distributor: HyperQual
3377 North Dakota, Chandler, AZ85224, USA

HyperQual version 4.3 (Mac)

This program has the usual features of other code and retrieve packages, except that hypercard software is necessary and data can be typed in directly. Automatic coding can occur (key codes [tags] are isolated and run through the data), and a memo function is present.

Distributor: HyperQual (see Hyperfocus)

KWALITAN version 4 (PC)

KWALITAN is menu driven and combines both code and retrieve and content analysis features. It has unlimited files (via floppy disks) that can cope with up to 25 codes per segment; has a memo function of up to 300 attached lines of text; and it conducts Boolean searches. The content analysis capacity counts word and code frequency, and key words in and out of context. Results of these can be displayed in matrix form.

Distributor: Qualitative Research Management (*see* The Ethnograph)

Martin version 2.0 (PC)

This targets phenomenological and hermeneutical analyses. Documents and inter-view texts and segments can be displayed, moved, tiled, resized or reduced to icons via a windows function. Notes can be attached or discarded. Hierarchies of folders can be developed. There is no coding capacity in this program, and it uses a lot of disk space.

Distributor: Martin c/- Robert Schuster
Simonds Center, School of Nursing, University of
Wisconsin–Madison
Room K6/152, 600 Highland Avenue, Madison, WI53792–2455,
USA

MAX International version 3.5 (PC) and WINMAX 3.1 (PC Windows)

Like The Ethnograph, the data in MAX can be linked to field notes, and both one-and two-step coding are possible. This program combines quantitative and qualitative data through an end-on statistical package. Both narrative and multiple choice data can be entered. The creator of MAX asserts that the program has the (very contentious) capacity to take open-ended responses from a qualitative database, turn them into multiple choice responses, then undertake second-order coding by trans-ferring codes to variables and running these through the statistical packages SPSS,

SAS or SYSTAT, thus quantifying the data. The contention here lies in the different sampling approaches and the lack of variable control in qualitative data collection.

WIN MAX for Windows, in addition to the above and in the presence of a graphic user interface, facilitates simple linguistic analysis. It has been suggested that this program is better at processing quantitative data (Weitzman and Miles, 1995). It has a limited search and retrieval function, and is not particularly useful for grounded theory data management.

Distributor: Qualitative Research Management (*see* The Ethnograph)

QUALPRO version 4.0 (PC)

This is the most basic of the code and retrieve programs. A two-step coding process is necessary. It cannot search for documents coded with more than two code words, and has no memory or annotating features. Data can be entered while the editing of other data is in process. Seven different templates are available for headings that provide brief file descriptions. Intercoder reliability measures are supported through the creation of tables of coder-identified coding categories and the estimation of percentages of agreement. This program is best used in conjunction with a word processor.

Distributor: Qualitative Research Management (*see* The Ethnograph)

Sonar version 7 (Mac)

This is a simple code and retrieve package with on-screen coding, nested Boolean searches, minimum file preparation, fast retrieval, and 'link files' or concept categories for searching the data. Files have to be indexed. There is no tagging facility, and the text is annotated through windows. Word frequency counts and synonym and phonetic searches are possible.

Distributor: Sonar Professional, Virginia Systems Software Services
5509 West Bay Court, Mid Lothian, VA23112, USA

SQL Text Retrieval version 2 (Mac, PC)

SQL is the most sophisticated of the code and retrieve packages, more suitable for a commercial or government environment than for individual researchers. It combines literature and data; searches for proximity, synonyms and wild cards; uses Boolean logic ('and', 'not', 'or'); and can cope with unlimited document size, pattern matching and fuzzy word matching. It has a large thesaurus and synonym index, and can call on the Oracle indexes.

Distributor: Oracle Corporation
50 Oracle Parkway, Box 659510, Redwood Shores, CA94065
415–506–7000, USA

Textbase Alpha (PC)

This simple program (up to 200 files) can cope with unlimited coding and code overlapping. Structured information (such as question numbers) can be automatically coded. Limited wild card searches are possible. Data matrices can be constructed for code frequency and sentence segmentation, and exported to SPSS files for cross-tabulation analysis. Tabular presentation of results is possible.

Distributor: Qualitative Research Management (*see* Ethnograph)

Theory-generating packages

AQUAD version 4.03 (PC)

AQUAD is a logic-based system that was developed to access *implicit theories* (a person's view of self) utilising the discipline of psychology. It has hypotheses, co-occurrence of codes, matrix displays, true–false dichotomies, fuzzy logic, and one-step and two-step coding. The data can be typed in directly, but it has no graphical interface. Qualitative/quantitative demographic variables can be entered to be cross-tabulated with conceptual codes. Twelve preformulated linkages (via Boolean searches) are offered, and others can be created. Memos can be attached, and hypotheses and causation can be explored. The limitations lie in line-by-line coding, few multiple or linked windows, and the capacity to work in only one module at a time.

Distributor: Qualitative Research Management (see The Ethnograph)
and
Dr Gunter Huber
Eberhard-Karls-University of Tübingen,
Institute for Erziehungs-Wissenschaft 1,
Arbeitsbereich Pädagogische Psychologie
Munzgasse 22–30, DW–7400 Tübingen, Germany

ATLAS/ti (PC)

ATLAS/ti is one of the most powerful of the theory-generating packages and, arguably, has the most potential. It has two systems (document and hermeneutic), coding and retrieval, memoing, graphical user interfaces and researcher-defined codes—the hermeneutic units can be converted into HTML format for display on the worldwide web. It also has wild card searches (all words starting with 'go-' or ending with '-ed', for example); semi-automatic coding (to specific criteria); links with hypertext and SPSS; a multiresearcher networking capacity; a thesaurus; unlimited coding; swarm searching (related words); and concept networks. The thesaurus allows for the development of taxonomies from conceptual frameworks, and it has a user friendly focus. The difference between ATLAS/ti and other theory-building packages lies in the conceptualising of grounded theory as a non-hierarchical and horizontal network, forming unbounded and unregulated connections that permit any element to be connected with any other.

Distributor: Scolari (*see* The Ethnograph, version 5)

HyperRESEARCH™ (Mac, PC Windows 3.1)

This program's emphasis is on textual, audio and video materials to which the computer can be mechanically connected. Data can be directly typed in, data files can be assigned to a 'case', and Boolean searches and co-occurrence of codes can be undertaken. Hypothesis testing is possible by combining codes in an 'if . . . then' format. Qualitative analysis of audiovisual materials is also possible. Theory building, through segregating 'cases' into meaningful subsets and by testing hypotheses, is one of the program's aims.

Distributor: Qualitative Research Management (*see* The Ethnograph)
and
Researchware Inc.
20 Soren Street, Randolph, MA02368–1945, USA
Tel. (617) 961 3909

Hypersoft (Mac)

This program's focus is on modelling tasks. Boolean searches, conceptual audits, links to SPSS and descriptive statistics, frequencies and cross-tabulation are possible. A dictionary allows the development of conceptual definitions.

Distributor: Ian Dey
Department of Social Policy and Social Work, University of Edinburgh
Adam Ferguson Building, George Square GB, Edinburgh, EHH9LL, UK

NUD*IST version 4 (Mac, PC)

Again, two systems (document and index) occur. An inverted, hierarchical tree system provides the base, in contrast with ATLAS/ti's non-hierarchical concept system. This tree structure is made up of stratified aspects with regulated and limited connections between components. There is an automatic coding function and multiple windows. An audit trail can record all researcher-initiated changes. The text unit can be any size from one word up. Matrix building is possible through cross-tabulation searches. Non-Boolean operators encourage the generation of new ideas. Statistics can be generated on proportions of files and text units.

Distributor: Qualitative Solutions and Research
PO Box 17, La Trobe University, Victoria 3085, Australia
or
Research and Development
Park Centre
2 Research Avenue, La Trobe University, Bundoora, Victoria 3083, Australia
and
Scolari (*see* The Ethnograph, version 5)

Qualog (PC Mainframe)

Logic programming using Lisp provides a deductive loop for text searching. The user interface in Qualog is very cryptic.

Distributor: E. Sibert and A. Shelley
4–116 cst School of Computer and Information Science, Syracuse University
Syracuse, NY13244–4100, USA

Content analysis packages

There are a number of these packages, most of which will carry out word frequencies and search for key word in context and key word out of context, as well as creating alphabetic word lists.

Textpack (Mac, PC)

Textpack carries out automatic reformatting and indexing, in addition to the above functions. It is very fast and reliable, but some preliminary time is needed to prepare the text.

Distributor: Zuma
Postfach 5969D–6800,
Mannheim 1, Germany 621–18004

WordCruncher version 4.5 (PC)

WordCruncher was originally designed for literary analysis. It will sort words by decreasing frequency (ranking); compare words from one file with those found in others; and create indexes. Marker codes can be used to organise the text into three specified levels (book, chapter and page). The 1995 version has windows.

Distributor: Electronic Text Corporation
560 North University Avenue, Provo, UT84604, USA

ZyIndex (PC Windows 5.14)

ZyIndex will attach key words to segments of text and entire files, as well as carrying out the usual functions of content analysis packages. Hypertext links exist, but files have to be indexed.

Distributor: Zy-lab Corporation
233E Erie Street, Chicago, IL60611, USA

World processing as an analytic tool

Despite this wide variety of computer-assisted analysis packages, it should be remembered that, although qualitative computer programs are useful for managing data, a good word processor can accomplish many of the same tasks. A word processor should, in fact, be tried first as an analytic aid (Stanley and Temple, 1995). Programs with windows, in particular Word for Windows or Word for Macintosh, can display several documents at once. ASCII files can be utilised. Some programs have good text search facilities and links to hypertext for inspection and editing. Words and phrases can be counted, memos can be added, and references and other data (such as films and videotapes) can be made accessible via icons in the text (Richards and Richards,

1994; Stanley and Temple, 1995). The tasks with which word processors currently have difficulties are the automatic grouping of coded passages; the undertaking of text searches for co-occurrences of codes; and the management of the codes used and their meanings (Richards and Richards, 1994). This form of clerical data has to be stored separately in word-processing packages.

Issues in qualitative computing

In contrast to the enthusiasm of the computer programs' developers, there have been rumblings of concern from qualitative 'watchers' and the programs' users. These rumblings have become focused into a whole range of issues, some of which are briefly addressed below.

Computer-based research

One issue is the concern that we have moved from computer programs that aid research to computer-'based' research, where the tools constructed for a particular program *impact* upon the data. Each tool creates artefacts and metaphors ('frames') that change our ways of seeing and thinking. 'Reality' has to be segmented, truncated and textured to prepare data to 'fit' a particular form of programming. These procedural aspects affect our views of the data as the data move from a 'complex reality' of intersecting aspects embedded in rich contexts, to a simplified, rational version of 'reality'.

Rule-based approaches

The rule-based approaches of computer programming have much in common with 'positivism'. Views of 'reality' are 'formal, discrete, reductionist, algorithmic, sequential, deterministic, mechanical, computational, atomised, digitalised, and logical' (Henman, 1992, p. 1). A close examination of qualitative computing packages can support this view. Firstly, some considerable time needs to be spent learning to manage the program. NUD*IST users have estimated (anecdotal information) that it takes three months to become proficient in the use of this program. This suggests that program proficiency, rather than data, handling may be the outcome for many. The emphasis on process rather than content may result in a loss of interaction with the data, which then becomes one step further removed from the researcher. This leads to the Gigo principle, Garbage In, Gospel Out (Roszak, 1986, p. 142), becoming the potential outcome.

Communication

Although networking facilities are available, especially for the more developed programs such as NUD*IST and ATLAS/ti, these structured forms of communication (person to computer, computer to computer) bear no resemblance to the more usual processes of collaborative research. These processes usually comprise spontaneous verbal arguments, hands-on data interaction and high level theoretical discussions, which lose not only speed but also flavour in the laborious type–send–wait–read–type–send–wait cycle of computer interaction.

Currently, the programming languages that have been used as a basis for qualitative computing packages are either the very basic first- and second-generation languages with mechanical functions, or the third- to fifth-generation languages incorporating Boolean logic ('and', 'or' and 'not') and true–false dichotomies. True–false dichotomies are based on the Boolean concept of *minimisation*, which 'corresponds to the variable orientated experimental design' (Huber and Garcia, 1993, p. 145) in which single cases are compared. These rigorous, mathematical approaches differentiate 'subjectivity' and foster the appearance of 'objectivity' (Guattari, 1984) through diagnosis and control. The units of data are treated as inert objects or 'input' (Murphy and Pardeck, 1988), reinforcing the abstract model of segmentation, categorisation, comparison and relinking of data. This model is not explicitly theoretical, however, and the search for an underpinning that would best fit this orientation has led to the incorporation of grounded theory approaches.

Grounded theory

Grounded theory is based in the interactionist perspective that has been widely criticised for its focus on the minutiae of microcosmic activity in small groups, to the detriment of the structural factors that may be impacting upon, or influencing, the settings and action under consideration. This focus is both a strength and a weakness of this approach, and many interactionists would counter criticism by asserting that they do not neglect overarching structural factors. Norman Denzin (1988, p. 432), an interactionist, has further criticised the grounded theory approach for its 'over-emphasis on discovering categories and indicators', its minimisation of thick description, and the location of theoretical explanations within the social worlds being studied. The potential for decontextualising, which is inherent in any process of segmentation and categorisation, tends to produce a semantically rather than socially constructed analysis (Manwar, Johnson and Dunlap, 1994).

The focus on segmented aspects inevitably results not only in a loss of context, but also in a 'sacrifice of resolution for scope' in the overall picture (Seidel, 1991, p. 107). The loss of process dimensions and the focus on what can be seen on screen at any one time leads to a 'snapshot approach to data analysis' (Catterall and MacLaren, 1997). John Seidel has also pointed to the 'infatuation' with data, which leads to 'more and more information, less and less meaning' (Dupuy and Dupuy, 1980, p. 3). The researcher tends to endlessly code and recode this information rather than interpreting it (Seidel, 1991, p. 109). Even when interpretation does occur, the frames placed continually over each piece of data tend to obscure its origin. The frames themselves become the centre of analysis, an analysis that is more enumerative than interpretive. The use of computer programs for data management have encouraged a tendency towards larger and larger projects. This begs the question of whether larger projects necessarily produce good qualitative research. Is it better to conduct 50, 500 or 5000 interviews? Clearly, the greater the number of interviews, the more superficial the analysis will tend to be.

Reification

The concept of reification emerges often within criticisms of qualitative computing packages. The first concern is the reification of the computer as a system of *self-regulation*: a preferred way of defining the social world (Dupuy and Dupuy, 1980) concisely and logically, where individuals become depersonalised and events neutralised. Jean Baudrillard (1980, p. 139) points to the development of the *hyper real*: the fantasy of simulated communication that disguises loss of meaning by becoming more real than the original 'reality', which then becomes destroyed in the process. The second concern with reification is the relationship between the researcher and the data (Seidel, 1991). Codes become objectified and reified as major explanatory foci through the processes of coding and enumeration, which are often products of this relationship.

The representations of 'reality' produced are primarily based on discrete objects, although fuzzy logic has been used in AQUAD version 4.1. This moves from the true–false dichotomy to the probability of truth (Zadeh, 1988), but this probability is still quantifiable. Such simplification of reality textures the world we see. Further texturing can be located in:

- the gendering of technology through 'masculine' logic (Wajcman, 1991);
- the promotion of procedural thinking (Roszak, 1986);
- the highlighting of rationality, data glut, and the continual coding and counting of meaningless information (Henman, 1992);
- the change in the nature of knowledge (Lyotard, 1984);
- the elevation of logic as authority (Nye, 1990); and
- the fragmentation of 'reality' (Henman, 1992; Bruhn and Lindberg, 1995).

It has been suggested that computer-aided qualitative research has lost its connection with the theoretical and methodological debates of the sociology, psychology and philosophy disciplines, and that these links are in urgent need of reconstruction (Boy, 1992).

Quantitative interface

The quantitative interface that has been developed in some programs through end-on SPSS programs has also produced considerable discussion (Laurie, 1992; Hesse-Biber, 1995), especially in relation to issues of different theoretical orientations, different sampling techniques and lack of variable control. Qualitative research's emphasis on diversity, non-representativeness, small numbers, minimal stratification and self-selection, and the focus on thick ethnographic description, suggests that quantification is a waste of energy, and that such a transformation produces unrealistic versions of the original.

Users' comments

Although many researchers have found these packages useful in assisting with larger databases, there is an ongoing discussion about their negative aspects. Users who have commented negatively on particular computing packages (see Fielding and Lee, 1991; Laurie, 1992) have pointed to the following concerns:

- These packages emphasise the common and shared properties of a large number, rather than variations in the minutiae of detail of small numbers (Agar, 1991).

- Considerable time is undertaken in setting up the data. The larger the sample, the more time will be required, with the outcome that project analysis and interpretation ultimately take the same amount of time as they would without computer assistance (Laurie, 1992).
- On-screen coding limits the researcher's view, resulting in a less complex coding pattern with fewer overlapping and nested codes (Laurie, 1992).
- The reification of codes has led to codes being regarded as variables to be looked at in terms of frequency of occurrence. This results in spurious theoretical conclusions (Seidel, 1991; Laurie, 1992).
- In general, users have been irritated or concerned by:
  — menu proliferation;
  — proliferation of dialogue boxes;
  — difficulties in file navigation;
  — graphical user interface (lack of);
  — the need for greater flexibility to move among programs;
  — coding problems;
  — epistemological doubts;
  — the impact of the software on the analytic process (encouraging commonality and quantification); and
  — the dominance of coding as the main purpose of the program (Fielding and Lee, 1992).

Other documented concerns include the following:

- Many programs are idiosyncratic in nature, having been originally developed by individual academic researchers to help manage their own databases (Fielding and Lee, 1991).
- The 'untypeable'—the fleeting notes and doodles that often encapsulate insight—are lost (Richards and Richards, 1994).
- There is an urgent need for a conversation regarding the theory of science within the processes of qualitative computing (Boy, 1992; Bruhn and Lindberg, 1995).
- It is very easy to move into quantitative mode in large databases, counting frequencies and undertaking variable analysis (Bruhn and Lindberg, 1995).
- The structure of the program influences analytic results, varying between labelling, pattern making and synthesis, and pattern searching leading to thick description (B. Walker, 1993).

- Cutting the text up interrupts the chain of reasoning. Utterances have multiple actions and events embedded in them, and segmentation disrupts the ethnographic process, completely changing this approach and tending to drive the research (Agar, 1991).
- The *etic* (outsider, 'objective') rather than the *emic* (insider, 'subjective') approach to interpreting meaning is fostered within the data (Manwar, Johnson and Dunlap, 1994).

Despite the proliferation of programs and texts written by developers to help in the management of qualitative data, considerable concern is now evident regarding the appropriateness of these programs.

Summary

This chapter has provided an overview of available computer program packages that can be used as an aid to qualitative research data analysis. It has presented a discussion of such programs' generation and the issues surrounding their use.

The major points to emerge from this chapter are that the history of qualitative computing comprises two generations of programs—systematisation and theory development—within which three types of packages are currently available:

- code and retrieve;
- theory generation; and
- content analysis.

Despite the proliferation of programs and their usefulness to some researchers, other users, together with critics, continue to express their concerns about these tools and their effects on qualitative data. These concerns include:

- the representations (or texturing of reality) being promoted by mathematically based programs;
- the reification of endless coding processes and the potential for overinterpretation;
- a focus on process and program management that distances researchers from their data;
- the limitations of the grounded theory method and its theoretical underpinning of symbolic interactionism;
- decontextualisation;

- the tendency to quantification through the addition of SPSS packages; and
- the lack of a critical analysis of the infiltration of these programs into the qualitative arena.

The single most important thing to remember is that the final process of interpretative analysis rests with the researcher.

This is the final discussion of data analysis in this book. The next chapter moves on to the last stage in the qualitative research process: presentation.

Further readings

Burgess, R. (ed.) (1995) *Computing and Qualitative Research*. Studies in Qualitative Methodology, 5. Greenwich: JAI Press.

Coffey, A. and Atkinson, P. (1996) *Making Sense of Qualitative Data Analysis: Complementary Strategies*. California: Sage.

Ihde, D. (1990) *Technology and the Life World: From Garden to Earth*. Bloomington: Indiana University Press.

Kelle, U. (ed.) (1995) *Computer Aided Qualitative Data Analysis: Theory, Methods and Practice*. London: Sage.

Pfaffenberger, B. (1988) *Microcomputer Applications in Qualitative Research*. Qualitative Research Methods, 14. California: Sage.

Qualitative Sociology Journal (1991) 14. (Special issue on computers in qualitative research.)

Ragin, C. and Becker, H. (1989) How the microcomputer is changing our analytic habits, in G. Blank et al. (eds), *New Technology in Sociology: Practical Applications in Research and Work*. New Jersey: Transaction.

Reid, A. (1992) Computer management strategies for text data, in B. Crabtree and W. Miller (eds), *Doing Qualitative Research*. California: Sage.

Tesch, R. (1990) *Qualitative Research: Analysis Types and Software Tools*. New York: Falmer Press.

Weitzman, E. and Miles, M. (1995) *Computer Programs for Qualitative Data Analysis: A Software Sourcebook*. California: Sage.

11 Presentation of data

A range of factors must be taken into consideration in presenting data. Those who read the research will dictate to a greater or lesser extent whether the researcher writes a closed report, or attempts an open experimental approach. The position taken by the researcher will impact on the tone taken, and the type of data collected will also limit the possible forms of presentation.

Data transformation

The processes of data analysis should result in a database that has been transformed into particular *groupings* that are relevant to the topic under investigation. In the case of a grounded theory approach, these will already have been abstracted to a higher level of interpretation through the constant comparison of data with theoretical concepts. In most other cases, the theoretical frame will have already permeated the design, questions and view of the collected data (theory-directed approach); or it will now be more actively utilised to provide a more abstract analysis (theory-generating and postmodern approaches) of data that have their basis in the empirical world.

The regrouping of data into more manageable segments through deconstruction and reconstruction, and the rewriting of these at an interpretive, theoretical level, provide the basis for the final writing up and presentation of results. The actual development of *subgroups* within a group can be seen in Barney Glaser and Anselm Strauss' (1971) work on 'awareness contexts', which formed part of the results in their study of 'status passage'. In analysing the interaction between doctors and patients to examine the awareness of dying, four subgroups were identified:

- open awareness—both openly discuss the fact that the patient is dying;
- closed awareness—the patient is unaware of his/her situation;

- suspicion awareness—the doctor has not told the patient, who is suspicious but unsure; and
- pretence awareness—both know, but the topic is not discussed.

These subcategories provide the basis for extensive writing up, including the presentation of case studies, vignettes, quotes and dramatic scenarios to creatively expose the collected data. Most studies will comprise up to six major groupings of outcomes, each of which will have several subgroupings to illustrate the complexity and diversity that has been discovered.

Multiple data sets are written up separately. Jan Garrard and Jeff Northfield's (1987) investigation of drug education in Victorian secondary schools provides an example. They combined a survey questionnaire with school-based case studies, focus groups and one-to-one interviews. The final report comprised five sections:

1   Literature review and methodology.
2   Survey of drug education in schools. This was further divided into subsections on: background; schools; resources; drugs; program initiation; issues; and future developments, all of which emerged from open- and closed-ended responses to the questionnaire.
3   Presentation of 18 school-based case studies, each of which displayed narrative, descriptive information on the school programs, and students' and teachers' views and experiences of these.
4, 5 Examination of students' perceptions of drugs and teachers' perspectives on drug education, both taken from a collation of the overall interview data.

Form of presentation

The form of presentation will depend on:

- the intended audience;
- the position of the researcher; and
- the styles which enhance the purpose of the research.

Intended audience

Reports for government, community and other *funding agencies* generally comprise a one- to two-page executive summary in bullet point format, printed on different-coloured paper from the rest of the text. This summary includes:

- the topic investigated;
- how it was investigated;
- the findings; and
- specific recommendations for change.

The remainder of the report comprises a brief introduction and literature review; a detailed methodology; results; analytic interpretation (either separate or interwoven); and an action plan/recommendations for change. These proportions vary depending on the targeted audience. If a management team is involved and a process of education is occurring, the literature review may be quite extensive, and the discussion section may be separate and detailed. When the funding authority requires only a brief 'report of progress' or a final report that highlights findings and recommendations, the format will be adapted to suit the occasion and the audience.

If the intended audience is an *examiner* or a *journal* readership, the general format would involve in the following order:

- an abstract;
- an introduction;
- methodology;
- results;
- discussion; and
- a conclusion.

Abstract

This is a summary of the question and the most important findings of the study. It outlines how these differ from those of previous studies, and gives some indication of the methodology undertaken. It is usually up to 200 words long (depending on the guidelines for specific journals and the thesis formats of the relevant university). The abstract serves to provide a potential reader with a quick overview of what the researcher has done and found. Clearly, an enthusiastic tone may draw in an uncertain reader, while an uninspired one may not. If, however, the topic area is of interest, nothing will stop the reader from continuing.

The following steps, clarified with examples (*in italics*), provide a general guideline for writing an abstract.

- Identification of the question. *This study investigated the resources used by home care givers of family members who were terminally ill with cancer.*

- The methodology used. *A qualitative investigation of 40 families, selected on the basis of maximum variation of cancer type, ages of patient and carer, and living situation, were followed during the last weeks of the care-giving process. A final interview took place six weeks after the death had occurred. A survey questionnaire was also administered to a larger group of families who had recently been involved in the home care-giving process.*

- The findings. *The results indicated that most families underwent considerable financial and personal stress; the resources utilised were largely limited to the palliative care nurse and doctor; and lack of resource use stemmed partly from lack of knowledge regarding availability, and partly from a preference to 'manage' without other supports, even when awareness existed.*

- Implications of the findings. *These findings suggest that a public campaign is needed to make families more aware of the processes of terminal care and of the supports that can be drawn upon.*

Introduction

The introduction serves to explain 'why' and 'how' the research problem came to be defined in this particular way. It critically reviews previous relevant *literature* (pointing out any limitations in findings, methodology or theoretical interpretation); and it provides a pathway to the methodology section by clarifying the urgent need for research to be undertaken in the chosen topic, especially with the methodological orientation or techniques chosen by the researcher.

A thesis requires an extensive *literature review*, while in a journal article the author only needs to cite the *major* pieces of work that are particularly relevant. Some new researchers tend to provide many detailed paragraphs on the methodology and results of individual studies. This practice should definitely be avoided. The researcher should focus instead on what can be gained from past research, asking her/himself: 'Do the theoretical and methodological orientations provide a very limited view of the topic, or is there a seminal study with important findings that now need updating in another culture and context (the researcher's, for example)?'

The researcher should highlight aspects of the theory, methodology or findings that provided a sound basis on which she/he could build. The researcher should also indicate which theoretical or conceptual positions were chosen to direct, underpin or inform her/his interpretation of the data she/he planned to collect.

Methodology

The methodology section must fully inform the readers of the step-by-step processes undertaken in conducting the study. A good formula for providing this information is to summarise answers to the following questions.

- Exactly how was this research carried out?
- How were people or documents accessed or selected? How many were used?
- What data were collected?
- Was sampling used? If not, why not?
- Why was one approach chosen and not others?
- What steps were taken to ensure dependable and trustworthy (or valid and reliable) data?
- What ethical or political issues were confronted?
- What agreements were made with participants or funding agents?
- What control did either of these groups have over the data? Did they have access to journal article drafts or transcripts? Did they have power of veto?
- How was (any) information recorded?
- How was information stored?
- How has the setting (if relevant) been described? If an ethnographic study was undertaken, how has the context been described?
- What forms of analysis and interpretation occurred?

It is also advisable to justify the analytic approach in sufficient detail for an uninformed reader to understand what was done.

Results

Results are usually presented as a separate section and displayed in a variety of ways. Some researchers interweave their results with the discussion (theoretical interpretation) section. They do this in one of two ways. The most common method is to interweave the results with the interpretation, leading to the production of a particular outcome. The other, less common, method is the reverse of this. The researcher presents an outcome (conceptual framework model) or theoretical proposition, then works backwards to explain how this was achieved. The categories, sections or groups of data mentioned earlier provide the basis of data display.

Discussion

When the discussion is a separate section, it incorporates an interpretive approach. This raises the results section to a more abstract plane by discussing the findings, or new theoretical propositions or models, in terms of existing theoretical or conceptual frameworks, then placing this new framework within the literature (research) previously identified in the introduction. Many readers consider this section to be the most important, as it separates information 'gatherers' from 'real' researchers who are capable of moving beyond personalised and biased analyses to broader theoretical interpretations.

Conclusion

This states a brief review of the final outcomes, along with any limitations of the study and implications for further research or action.

Variations in format

Other variations in writing-up formats can be seen in:

- grounded theory, which interweaves data and theoretical concepts from the earliest point of data collection;
- phenomenology, in which a narrative account dominates, ending with the hypotheses and theoretical propositions to be tested further; and
- postmodern and feminist narratives, which may display the interwoven stories in the voices of researcher and researched, and in which these stories are interpreted either minimally or not at all.

Trinh T. Minh-ha (1989) terms writing as a mirror that catches reflections from other mirrors (other writings).

Patti Lather (1989) has presented some exemplars of postmodern feminist research that reflect the complexity of research within this tradition. These exemplars include a dialogical approach that uses free verse to centre the interviewee, and incorporates pauses and the reflections within the voice to produce polyvocal, non-linear, multilevelled explorations.

Another example involves self-interrogation, where dialogues between those in a research team document their responses to particular programs. In this approach, 'self' is both subject and object.

Data can also be presented in different voices and different writing styles within one study. For example:

- a realist tale (formal author-voiced description of research design and method);
- a critical tale (a critical author-voiced interpretation of questions relating to emancipation and the deconstruction of authority in the setting); and
- a self-reflexive tale (the interplay of student voices in a mini dramatic presentation as they work with journal data).

Margery Wolf (1992) has used a similar presentation technique in her *Thrice Told Tale*, in which she uses three separate formats to present data collected on a particular incident 30 years previously. The data are presented firstly as a short story, secondly as field notes, and thirdly as a journal article.

Position of the researcher

The researcher's position also will influence the forms of presentation, regardless of whether it is centred or decentred, voiceful or voiceless. The researcher has more traditionally adopted a distant position. The first sentence of the research report *Drug Education in Victorian Post Primary Schools* (Garrard and Northfield, 1987) is in typical third-person voice:

> Since the commencement of concerted attempts at drug education in Australian schools in the early 1970s debate has simmered over what should be taught in drug education and what students should actually learn from drug education programs.

The research team's voices remain largely invisible. Their names are appended to case studies displayed as third-person accounts. Only in the conclusion is an echo of opinion vouchsafed, and the 'we' of the group emerges:

> *The findings of this study are considerable but we will need the support and cooperation of teachers to see what can be implemented into school programs in the future* (p. 228).

In *The Mirror Dance* (Krieger, 1983) the researcher's voice is submerged in past tense, third-person reportage of individuals' responses to each question. This can be seen in the display of responses to a question regarding the issue of privacy:

> 'It was a self indulging aloneness', said Frances.
> 'It was something some people seemed to need more than others', said Leslie. (p. 165)

The 'I' of the researcher emerges in a postscript: an appendix that discusses and justifies the approach taken. This austere presentation of participants' voices without integrative narrative allows for orchestration of presentation, but nothing more (p. 191).

More recently, the 'I' of the researcher can be seen moving in and out of the text to suit different emphases. Elizabeth Turnbull's (1992) investigation of transformation and the writing-up of this, using the recovery experiences of adult children of alcoholics in Alcoholics Anonymous programs, present the stories told at these meetings in the third person, using storytelling format. The researcher retains the first-person voice to directly address the reader: 'You may find it disturbing' (p. 1). Whenever her personal opinion intrudes it is encapsulated in her own voice: 'As I took it, she was referring to the ambiguities . . .' (p. 2). The first person is also used to explain the processes of, and approaches to, her topic: 'My thesis concerns transformation . . .'. She slips back into the third person for more theoretically oriented discussions: 'From Derrida one can understand . . .'. Participation and intersubjectivity are emphasised, and methodological and theoretical issues, plus the researcher's views, are interwoven in the presentation and analysis of the stories.

The researcher's position emphasises the power she/he has to privilege certain stories and to filter, transform and present respondents' voices so that particular interpretations dominate. Bronwyn Davies (1992) refers to the *'positionless' researcher*, the mythical being within science who, in presuming to speak for all, has made all those who are not middle class, male academics voiceless and invisible. Davies (1992, pp. 66–68) claims that, through poststructural approaches, the advent of feminist subjectivity has the capacity to burst open this previous positioning: to fragment 'reality', and to reposition people in such a way that they can understand how the narrow confines of previous positionings constructed a particular view of 'reality'.

Styles enhancing the purpose and the research

Some methodologies (grounded theory and phenomenology) and some purposes (formal reports) have tended in the past towards fairly specific forms of data presentation. These techniques are currently being challenged and the researcher can now select from the following the forms of display most suited to the research purpose and the intended readership.

Graphic displays

In the past, qualitative research has favoured such formal techniques of display as:

- descriptive statistics;
- bar graphs;

- pie charts;
- tables; and
- matrix displays (Miles and Huberman, 1984, 1994).

An example of mixed graphic display can be seen in the presentation of the results of a study that evaluated the use of a simplified medical manual that had been provided for indigenous health workers in remote health centres in the desert areas of Central Australia (Williams, 1994). Twenty-three health centres were visited. Observations of 78 indigenous health workers were conducted. Fifty-eight of these workers were also interviewed regarding their use of the manual. Their responses were graphically represented in a pie chart, under the categories of 'active manual usage', 'aware of the manual and reference usage' and 'non-usage'. Further details of the numbers and percentages of these categories were displayed in a table. The pie chart and table are presented below.

Other graphic forms of display include hierarchical models of departmental and other relationships within organisations or groups, and diagrammatic representations. William Foote Whyte (1955, p. 13) provides an example of the former in *Street Corner Society*, where he draws the lines of power between Doc (the head of the group) and

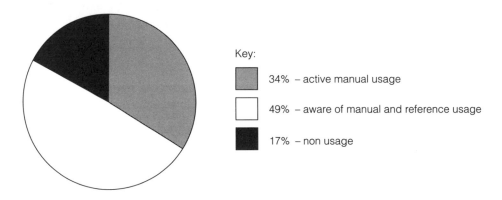

Key:

34% – active manual usage

49% – aware of manual and reference usage

17% – non usage

Indigenous health workers' (AHW's) reported use of the manual

	Number	%
AHWs interviewed	58	100
AHWs who said that they were actively using the manual	20	34
AHWs who said that they were 'aware' of, or were referring actively to, the manual	28	49
AHWs who said that they were not using the manual	10	17

Source: Adapted from Williams (1994, p. 63).

the rest of the group. It is interesting to note here that age and position in the hierarchy are related. Sherri Cavan's (1978) study of a rural settlement is an example of the use of diagrammatic representations. She uses these to demonstrate the places where locals, hippies and tourists meet. She also uses diagrams to demonstrate interpersonal relationships within the setting and to explore institutional constellations.

Writing styles

These formal techniques of display (statistics, graphs, diagrams, pie charts, tables and matrix displays) can be interspersed with a range of more recent literary forms:

- vignettes (researcher-constructed narratives);
- anecdotes;
- layers of information;
- pastiche;
- quotes of larger segments of interview data; and
- thick ethnographic description.

Vignette

A *vignette* (a compressed story, narrating what the researcher has learned over a period) can be included to illustrate a problem more clearly. In this instance, the subjective 'I' of the author was used:

> At one health centre I asked the indigenous health workers to show me an example of the 'hard words'. An experienced male health worker opened the page to 'conjunctivitis'. We discussed the fact that 'conjunctivitis' could be changed to 'pussy red eye'. He however was referring to the next line in the manual which stated 'document visual acuity'. It was obvious that this style of language is not generally used in conversation and is an example of the concise nature of the written medical word. Over the phone during a medical consult the doctor is far more likely to say, 'have you checked the vision with the eye chart?' It was this type of 'complicated jargon' that indigenous health workers found difficult to understand and it discouraged them from reading the manual. (Williams, 1994, p. 65)

It is possible to segment the total text into three or four vignettes that operate rather like case studies, instead of distributing small vignettes throughout the text. A study examining gender and sexuality in women's bodies through the experience of

DES-related cancer (Bell and Apfel, 1995) presented three vignettes, each representing a different social or political context. One vignette is overtly political and is taken from the transcript of a presentation given by a feminist health activist at a DES conference. The second is a clinically oriented workshop presentation given by a gynaecologist (male) on DES cancer cases. The third vignette is taken from an interview account with a woman DES sufferer. It focuses on sexuality and sexual experiences, but the researcher presents the gained information in poetic form. Bell and Apfel contrast the voices, constructions, attitudes and beliefs represented in these three vignettes to illustrate the complexity of perspectives on this topic.

Anecdote

Anecdotes are written recordings of incidents, seen as significant by the researcher, that took place within the data collection. One example of this can be drawn from my own study of the integration of young people with severe intellectual disabilities into regular classroom settings (Grbich and Sykes, 1989). I had collected extensive information, recording parents' and teachers' positive views as to the outcomes of this process. It was a chance comment from a regular school student, who said she viewed the presence of students with disabilities as 'like having rather cute toys around', that led me to change my observation patterns. From then on, I undertook a much closer observation of playground interaction and classroom learning potential for the students with disabilities, in order to pursue this 'othering' tendency.

Layers of information

The *layered approach* to data presentation can take two forms: either over time, where the researcher spaces his/her own perceptions and those of others to demonstrate transition and change; or by presenting the perceptions of many people regarding a single event or situation. In this way, story after story can open different windows on a situation, a person or an incident. This technique can also be used to provide a dialogue with the self, where different aspects or tones are taken in a monologue (Ely et al., 1997, pp. 91–92).

Pastiche

Pastiche is a method of presenting a range of perspectives (by either one person, or a range of voices), using two or three columns to a page, different-sized fonts, and variations on bold and italic type. This enables the juxtaposition of large chunks of quoted material. A pastiche weaves related meanings across texts (*intertextuality*) in processes of construction, deconstruction and transformation. Poems, researcher comments, dramatic dialogue and vignettes, as well as direct quotes from interviewees can be creatively interwoven. Derrida's *Glas* (1986 [1972]) provides an excellent example of pastiche with its letters, poetry, interpretations, different languages, quotes from other texts and author's commentary.

Quotes of interview data

Another technique used to display the data and illustrate cross-referencing of opinion involves listing *quotes* from participants. Williams used a display of typical comments made by indigenous health workers regarding their health manual:

> Too many hard words.
> Too many words.
> Too many big medical words—too complicated for us.
> All these western medical words are like white-fella secrets.
> (Williams, 1994, p. 65)

Ethnographic description

There is enormous variation in descriptive writing, from thin factual accounts, to accounts that use literary genres to access emotion and meaning as a demonstration of this diversity. The following examples show how the same information can be rewritten using different presentation styles/formats.

Factual third person (thin description):

> Jane went into labour at 7.30 am. By 9 am her contractions were coming every five minutes, so they set off for the hospital. Jane was delivered of a baby girl at 10.45 am.

Third-person, thick ethnographic description: This is still factual and is delivered in the researcher's voice, but it includes context, intentions and meanings, and the processes of experience:

> Jane woke at seven o'clock. Her stomach felt uncomfortable and labour started half an hour later. She woke Jim who reassured her that there was no rush, that he and Jill (their two year old) needed breakfast before embarking on the trip to the city. Jane did not eat but half sat, half lay on a bean bag while the others breakfasted. Between 8.30 and 9 am she realised her contractions were increasing and she indicated she would like to get moving, that the hospital was an hour's drive away, that they would also have to drop their dog off at Jim's parents' place, that second babies often come quite fast

and that she was not anxious to deliver in the van. By 9 am they were on the road, Jill and Jim up front chatting and singing while Jane lay on a mattress in the back on her left hand side with the labrador lying with his back against hers. They left the dog tied up at Jim's parents' place. By the time they were approaching the hospital Jane was well into labour and as they drew up at the hospital door the baby's head shot out then slipped back. Jim raced into the hospital and found the midwife. They both ran to the van carrying an emergency delivery tray. As Jane was managing to hold on, the midwife ran for a wheelchair and helped Jane in. All the way up to the delivery suite Jane could feel the head of her baby trying to force its way out. Jane reached the delivery room, climbed onto the bed and the baby was born a few minutes later.

Polyphonic, dramatic, layered presentation: This lies within the mode of thick ethnographic description, but uses the participants' voices and thoughts to get closer to the contexts, meanings, processes and emotions of their experiences:

Jane: I woke around seven o'clock. Early morning winter light was trickling through the gaps between the burgundy velvet curtains. Ten days overdue. If it isn't born in the next four days they'll pressure me for an induction. I'm feeling pre-menstrual, better go to the loo. Brr, it's cold, back to bed. Ouch, that was definitely a contraction—better wait, no point in waking everyone if it's a false alarm. Two contractions later I woke Jim.

Jim: I could sense she was awake and moving, first to the toilet, then turning over and sighing. I knew what was happening even before she touched my face, her eyes wide and anxious. I guess she's remembering the first one—induced, no control. Well this will be different—birth centre and we're more experienced. Wonder what it will be, maybe a boy? Well, whatever, two girls would be great, just a healthy baby and everything going smoothly—yes that's it. Well, up and at it, breakfast and then off. Have to drop off the dog or he'll wander if we're not around.

Jane: God, I'm sweltering, must be the contractions. I don't want to scare anyone but things seem to be moving, distinct descending feeling like an elevator slipping slowly down. These contractions are changing. Where's my watch. Let's see, five minutes, two minutes, three minutes, five minutes. It's not bad, I can cope but I can't work it out, is it five minutes? Or less, varying in intensity, almost like one strong, one weak. If both are contractions I'm down to 2–3 minutes—ye Gods, we're an hour away, and the dog, and, they've just started eating. Christ, how'm I going to get this lot moving before the baby takes over? 'Jim, I think we'd better move.'

Jim: 'Oh, no hurry, it'll be ages yet, Jill's just started her egg, sure you don't want . . . no, guess not, eat later, eh?'

Jane: 'No seriously, I don't think I'm going to be long, unless you want to deliver in the van . . . ?'

Jim: 'No, no.' I went over and stroked her head—it felt hot. I put a hand on her stomach and gently massaged her for a few minutes. I thought I counted two contractions. OK. Quick revision of priorities. Don't panic, take it slow, collect Jill's stuff, new baby's stuff, dog into van with mattress—dog immediately stretched out—pleased at such unexpected comfort. Jill onto toilet, then into car with bottle and a bag of fruit for later. Helped Jane into van, turned off heater, locked up and off—ten minutes—not bad.

Jane: Dog feels great, my back pushes against his—takes the pain—not bad, quite bearable in fact—lying down seems to have slowed things down a bit—might just make it. Feel a bit lonely back here, glad to have dog, others chatting and singing with occasional 'How are you going?' 'Fine, fine.' What else can I say? I'm lonely back here, want someone to hold me, rub my back, talk to me, after all *I'm* having the baby . . . Pause to drop off dog, I begin to panic—where is he, why so long . . . ?

Jim: 'Sorry about that, Mum and Dad are out, I had to find something to tie him up with. As soon as they see him they'll realise we've gone to the hospital. Off we go—we'll be there in 40 minutes.' She seems calm, no rush, we'll make it OK.

Jane: Blue sky, white clouds, breathe in, pant gently, in, out, keep calm, there it goes, break, now we're off again—breathe in air. Ah city buildings. 'Hey Jim, help I think it's coming, I think you're going to have to stop . . .'

Jim: Oh no, this is not a good idea. 'Hold on, just two more blocks, nearly there, hold on, we're just entering the hospital.' Christ I took that bump too fast. 'You OK?'

Jane: 'No-oo, the head's coming, I can't hold it, a . . . ahh, it's gone back.'

Jim: 'Right, hang on, I'll get someone.'

Jane: 'Jesus, make it fast . . .'

Jim: Running, faces in outpatients—lift—no too slow, stairs, hallway, office—oh thank God she's there, 'Quick, Jane's in the van, she's about to deliver . . .'

Margaret: 'Right, I'm coming.' Tray, right. Ah, a bit of excitement in a quiet morning, it's a while since I've delivered in a car. I wonder if we can get her up here—more hygienic and easier. 'Here, you take the wheelchair.' Ah, the lift's here—down and out. Van. 'Hi, you're doing fine.' Seems to be holding. 'Let's get you into the wheelchair.'

Jane: Oh no, this is not good, sitting up and each bump is bringing it down—poor bloody baby, I'm sitting on its head. God, I wish they wouldn't stare. Oh no! We'll have to wait for the lift—hands clenched and teeth clamped together—oh, up we go, corridor and bedroom, am I glad to see this bed, I thought we'd never make it. Stand up, roll onto bed—half sit—now baby you're on your own. 'No thank you, I don't want the mirror.' I just need to concentrate, breathe slowly, relax, breathe—head, shoulders and oh, how beautiful, all vernixy, white, that grunt of disapproval, a quick and rather disgruntled look and she curls up on my stomach and chest and sleeps. I gently stroke her back—beautiful, beautiful baby, ah how clever we are to make such a perfect thing . . .

Jim: Made it, thank God—I'm sure I could have managed, the string for the cord might have been a problem—not sure if we had any thin enough and no Dettol—hm, not very organised, I should have prepared—didn't think she'd go so fast. 'Look Jill, there's our new baby's head coming out.' Mm . . . black hair, lots of cream on the skin. Oh . . . pretty little face—eyes closed, shoulders, here comes the body—ah perfect, beautiful baby, another girl— great. 'Look Jilly, you've got a baby sister . . . let me touch her, hey baby it's me look, it's your dad, oh I must hold her—my baby . . . my baby . . .

This account, derived from interviews with both parents and the midwife, takes the reader much closer to the participants' experiences and constructions. These three versions of the same event demonstrate the involvement levels demanded of both the reader and researcher in delving below superficial accounts to the emotional levels of meaning.

Other styles

Postmodernism, poststructuralism and some feminist approaches have generated critiques of 'objective', 'linear' and 'researcher-dominated' forms of representation. These critiques allow the emergence of a variety of genres that are capable of presenting qualitative data in a manner that reflects the emphasis on emotion, subjectivity and the decentring of the researcher's voice. These genres have included:

- *ethnographies of the self*, such as Carol Ronai's (1992) account of being employed as an erotic dancer, in which she uses personal narrative to meticulously document her experiences, reactions and emotions within and beyond this role;
- *fiction* where the account is firmly based within the research that has been undertaken, but allows for compression of events and consolidation of characters from many to few, providing a powerful focus and a strong story line (Frohock, 1992); and

- *poetry* that has also been used to capture the essence of interviews, events and observations, and to reflect the study environment's underlying patterns of movement and language emphases—Laurel Richardson (1992) has explored the process, responses and consequences to the self of turning a 36-page typed transcript of another person's life into a three-page poem.

Capturing the essence of another person's life has consequences for the (re)writing of the self. The utilisation of dramatic approaches provides the author with new insights, as well as having the capacity to display both the inside (thoughts) and outside (vocalisations), contrasting an individual's responses to a situation or set of events. Carolyn Ellis and Art Bochner's (1992) dialogue between a woman (who undergoes an abortion) and her partner provides a powerful example of what can be achieved using this medium. Polyphonic texts are other examples. Krieger's *Mirror Dance* (1983) illustrates how the respondents' voices interweave in reflections of different points of view, and comedy and satire provide an entertaining way of polyphonically exposing the debates in which researchers often involve themselves within the research setting. Krieger (1985) also describes the issues involved in locating one's own voice (in an attempt to come to terms with one's own performance and reactions in the data collection phase), then decentring it so that participants' voices take front stage.

Visual, aural and interactive presentations

Other forms of presentation include:

- *visual* representations on film, video, computer or paintings;
- *aural* representations using audiotape, or compact disc and musical representation; and
- *interactive* readings that invite reader involvement—these use breaks in the text to present the reader with a choice of different endings, or an ending with a climax that is so convoluted or unexpected that the reader is obliged to trace back to find clues and explanations. (See Eco, 1979, Appendices 1 and 2.)

The idea that *multiple perspectives* provide the best view/s of any situation emphasises the appropriateness of using a combination of the above techniques, while also including the more traditional representations of quasi-statistical information and quotes. Linden (1992) and Wolf (1992) provide examples of mixed genres.

Language

Language is very important in writing up research. Language should be non-discriminatory, non-stereotypical, inclusive, neutral, equal and consistent. *Sexism* is not accepted. The 'he/she' pronouns should be equally alternated with 'she/he' to avoid any criticism of gender bias; and the neutral 'they', 'us' or 'we' can be used to replace 'she/he' and 'he/she'. Other points to consider include:

- The term 'aboriginal people' refers to indigenous people worldwide, while 'Aboriginal' refers to one group of indigenous people within Australia.
- Terms such as 'part' or 'half-caste' should be avoided.
- Where people of ethnic extraction are discussed, their cultural identity should be mentioned first: Vietnamese-born . . .; men/women/person of non-English-speaking background.
- The word 'partner' is a neutral term that encompasses husbands, wives, defacto relationships, and lesbian and homosexual couples.
- Words to avoid include: 'man'—use human, human being, or man and woman; 'man-made'—use synthetic, artificial, handmade or constructed; 'mankind'—use humankind; 'sportsmanlike'—use fair or sporting; 'manpower'—use staff, labour/workforce; 'chairman'—use chairperson; and 'manhole—use service hole or access point.
- Changes in occupational terminology include: 'actress'—actor; 'air hostess'—flight attendant; 'manageress'—manager; 'cleaning lady'—cleaner; 'lady doctor'—doctor; 'workman'—worker; and 'groundsman'—ground staff/gardener.
- With regard to sexuality, the following terms are currently acceptable: lesbian, gay man, bisexual woman, heterosexual woman, transgender people and transsexual.
- People with disabilities or particular medical conditions should be referred to as 'people who are blind' or 'people who are HIV positive', and so on.

Politically correct terminology is creeping into our writing, and individual decisions need to be debated. In a study of older women and their experiences with medication (Grbich et al., 1997), the alternatives were 'old', 'older', 'aged' and 'mature'. The team felt that although 'mature' was the most politically correct, it had uneasy connections with cheese-making processes. 'Chronologically gifted' and 'matriarchically wise' were too much of a mouthful, so 'women who are older' was adopted as being more neutral.

Other 'politically correct' terminology that may need consideration is:

- 'person' rather than 'male' or 'female';
- 'matriarch' or 'patriarch', to avoid the negative connotations of 'old' or 'aged', and to incorporate the respectful concept of wisdom;
- 'optically challenged' for 'of limited vision' or 'blind';
- 'aurally challenged' for 'having hearing deficits' or 'deaf';
- 'vertically challenged' or 'a person of non-standard height' for persons below the average height for their culture;
- 'decorum-impaired' for a person who is socially inept or behaving antisocially;
- 'abusing alcohol or other drugs' rather than 'getting rotten' with drink or drugs;
- 'invading personal space' rather than 'assaulting' or 'harassing';
- 'wisdom-challenged', 'cerebrally constrained' or 'differently abled', rather than 'stupid' or 'ill-informed';
- 'testosterone-heavy' rather than 'macho';
- following a 'clothing-optional lifestyle' rather than 'naked' or 'strangely dressed';
- 'economically disadvantaged' rather than 'poor';
- 'cognitively advanced' rather than 'cognitively competent';
- 'liberated' rather than 'stole';
- 'kindness impaired' rather than 'nasty' or 'unpleasant'; and
- 'co-dependency problem' rather than 'infatuation'.

These examples come from a range of official sources and are presented as indicators only of politically correct language. Although some may sound 'over the top', it is assumed that researchers *can* manage to write about others in a respectful manner without seeming ridiculous to some readers. Garner (1994) provides many more examples.

Assessing qualitative research

What does a 'good' piece of qualitative research look like? Clearly, this is highly contentious, but certain positions can be documented. At the more conservative end of the spectrum, a good piece of qualitative research is worthy of the term if it:

- produces findings that can be transferred to or have relevance to other similar contexts by another researcher;
- is grounded in the empirical world;
- is critically reflexive regarding the researcher's impact on the setting; and
- is designed to produce verified and triangulated (or trustworthy and dependable) data.

Researchers may also need to demonstrate:

- minimisation of power relations between researcher and researched;
- the capacity to incorporate theory with interpretation;
- insider access to emotions;
- subjectivity; and
- the capacity to gain and maintain long term relationships that feature account-ability. Feminist research would further require exposure of the power structures that oppress women, and the emancipatory action needed to remedy this.

At the other end of the spectrum, postmodernism would see 'good' research as avoiding any single interpretive 'truth', and decentring the researcher in favour of multivocal and other representations. The crystals and mirrors that provide the image of 'validity', with their capacity for 'reflection, refraction, light and shade, motion and change, combining symmetry and substance with an infinite variety of shapes, substances, transmutations, multi dimensionalities and angles of approach' (Richardson, 1994, p. 533), are a far cry from the limited structures favoured in triangulation.

Summary

This chapter has offered an insight into the diverse presentation modes that can be used for data display. The major points made in this chapter are that:

- Data are transformed into manageable segments or formats through the processes of construction or deconstruction.
- Data presentation will vary depending on the intended audience, the researcher's position, and the style which enhances the purpose of the research.
- Writing styles vary from thin and thick description to polyphonic, dialogical, dramatic and visual presentations.
- Non-sexist and politically correct language forms must be addressed.

It is hoped that this chapter will be useful in helping the researcher to decide the most appropriate presentation format when undertaking a qualitative research study.

Further readings

Madsen, O. (1990) *Successful Dissertations and Theses*. San Francisco: Jossey Bass.

Meloy, J. (1994) *Writing the Qualitative Dissertation: Understanding by Doing*. New Jersey: Lawrence Erlbaum Associates.

Richardson, L. (1990) *Writing Strategies. Reaching Diverse Audiences*. California: Sage.

Conclusion

This book has presented a brief overview of the history, theoretical bases, concepts, methodologies, processes and techniques of, and approaches to, qualitative research, with particular reference to its use in the area of health.

It has also discussed issues surrounding the use of qualitative research, including the ongoing qualitative versus quantitative debate; ethical dilemmas raised in relation to data-collection techniques (overt versus covert) and to the ownership, documentation and presentation of data; and the importance of the position adopted by the researcher, which has the capacity to impact on every stage of the research process from the initial choice of a research topic, through project design, data gathering, evaluation and interpretation, to modes of presentation.

The issue of researcher bias has been highlighted to ensure that all researchers, whether novice or experienced, are aware of its existence and possible impact on a research project. This issue is inextricably interwoven with issues of 'objectivity', 'subjectivity', 'validity', 'reliability', 'generalisability' and 'rigour'.

Definitions of these and other terminologies commonly used in qualitative research have been included in the text to enable the novice researcher/student to understand such concepts in the context of everyday language. Significant attention has also been given to postmodern/poststructuralist and feminist approaches to qualitative research, and their contribution to the overall qualitative versus quantitative debate.

Throughout, the advantages, criticisms and limitations of each theory, approach, methodology and technique have been presented to give the reader as balanced and unbiased a view as possible of qualitative research, while highlighting its capacity to provide important insights into different perceptions of 'reality' in the search for 'truth' in social research.

It is hoped that this book will provide a useful introduction to qualitative research for those starting out in research, as well as an extensive reference resource for those already in the field. It is intended to be used as a basis on which individuals can build a deeper understanding of qualitative research.

Appendix: qualitative research resources

Journals

Australian and New Zealand Journal of Sociology
Health
International Journal of Qualitative Studies in
    Education
Journal of Contemporary Ethnography
Journal of Health and Illness
Journal of Primary Health Interchange
Qualitative Health Research
Qualitative Sociology
Studies in Symbolic Interaction
Symbolic Interaction
Visual Anthropology Review
Visual Sociology

Websites

Qualitative Report
    (http://www.nova.edu/sss/qr/index.html)
    An online journal of qualitative research.
Qualitative Research Base, Qualitative Resources
    on the Internet
    (http://www.nova.edu/ssss/qr/qualres.html)
    Contains links to qualitative research
    websites, online papers, collections of
    papers, syllabi and announcements.

Qualitative research email discussion groups

ATLAS-TI@tubvm.cs.tu-berlin.de *Topics on
the text analysis, text management and
theory-building program ATLAS/ti.* To
subscribe send this one-line message (no
subject, no signature) to

listserve@tubvm.cs.tu-berlin.de: sub
atlas-ti <your firstname your lastname
more stuff up to 32 letters>. For help
contact Thomas Muhr
(thomas.muhr@tu-berlin.de or
muhr@cs.tu-berlin.de).

qsr-forum@qsr.latrobe.edu.au *Qualitative
Solutions and Research, for the qualitative
analysis program* NUD*IST. To subscribe,
send this message to
mailing-list-request@qsr.com.au: subscribe
qsr-forum <your name>. For help contact
Dianne Goeman (dianne@qsr.com.au).

qual-l@scu.edu.au *Qualitative Research List,
which initiated to serve people at
Pennsylvania State University, but
immediately attracted a broader audience.* To
subscribe, send this message to
listproc@scu.edu.au: subscribe qual-l
<your name>. For help contact Bob Dick
(bd@psy.uq.oz.au).

QUALNET@listserv.bc.edu *Qualitative
Research in Management and Organisation
Studies.* To subscribe, send this message to
majordomo@listserv.bc.edu: subscribe
qualnet. For help contact Ted Gaiser
(gaiser@bcvms.bc.edu).

QUALRS-L@uga.cc.uga.edu *Qualitative
Research for the Human Sciences.* To
subscribe, send this message to
listserv@uga.cc.uga.edu: subscribe qualrs-1
<your name>. For help contact Judith
Preissle (jude@uga.cc.uga.edu).

qual-software@mailbase.ac.uk *A list on
qualitative analysis computer programs.* To
subscribe, send this message to
mailbase@mailbase.ac.uk: join

qual-software <your name>. For help contact Ann Lewins (qual-software-request@mailbase.ac.uk).

Other resources for qualitative research in the human sciences

ANTHRO-DESIGN-L@lists.teleport.com *Qualitative methods in industrial design and connections between anthropology and other social sciences and user-centred product design and development.* To subscribe, send this message to majordomo@teleport.com: subscribe anthro-design-l. For help contact Mark Dawson (anthro@teleport.com).

arlist-1@scu.edu.au *Action Research Mailing List.* To subscribe, send this message to listproc@scu.edu.au: subscribe arlist-1 <firstname lastname>. For help contact Bob Dick (bd@psy.uq.oz.au).

ethno@vm.its.rpi.edu *Ethnomethodology/conversation analysis.* To subscribe, send this message to comserve@vm.its.rpi.edu: join ethno <your name>. For help contact support@vm.its.rpi.edu.

evaltalk@ua1vm.ua.edu *American Evaluation Association Discussion List.* To subscribe, send this message to listserv@ua1vm.ua.edu: subscribe evaltalk <your name>. For help contact the Evaluation and Assessment Laboratory at the University of Alabama (eal@ua1vm.ua.edu).

GOVTEVAL@jaring.my *Public Sector Program Evaluation.* To subscribe, send this message to listserver@jaring.my: subscribe govteval <your name>. For help contact Dr Arunaselam Rasappan (aru@intanbk.intan.my).

IVSA@pdomain.uwindsor.ca *International Visual Sociology Association.* To subscribe, send this message to listserv@pdomain.uwindsor.ca: subscribe ivsa <your name>. For help contact Dr Veronica Mogyorody (mogy@uwindsor.ca).

METHODS@cios.llc.rpi.edu *A list for instructors of social science research methods.* To subscribe, send this message to comserve@cios.llc.rpi.edu: subscribe methods <your name>. For help contact support@cios.llc.rpi.edu.

OHA-L@lsv.uky.edu *Oral History Association Discussion List.* To subscribe, send this message to listserv@lsv.uky.edu: subscribe oha-l <your name>. For help contact Mary Molinaro (molinaro@ukcc.uky.edu).

partalk-1@cornell.edu *Participatory Action Research Network.* To subscribe, send this message to listproc@cornell.edu: subscribe partalk-1 <your name>. For help contact Carla Shafer (cs13@cornell.edu).

PSYCH-NARRATIVE@massey.ac.nz *A discussion of narrative in everyday life.* To subscribe, send this message to majordomo@massey.ac.nz: subscribe psych-narrative. For help contact Andy Lock (A.J.Lock@massey.ac.nz).

VISCOM@vm.temple.edu *Visual Communications Discussion List.* To subscribe, send this message to listserv@vm.temple.edu: subscribe viscom <your name>. For help contact Jay Ruby (v5293e@vm.temple.edu).

XTAR@lester.appstate.edu *Teacher Researchers List.* To subscribe, send this message to listserve@lester.appstate.edu: subscribe xtar <your name>. For help contact William E. Blanton (blantonwe@conrad.appstate.edu).

Social and professional sciences discussion lists

AERA-G@asu.edu *Social Context of Education, Division G of the American Educational Research Association.* To subscribe, send this message to listserv@asu.edu: subaera-g <your name>. For help contact Gene Glass (glass@asu.edu).

ANTHAP@oakland.edu *Society for Applied Anthropology.* To subscribe, send this message to majordomo@oak.oakland.edu:

subscribe anthap <your name>. For help contact James Dow (dow@argo.acs.oakland.edu).

Anthro-L@ubvm.cc.buffalo.edu *A general anthropology bulletin board.* To subscribe, send this message to listserv@ubvm.cc.buffalo.edu: subscribe anthro-l <your name>. For help contact Patrick Miller (psmiller@acsu.buffalo.edu).

CAE-L@lmrinet.gse.ucsb.edu *Council on Anthropolgy and Education Discussion List.* To subscribe, send this message to listproc@lmrinet.gse.ucsb.edu: subscribe cae-l <your name>. For help contact Susan Florio-Ruane (suanfr@msu.edu) or Linguistic Minority Research Institute (lmri@lmrinet.gse.ucsb.edu).

COCTA-L@nosferatu.cas.usf.edu *Concepts and methods in the social and human sciences and the philosophy of the social sciences.* To subscribe, send this message to listserv@nosferatu.cas.usf.edu: subscribe cocta-l <your name>. For help contact turner@chuma.cas.usf.edu.

h-net@uicvm.uic.edu *Humanities On-Line, a large collection of lists for history, social science and humanities interests.* For information send this message to listserv@uicvm.uic.edu: get h-net whatis. For help contact h-Net@uicvm.uic.edu.

INTERACT@sun.soci.niu.edu *Discussion list on social interaction.* To subscribe, send this message to listproc@sun.soci.niu.edu: sub interact <your name>. For help contact the listowner (epstein@ufu.edu).

NATIVE-L@tamvm1.tamu.edu *Discussion lists for and on indigenous peoples.* To subscribe, send this message to listserv@tamvm1.tamu.edu: subscribe native-l <your name>.

ORGCULT@commerce.uq.edu.au *Organizational Culture Caucus.* To subscribe, send this message to listproc@commerce.uq.edu.au: subscribe orgcult <your name>. For help contact Neal Ashkanasy (nxa6@email.psu.edu).

pcp@mailbase.ac.uk *Personal Construct Psychology List.* To subscribe, send this message to mailbase@mailbase.ac.uk: join pcp <your name>. For help contact David Nightingale (d.j.nightingale@hud.ac.uk).

postcolonial@jefferson.village.virginia.edu *Discussion list on postcolonial literature, film and theory run by the Spoon Collective.* To subscribe, send this message to majordomo@jefferson.village.virginia.edu: subscribe postcolonial <your name>. For help contact the Spoon Collective (spoons@jefferson.village.virginia.edu).

radical-psychology-network@mailbase.ac.uk To subscribe, send this message to mailbase@mailbase.ac.uk: join radical-psychology-network <your name>. For help contact David Nightingale (d.j.nightingale@hud.ac.uk).

social-theory@mailbase.ac.uk To subscribe, send this message to mailbase@mailbase.ac.uk: join social-theory <your name>. For help contact David Nightingale (d.j.nightingale@bolton.ac.uk).

sssitalk@sun.soci.niu.edu *Society for the Study of Symbolic Interaction.* To subscribe, send this message to listproc@sun.soci.niu.edu: sub sssitalk <your name>. For help contact Jim Thomas (jthomas@sun.soci.niu.edu).

virtpsy@sjuvm.stjohns.edu *St Johns University Virtual Psychology List on the interaction of people in electronic environments.* To subscribe, send this message to listserv@sjuvm.stjohns.edu: subscribe virtpsy <your name>. For help contact Sheila Rosenberg (shrose@sjuvm.stjohns.edu).

Bibliography

Abrahamson, P. (1992) *A Case for Case Studies: An Immigrant's Journal*. California: Sage.

Achanfuo-Yeboah, D. (1995) Problems in indigenous health research: issues for Australia. *Australian Journal of Social Research*, 1 (1) pp. 3–20.

Agar, M. (1991) The right brain strikes back, in N. Fielding and R. Lee (eds), *Using Computers in Qualitative Research*. London: Sage.

Alasuutari, P. (1995) *Researching Culture: Qualitative Method and Cultural Studies*. California: Sage.

Albrecht, G. (1985) Videotape safaris: entering the field with a camera. *Qualitative Sociology*, 8 (4) Winter, pp. 325–344.

Allbutt, H., Amos, A. and Cunningham-Burley, S. (1995) The social image of smoking and young people in Scotland. *Health Education Research*, 10 (4) pp. 443–454.

Altheide, D. (1987) Ethnographic content analysis. *Qualitative Sociology*, 10 (1) pp. 65–77.

Althussar, L. and Balibar, E. (1975) *Reading Capital*. Translated by B. Brewster. London: NLB. First published 1968.

——(1977) *Systematically Distorted Communication*. London: NLB.

Anderson, J. (1996) Aboriginal wellbeing, in C. Grbich (ed.), *Health in Australia: Sociological Concepts and Issues*. Sydney: Prentice Hall.

Appiganesi, R. and Garratt, C. (1995) *Postmodernism for Beginners*. Cambridge: Icon Books.

Aroni, R. (1992) Looking at the media, in E. Timewell, V. Minichiello and D. Plummer (eds), *AIDS in Australia*. Melbourne: Prentice Hall.

Asch, A. and Fine, M. (1992) Beyond pedestals: revisiting the lives of women with disabilities, in M. Fine (ed.), *Disruptive Voices: The Possibilities of Feminist Research*, pp. 139–171. Ann Arbor: University of Michigan Press.

Asch, T. (1988) Collaboration in ethnographic film making: a person with a view, in J. Rollwaggon (ed.), *Anthropological Film Making*. London: Harwood Academic.

Ashworth, P. (1995) The meaning of 'participation' in participant observation. *Qualitative Health Research*, 5 (3) pp. 366–387.

Atkinson, P. (1992) The ethnography of a medical setting: reading, writing and rhetoric. *Qualitative Health Sociology*, 2 (4) pp. 451–474.

——(1995) Some perils of paradigms. *Qualitative Health Research*, 5 (1) pp. 117–124.

Australian Health Ethics Committee of the National Health and Medical Research Council, (1996) *Assessment of Qualitative Research*. Final Report. Canberra: AGPS.

Australian Health Technology Advisory Committee (1996) *Prostate Cancer Screening*. Commonwealth Department of Health and Family Services Canberra: AGPS.

Bach, C. and McDaniel, R. (1995) Techniques for conducting research with quadriplegic adults residing in the community. *Qualitative Health Research*, 5 (2) pp. 250–257.

Bailey, K. (1987) *Methods of Social Research*, 3rd edition. London: Collier.

Barley, N. (1986) *Ceremony: An Anthropologist's Misadventures in the African Bush*. New York: Henry Holt.

Barthes, R. (1968) *Elements of Semiology*. New York: Hill and Wang.

——(1972) *Mythologies*. New York: Hill and Wang.

Bateson, G. (1973) A theory of play and fantasy, in G. Bateson (ed.), *Steps to an Ecology of Mind: Collected Essays in Anthropology, Psychiatry, Evolution and Epistemology*. St Albans: Paladin.

Bateson, G. and Mead, M. (1942) *Balinese Character: A Photographic Analysis*. New York: New York Academy of Sciences.

Baudrillard, J. (1980) The implosion of meaning in the media and the implosion of the social in the masses, in K. Woodward (ed.), *The Myths of Information Technology and Post Industrial Culture*. London: Routledge and Kegan Paul.

Baudrillard, S. (1988) *Selected Writings*. M. Foster (ed.). Cambridge: Polity Press.

Bauman, Z. (1992) *Limitations of Postmodernity*. London: Routledge.

Becker, H. (1962) *Outsiders: Studies in the Sociology of Deviance*. London: Free Press of Glencoe.

——(1963) *Outsiders: Studies in the Sociology of Deviance*. London: Free Press of Glencoe.

——(1978) Do photographs tell the truth? in T. Cook and C. Reichardt (eds), *Qualitative and Quantitative Methods in Evaluation Research*. Beverley Hills: Sage.

Becker, H., Geer, B., Hughes, E. and Strauss, A. (1961) *Boys in White: Student Culture in a Medical School*. Chicago: University of Chicago Press.

Bedolla, M. (1992) Historical method: a brief introduction, in B. Crabtree and W. Miller (eds), *Doing Qualitative Research: Multiple Strategies*. California: Sage.

Bell, M. and Smith, G. (1992) Analyzing visual data. *Qualitative Research Methods*, 24. California: Sage.

Bell, S. and Apfel, R. (1995) Looking at bodies: insights and inquiries about DES related cancer. *Qualitative Sociology*, 18 (1) pp. 3–20.

Bell, T. (1993) *Curriculum guidelines for the communication technology area of technology education: teacher preparation programs*. Paper presented at the International Technology Education Association Conference, North Carolina.

Berg, B. (1989) *Qualitative Research Methods*. Boston: Allyn and Bacon.

——(1995) Focus group interviewing, in B. Berg (ed.), *Qualitative Research Methods for the Social Sciences*. Bloomington: Indiana University Press.

Berger, J. (1978) Ways of remembering. *Camerawork*, 10. London: Half Moon Gallery.

Berliner, D. (1988) *The Development of Expertise in Pedagogy*. Unpublished manuscript.

Bernard, R. (1994) *Research Methods in Anthropology: Qualitative and Quantitative Approaches*, 2nd edition. California: Sage.

Bertaux, D. (ed.) (1981) *Biography and Society: The Life History Approach in the Social Sciences*. California: Sage.

Blaikie, N. (1991) A critique of the use of triangulation in social research. *Quality and Quantity*, 25, pp. 115–136.

Blane, D. (1985) An assessment of the Black Report's explanations of health inequalities. *Sociology of Health and Illness*, 7 (3) pp. 423–445.

Blauner, R. (1987) Problems of editing 'first-person' sociology. *Qualitative Sociology*, 10 (1) pp. 46–64.

Bloom, H. (1976) *Poetry and Repression*. New Haven: Yale University Press.

Bloom, R., Obler, L., De Santi, S. and Ehrlich, J. (1994) *Discourse Analysis Applications: Studies in Adult Clinical Regulations*. Hillsdale, New Jersey: Lawrence Erlbaum.

Bloor, D. (1991) *Knowledge and Social Imagery*, 2nd edition. Chicago and London: the University of Chicago Press. First published 1976.

Blumer, H. (1978) Social unrest and collective protest, in N. Denzin (ed.), *Studies in Symbolic Interaction*, vol. 1. Greenwich: SAI Press.

Bogdan, R. (1974) *Being Different: The Autobiography of Jane Fry*. London: John Wiley.

Bogdan, R. and Biklen, S. (1982) *Qualitative Research for Education: An Introduction to Theory and Methods*. New York: Allyn and Bacon.

Bogdan, R. and Taylor, S. (1975) *Introduction to Qualitative Research Methods: A Phenomenological Approach to the Social Sciences*. New York: John Wiley.

——(1982) *Inside Out: The Social Meaning of Mental Retardation*. Toronto: University of Toronto Press.

Bond, M. (1996) *Medication Matters: Improving Medication Practices in Residential Homes for Older People*. Coventry: University of Warwick.

Bottoroff, J. (1994) Using videotaped recordings in qualitative research, in J. Morse (ed.), *Critical Issues in Qualitative Research Methods*. California: Sage.

Boy, P. (1992) *Introductory remarks: Current trends in computer-aided qualitative analysis*. Paper presented at the Qualitative Research Process and Computing Conference, Bremen, Germany, October.

Boyne, R. and Ratanis, A. (eds) (1990) *Postmodernisms and Society*. New York: St Martins Press.

Braden, S. (1983) *Committing Photography*. London: Pluto Press.

Bray, J., Powell, J., Lovelock, R. and Philip, I. (1995) Using a softer approach: techniques for interviewing older people. *Professional Nurse*, March, pp. 350–353.

Breitmayer, B., Ayres, L. and Knafl, K. (1993) Triangulation in qualitative research: evaluation of completeness and confirmation purposes. *IMAGE: Journal of Nursing Scholarship*, 25, pp. 237–243.

Brewer, J. and Hunter, A. (1989) *Multimethod Research: A Synthesis of Styles*. California: Sage.

Brown, G. (1973) Some thoughts on grounded theory. *Sociology*, 7, pp. 1–16.

Brown, G. and Harris, T. (1978) *Social Origins of Depression*. London: Tavistock.

Bruhn, A. and Lindberg, O. (1995) *Computer aided qualitative data analysis: some issues from a Swedish perspective*. Paper presented at the Australian Association of Social Research Conference. La Trobe University, Melbourne, Victoria, December.

Bryman, A. (1984) The debate about quantitative and qualitative methods: a question of method or epistemology? *British Journal of Sociology*, 35, pp. 75–92.

——(1988) *Quantity and Quality in Social Research*. Boston: Unwin Hyman.

Bulmer, M. (ed.) (1984) *Sociological Research Methods: An Introduction*. London: Macmillan.

Bunuel, L. (1974) *La Fantome de la Liberté* (motion picture). Greenwich: Fox-Rank.

Burdess, N. (1996) Class and health, in C. Grbich (ed.), *Health in Australia: Sociological Concepts and Issues*. Sydney: Prentice Hall

Burgess, R. (1984) Keeping a research diary, in J. Bell (ed.), *Conducting Small Scale Investigations in Educational Management*. London: Harper & Row.

——(ed.) (1988) *Conducting Qualitative Research*. Studies in Qualitative Methodology, vol. 1. London: JAI Press.

Burgess, R., Pole, C., Evans, K. and Priestley, C. (1994) Four studies from one or one study from four? Multisite case study research, in A. Bryman and R. Burgess (eds), *Analyzing Qualitative Data*. London: Routledge.

Buroway, M. (1991) *Ethnography Unbound: Power and Resistance in the Modern Metropolis*. Berkeley: University of California Press.

Butler, S. and Rosenblum, B. (1991) *Cancer in Two Voices*. San Francisco: Spinsters Book Co.

Callaway, H. (1992) Ethnography and experience: gender implications in field work and texts, in J. Okely and H. Callaway (eds), *Anthropology and Autobiography*. New York: Routledge.

Carey, J. (1993) Linking qualitative and quantitative methods: integrating cultural factors into public health. *Qualitative Health Research*, 3, pp. 298–318.

Carey, M. and Smith, M. (1994) Capturing the group effect in focus groups: a special concern in analysis. *Qualitative Sociology*, 4 (1) pp. 123–127.

Carr, W. (1994) Whatever happened to action research? *Educational Action Research*, 2 (3) pp. 427–436.

Carr, W. and Kemmis, S. (1986) *Becoming Critical: Education, Knowledge and Action Research*. London: Falmer Press.

Cartwright, A. and O'Brien, M. (1976) Social class variations in health care and in the nature of general practitioner consultations, in M. Stacy (ed.), *The Sociology of the NHS*, Sociological Review Monograph 22. Keele: University of Keele.

Casey, K. (1996) The new narrative research in education, in M. Apple (ed.), *Review of Research in Education*, vol. 2. Itasca, Illinois: F.E. Peacock.

Cassell, J. (1988) The relationship of the observer to the observed when studying up, in R. Burgess (ed.), *Conducting Qualitative Research*. London: JAI Press.

Cavan, S. (1978) Seeing social structure in a rural setting, in N. Denzin, *Sociological Methods: A Source Book*. New York: McGraw Hill.

CERE (Tulane/Xavier Consortium for Environmental Risk Evaluation) (1997) *Health and Ecological Risks Report Summary*. http//www.esarl.tulane.edu/report.html.

Chalfen, R. (1981) A socio-vidistic approach to children's filmmaking. *Studies in Visual Communication*, 7 (1) pp. 2–32.

Cheek, J. and Rudge, T. (1994) Webs of documentation: the discourse of case notes. *Australian Journal of Communication*, 21 (2), pp. 41–52.

——(1996) Health for all? The gendered construction of health and health care, in C. Grbich (ed.), *Health in Australia: Sociological Concepts and Issues*. Sydney: Prentice Hall.

Clancy, S. and Dollinger, S. (1993) Photographic depictions of the self: gender and age differences in social correctness. *Sex Roles*, 29, pp. 477–495.

Clay, M. (1982) *Observing Young Readers: Selected Papers*. London, Auckland: Heinemann.

Clifford, J. and Marcus, G. (eds) (1986) *Writing Culture: The Poetics and Politics of Ethnography*. Berkeley: University of California Press.

Coffey, A. and Atkinson, P. (1996) *Making Sense of Qualitative Data: Complementary Research Strategies*. California: Sage.

Collier, J. and Collier, M. (1986) *Visual Anthropology: Photography as a Research Method*. Albuquerque: University of New Mexico Press.

Comaroff, J. and Comaroff, J. (1992) *Ethnography and the Historical Imagination*. Boulder: Westview Press.

Comte, A. (1974) *The Positive Philosophy*, trans. H. Martineau. New York: Ams Press. First published 1830–42.

Cook, T. and Reichardt, C. (1979) *Qualitative and Quantitative Methods in Evaluation Research*. California: Sage.

Corbin, J. and Strauss, A. (1985) Managing chronic illness at home: three lines of work. *Qualitative Sociology*, 8 (3) pp. 224–247.

——(1988) *Unending Work and Care: Managing Chronic Illness at Home*. San Francisco: Jossey Bass.

Corfield, P. (ed.) (1991) *Language. History and Class*. Oxford: Basil Blackwell.

Cortazzi, M. (1993) *Narrative Analysis*. Social Research and Education Studies, 12, R. G. Burgess (ed.). London: Falmer Press.

Crabtree, B. and Miller, W. (1992) Doing qualitative research. *Research Methods for Primary Health Care*, vol. 3. California: Sage.

Cresswell, J. (1994) *Research Design: Qualitative and Quantitative Approaches*. California: Sage.

Crook, S., Paluski, J. and Waters, M. (1992) *Postmodernization: Change in Advanced Societies*. Newbury Park: Sage.

Cronbach, L. (1975) Beyond the two disciplines of scientific psychology. *American Psychologist*, 30, pp. 116–127.

Crosby, A. (1997) *The Measure of Reality: Quantification and Western Society 1250–1600*. New York: Cambridge University Press.

Crotty, M. (1996) *Phenomenology for Nursing*. South Melbourne: Pearson Press.

Culler, J. (1988) *Framing the Sign*. London: Basil Blackwell.

Dalton, M. (1959) *Men Who Manage*. New York: John Wiley.

Daly, J. and McDonald, I. (1992) Covering your back: strategies for qualitative research in clinical settings. *Qualitative Health Research*, 2 (4) pp. 416–438.

Davies, B. (1990) *Menstruation and women's subjectivity*. Paper presented at TASA Conference, University of Queensland, Brisbane.

——(1992) Women's subjectivity and feminist stories, in C. Ellis and M. Flaherty (eds), *Investigating Subjectivity: Research on Lived Experience*. California: Sage.

Davis, K. (1988) Paternalism under the microscope, in A. Todd and S. Fisher (eds), *Gender and Discourse: The Power of Talk*. Norwood, New Jersey: Ablett.

——(1995) *Avoiding the discrepancy between moral theory and social reality in the context of health research*. Paper presented at the 4th Australian Bioethics Association National Conference, Brisbane.

de Man, P. (1979) *Allegories of Reading: Figural Language in Rousseau, Nietzsche, Rilke and Proust*. New Haven: Yale University Press.

de Saussure, F. (1983) *Course in General Linguistics*, trans. by Ray Harris. C. Bally and A. Sechehaye (eds). London: Duckworth. First published 1916, Paris: Payot.

Denzin, N. (1978) *The Research Act: A Theoretical Introduction to Sociological Methods*. Chicago: Aldine.

——(1984) *On Understanding Emotion*. San Francisco: Jossey Bass.

——(1986) Interpreting the lives of ordinary people: Heidegger, Sartre, and Faulkner. *Life Stories/Recits de Vie*, 2(9), pp. 6–20.

——(1988) Book review of qualitative analysis for social scientists. *Contemporary Sociology*, 17 (3) May, pp. 430–432.

——(1989) *The Research Act: A Theoretical Introduction to Sociological Methods*, 3rd edition. New Jersey: Prentice Hall.

——(1994) The art and politics of interpretation, in N. Denzin and Y. Lincoln (eds), *Handbook of Qualitative Research*. California: Sage.

Denzin, N. and Lincoln, Y. (1994) *Handbook of Qualitative Research*. California: Sage.

Derrida, J. (1982) *Margins of Philosophy*. Translated by A. Boss. Chicago: University of Chicago Press.

——(1986) *Glas*, trans. J. Leavey Jnr & R. Rand. Lincoln: University of Nebraska Press. First published 1972.

Descartes, R. (1968) *Discourses on Method and Other Writings*. Harmondsworth: Penguin. First published 1637.

Dewey, J. (1934) *Arts as Experience*. New York: Minton Baloch and Co.

——(1937) *Logic: The Theory and Inquiry*. New York: John Wiley.

Dex, S. (ed.) (1991) *Life and Work History Analysis: Qualitative and Quantitative Developments*. London: Routledge.

di Giacamo, S. (1988) Metaphor as illness: postmodern dilemmas in the representation of body, mind and disorder. *Medical Anthropology*, 14, pp. 109–137.

Dilthey, W. (1976) *Selected Writings*. Translated by H. Rickman (ed.). London: Cambridge University Press.

Dingwell, R. (1992) Don't mind him, he's from Barcelona: qualitative methods in health studies, in J. Daly, I. McDonald and E. Willis (eds), *Researching Health Care: Designs, Dilemmas, Disciplines*. London: Tavistock, Routledge.

Dolby-Stahl, S. (1985) A literary folkloristic methodology for the study of meaning in personal narrative. *Journal of Folklore Research*, 22, pp. 5–70.

Domarad, B. and Buschmann, M. (1995) Interviewing older adults: increasing the credibility of interview data. *Journal of Gerontological Nursing*, September, pp. 14–20.

Donmeyer, R. (1990) Generalisability and the single case study, in E. Eisner and A. Peshkin (eds), *Qualitative Inquiry in Education: The Continuing Debate*. New York: Teachers College Press, Columbia University.

Dootson, S. (1995) An in-depth study of triangulation. *Journal of Advanced Nursing*, 22, pp. 183–187.

Douglas, J. (1976) *Investigative Social Research: Individual and Team Research*. California: Sage.

Douglas, J. and Rasmussen, P. , with Flanagan, C. (1977) *The Nude Beach Study*. California: Sage.

Dovey, K. and Graffam, J. (1987) *The Experience of Disability: Social Construction and Imposed Limitation*. Melbourne: Victoria College Press.

Dowdall, G. and Golden, J. (1989) Photographs as data: an analysis of images from a mental hospital. *Qualitative Sociology*, 12 (2) pp. 183–212.

Downe-Wamboldt, B. (1992) Content analysis: method, applications and issues. *Health Care for Women International*, 13, pp. 313–321.

Dressler, W. (1991) *Stress and Adaptation in the Context of Culture Depression in a Southern Black Community*. Albany: State University of New York Press.

Dupuy, J. and Dupuy, P. (1980) Myths of the informational society, in K. Woodward (ed.), *The Myths of Information Technology and Post Industrial Culture*. London: Routledge and Kegan Paul

Durkheim, E. (1951) *Suicide: A Study in Sociology*. Glencoe: Free Press. First published 1897.

Eco, U. (1976) *A Theory of Semiotics*. Basingstoke: Macmillan.

——(1979) *The Role of the Reader: explanations in the semiotics of texts*. Bloomington: Indiana University Press.

——(1987) *Travels in Hyper Reality*, trans. W. Weaver. London: Pan Books.

——(1992) *Interpretation and Overinterpretation*. New York: Cambridge University Press.

——(1993) *Mis-readings*. Translated by W. Weaver. London: Picador.

Eichler, M. (1988) *Non-sexist Research Methods: A Practical Guide*. Boston: George Allen & Unwin.

Eisner, E. (1981) On the differences between scientific and artistic approaches to qualitative research. *Educational Researcher*, 10 (4) pp. 5–9.

——(1991) *The Enlightened Eye: Qualitative Inquiry and the Enhancement of Educational Practice*. New York: Macmillan.

Eisner, E. and Peshkin, A. (eds) (1990) *Qualitative Inquiry in Education: The Continuing Debate*. New York: Teachers College Press, Columbia University.

Elden, M. and Levin, M. (1991) Cogenerative learning, in W. Foote Whyte (ed.), *Participatory Action Research*. Newbury Park: Sage.

Ellis, C. (1991) Sociological introspection and emotional experience. *Symbolic Interaction*, 14, pp. 23–50.

——(1993) There are survivors: telling a story of sudden death. *Sociological Quarterly*, 34, pp. 711–730.

——(1995a) *Final Negotiations: A Story of Love, Loss and Chronic Illness*. Philadelphia: Temple University Press.

——(1995b) Speaking of AIDS: an ethnographic short story. *Symbolic Interaction*, 18, pp. 73–81.

Ellis, C. and Bochner, A. (1992) Telling and performing personal stories: the constraints of choice in abortion, in C. Ellis and M. Flaherty (eds), *Investigating Subjectivity: Research on Lived Experience*. California: Sage.

Ellis, C. and Flaherty, M. (1992) *Investigating subjectivity: Research on Lived Experience*. California: Sage.

El-or, T. (1992) Do you really know how they make love? The limits on intimacy with ethnographic informants. *Qualitative Sociology*, 15 (1) 53–72.

Elton, B. and Associates (1995) *Client Information and Referral Record (CIARR): National Review of the Progress of Implementation*. Canberra: Department of Human Services and Health.

Ely, M., Anzul, M., Freidman, T., Garner, D. and Steinmetz, A. (1991) *Doing Qualitative Research: Circles within Circles*. London: Falmer Press.

Ely, M., Vine, R., Downing, M. and Anzul, M. (1997) *On Writing Qualitative Research: Living by Words*. London: Falmer Press.

Fagerhaugh, S. (1993) Routing: Getting around with emphysema, in B. Glaser (ed.), *Examples of Grounded Theory: A Reader*. California: Sociology Press.

Fairclough, N. (1989) *Language and Power*. Essex: Longman.

——(1992) *Discourse and Social Change*. Cambridge: Polity Press.

——(1993) Critical discourse analysis and the marketisation of public discourse: the universities. *Discourse and Society*, 4 (2) pp. 133–168.

Farran, D. (1990) Analysing a photograph of Marilyn Monroe, in L. Stanley (ed.), *Feminist Praxis: Research Theory and Epistemology in Feminist Sociology*. London: Routledge.

Feagin, J., Orum, A. and Sjoberg, G. (1991) *A Case for the Case Study*. North Carolina: University of North Carolina Press.

Featherstone, M. (ed.) (1988) *Postmodernism*. London: Sage.

Fetterman, D. (1989) *Ethnography: Step by Step*. California: Sage.

Fielding, N. and Fielding, J. (1986) *Linking Data: The Inter-relation of Qualitative and Quantitative Methods in Social Research*. California: Sage.

Fielding, N. and Lee, R. (1991) *Using Computers in Qualitative Research*. London: Sage.

——(1992) *User experiences with computer-assisted qualitative analysis*. Paper presented at the Qualitative Research Process and Computing Conference, Bremen, Germany, October.

Fields, E. (1988) Qualitative content analysis of television news: systematic techniques. *Qualitative Sociology*, 11 (3) pp. 183–193.

Fine, G. and Kent, L. (1988) *Knowing Children: Participant Oberservation with Minors*. Quali-

tative Research Methods, 15. J. Van Maanen (ed.). Beverly Hills: Sage.

Fine, M. (1992) *Disruptive Voices: The Possibilities of Feminist Research*. Ann Arbor: University of Michigan Press.

Finke, A. (1984) Consensus methods: characteristics and guidelines for use. *American Journal of Public Health*, 74, pp. 979–983.

Fiske, J. (1990) *Introduction to Communication Studies*, 2nd edition. London: Routledge.

Focus groups as a qualitative method for cross-cultural research (1995) *Social Gerontology: Journal of Cross-cultural Gerontology*, 10, April, pp. 7–20.

Foucault, M. (1977a) *Discipline and Punish: The Birth of the Prison*, trans. Alan Sheridan. New York: Vintage Books.

——(1977b) *The Archaeology of Knowledge*. London: Tavistock.

——(1980) *Power/Knowledge: Selected Interviews and Other Writings, 1972–1977*, ed. and trans. Colin Gordon. New York: Pantheon Books.

——(1988) Technologies of the self, in L. Martin et al. (eds), *Technologies of the Self*. London: Tavistock.

Fowles, J. (1969) *The French Lieutenant's Woman*. London: Cape.

Fox, N. (1993) *Postmodernism, Sociology and Health*. Buckingham: Open University Press.

——(1994) Anaesthetists, the discourse on patient fitness and the organisation of surgery. *Sociology of Health and Illness*, 16 (1) pp. 1–18.

Freeman, D. (1983) *Margaret Mead and Samoa: The Making and Unmaking of an Anthropological Myth*. Canberra: Australian National University Press.

Freire, P. (1972) *Pedagogy of the Oppressed*, trans. M. Ramos. Harmondsworth: Penguin.

Friedson, E. (1970) *Profession of Medicine: A Study of the Sociology of Applied Knowledge*. New York: Harper and Row.

——(1986) *Professional Powers: A Study of the Institutionalization of Formal Knowledge*. Chicago: University of Chicago Press.

Frohock, F. (1992) *Healing Powers*. Chicago: University of Chicago Press.

Gadamer, H. (1989) *Truth and Method*. Translated by J. Weinsheimer and D. Marshall. New York: Crossroad.

Gagnon, J. (1992) The self, its voices and their discord, in C. Ellis and M. Flaherty (eds), *Investigating Subjectivity: Researching Lived Experience*. California: Sage.

Gans, H. (1982) in R. Burgess (ed.), *Field Research: Sourcebook and Field Manual*. London: George Allen & Unwin.

Garfinkel, H. (1967) *Studies in Ethnomethodology*. New Jersey: Prentice Hall.

Garner, J. (1994) *Politically Correct Bedtime Stories*. New York: Macmillan.

Garrard, J. and Northfield, J. (1987) *Drug Education in Victorian Post Primary Schools*. Melbourne: Monash University.

Gee, J., Michaels, S. and O'Conner, M. (1992) Discourse analysis, in M. Le Compte, W. Millroy and J. Preissle Goetz (eds), *The Handbook of Qualitative Research in Education*. New York: Academic Press.

Gerhardt, U. (1989) *Ideas about Illness: An Intellectual and Political History of Medical Sociology*. New York: New York University Press.

Gerson, E. (1991) Supplementary grounded theory, in D. Maines (ed.), Social Organisation and Social Process: Essays in Honour of Anselm Strauss. New York: Aldine de Gruyter.

Giddens, A. (1976) New Rules of Sociological Method: A Positive Critique of Interpretive Sociologies. London: Hutchinson.

——(1987) *Social Theory and Modern Sociology*. Cambridge: Polity Press.

——(1993) *Sociology*, 2nd edition. Cambridge: Polity Press.

Gilligan, C. (1982) *In a Different Voice: Psychological Theory and Women's Development*. Cambridge: Harvard University Press.

Giorgi, A. (1988) Validity and reliability from a phenomenological perspective, in W. Baker, M. Rappard and H. Stam (eds), *Recent Trends in the Theoretical Psychology*. Proceedings from the second biennial conference of the International Society for Theoretical Psychology. New York: Springer-Verlag.

Glaser, B. (1967) *The Discovery of Grounded Theory: Strategies for Qualitative Research*. New York: Aldine.

——(1978) *Theoretical Sensitivity*. California: Sociology Press.

——(1992) *Basics of Grounded Theory Analysis*. California: Sociology Press.

——(1993) *Examples of Grounded Theory: A Reader*. California: Sociology Press.

——(1994) *More Grounded Theory Methodology: A Reader*. California: Sociology Press.

Glaser, B. and Strauss, A. (1965) *Awareness of Dying*. Chicago: Aldine.

——(1971) *Status Passage*. London: Routledge and Kegan Paul.

Glesne, C. and Peshkin, A. (1992) *Becoming Qualitative Researchers: An Introduction*. New York: Longman.

Goffman, E. (1959) *The Presentation of Self in Everyday Life*. New York: Doubleday.

——(1961) *Asylums: Essays on the Social Situations of Mental Patients and Other Inmates*. New York: Anchor.

——(1974) *Frame Analysis: An Essay on the Organisation of Experience*. New York: Harper & Row.

——(1976) *Gender Advertisements*. London: Macmillan.

Goltz, K. and Buni, N. (1995) Health promotion discourse: language of change, in H. Gardner (ed.), *Politics of Health: The Australian Experience*, 2nd edition. Melbourne: Churchill Livingstone.

Goode, E. (1996) The ethics of deception in social research: a case study. *Qualitative Sociology*, 19 (1) pp. 11–33.

Goodman, N. (1983) *Fact, Fiction and Forecast*, 4th edition. Cambridge: Harvard University Press.

Goodwin, L. and Goodwin, W. (1984) Are validity and reliability relevant in qualitative evaluation research? *Evaluation of the Health Professions*, 7 (4) pp. 413–426.

Gordon, D. (1988) Writing culture, writing feminism: the poetics and politics of experimental ethnography. *Inscriptions*, 3 (4) pp. 7–24.

Gouldner, A. (1970) *The Coming Crisis of Western Sociology*. New York: Basic Books.

Graham, H. and Oakley, A. (1981) Competing ideologies of reproduction: medical and maternal perspectives on pregnancy, in H. Roberts (ed.), *Women, Health and Reproduction*. London: Routledge and Kegan Paul.

Grant, M. (1995) *Memory work: an emancipatory methodology*. Paper given at the conference of the Australian Association of Social Researchers, La Trobe University, Melbourne, December.

Gray-Vickrey, P. (1993) Gerontological research: use and application of focus groups. *Journal of Gerontological Nursing*, May, pp. 21–27.

Grbich, C. (1987). *Male Primary Care Givers: A Role Study*. PhD dissertation, Monash University, Melbourne.

Grbich, C., de Crespigny, C. and Watson, J. (1997) Women who are older and access to medication information. *Australian Journal of Primary Health—Interchange*, 3 (1) pp. 16–25.

Grbich, C. and Sykes, S. (1989). *'What about Us?' Access to School and Work of Young Women with Severe Intellectual Disabilities*. Melbourne: Krongold Centre, Monash University.

Greenbaum, T. (1993) *The Handbook for Focus Group Research*. New York: Lexington Press.

Greene, J., Caracelli, V. and Graham, W. (1989) Toward a conceptual framework for mixed-method evaluation designs. *Educational Evaluation and Policy Analysis*, 11, pp. 255–274.

Grosby, S. (1995) Introduction: the tasks of historical sociology. *Qualitative Sociology*, 18 (2) Summer, pp. 139–145.

Grumet, M. (1990) On daffodils that come before the swallow dares, in E. Eisner and A. Peshkin (eds), *Qualitative Inquiry in Education: The Continuing Debate*. New York: Teachers College Press, Columbia University.

Guattari, F. (1984) *Molecular Revolution*. Harmondsworth: Penguin.

Guba, E. (1990) *The Paradigm Dialog*. California: Sage.

——(1996) Foreword to E. Stringer, *Action Research: A Handbook for Practitioners*. California: Sage.

Guba, E. and Lincoln, Y. (1989) *Fourth Generation Evaluation*. California: Sage.

Gummesson, E. (1991) *Qualitative Methods in Management Research*. California: Sage.

Gunther, H. (1991) Interviewing street children in a Brazilian city. *Journal of Social Psychology*, 132 (3) pp. 359–367.

Haack, S. (1993) *Evidence and Inquiry*. Oxford: Basil Blackwell.

Habermas, J. (1970) On systematically distorted communication. *Inquiry*, 13, pp. 205–218.

——(1972) *Knowledge and Human Interests*, trans. J. Shapiro. London: Heinemann.

——(1976) *Legitimation Crisis*. London: Heinemann.

——(1984) *Theory of Communicative Action, Reason and the Rationalisation of Society*, vol. 1, trans. T. McCarthy. Boston: Beacon Press.

Hagaman, D. (1995) *How I Learned Not to be a Photojournalist*. Kentucky: Kentucky University Press.

Halloran, J. and Grimes, D. (1995) Application of the focus group methodology to educational program development. *Qualitative Health Research*, 5 (4) pp. 444–453.

Hamel, J., Dufour, S. and Fortin, D. (1993) *Case Study Methods*. California: Sage.

Hammersley, M. (1983) *Ethnography: Principles in Practice*. London: Tavistock.

——(1989) *The Dilemma of Qualitative Method: Herbert Blumer and the Chicago Tradition*. London: Routledge.

——(1992) *What's Wrong with Ethnography?* London: Routledge.

Hammersley, M. and Atkinson, P. (1995) *Ethnography: Principles in Practice*. London and New York: Routledge.

Hansen, K. and MacDonald, C. (1995) Surveying the dead informant: Qualitative analysis and historical interpretation. *Qualitative Sociology*, 18 (2) pp. 227–236.

Harding, S. (1987) *Feminism and Methodology*. Bloomington: Indiana University Press.

Harper, D. (1988) Visual sociology: expanding the sociological vision. *American Sociologist*, 19 (1) pp. 54–70.

Hart, E. and Bond, M. (1995) *Action Research for Health and Social Care: A Guide to Practice*. Buckingham: Open University Press.

Hartshorne, C., Weiss, P. and Bucks, A. (eds) (1958) *Collected Papers of Charles Pierce*. Cambridge: Harvard University Press.

Harvey, K. and Murray, M. (1995) Medicinal drug policy, in H. Gardner (ed.), *Politics of Health: The Australian Experience*, 2nd edition. Melbourne: Churchill Livingstone.

Hassan, R. (1983) *A Way of Dying: Suicide in Singapore*. Kuala Lumpur: Oxford University Press.

Hatch, J. and Wisniewski, R. (eds) (1995) *Life History and Narrative*, vol. 1. Qualitative Studies. London: Falmer Press.

Haug, F. (1987) *Female Sexualization: A Collective Work of Memory*, trans. E. Carter. London: Verso.

——(1992) *Beyond Female Masochism: Memory Work and Politics*. London: Verso.

Hayano, D. (1979) Auto-ethnography: paradigms, problems and prospects. *Human Organisation*, 38, pp. 99–104.

Hayes, T. and Tatham, C. (1996) Focus group interviews: A reader. *Health Transition Review*, 6 (2) October, pp. 179–201.

Health Transition Review (1994) 4 (1) April. (Whole issue on focus groups.)

Heidegger, M. (1972) *On Time and Being*, trans. J. Stombaugh. New York: Harper & Row. First published 1964.

——(1982) *Basic Problems of Phenomenology*, trans. A. Holfstadter. Bloomington: Indiana University Press.

Henman, P. (1992) *Grounding social critiques of computers: the world-view embodied in computers*. Paper presented at the Australian Sociological Association (TASA) Conference, Adelaide, December.

Henriques, J., Holloway, W., Urwin, C., Venn, C. and Walkerdine, V. (1984) *Changing the Subject: Psychology, Social Regulation and Subjectivity*. London: Methuen.

Hepworth, J. (1994) *Reconceptualising anorexia nervosa: medical discourse and feminist analyses*. Paper presented at the Discourse Construction of Knowledge Conference, Adelaide, February.

——(1997) Evaluation in health outcomes research: linking theories, methodologies and practice in health promotion. *Health Promotion International*, 12 (3) pp. 233–238.

Hepworth, J. and Griffith, C. (1990) The 'discovery' of anorexia nervosa: discourses of the late 19th century. *Text*, 10 (4) pp. 321–338.

Hertz, R. and Imber, J. (1995) *Studying Elites Using Qualitative Methods*. California: Sage.

Hesse-Biber, S. (1995) Unleashing Frankenstein's monster? The use of computers in qualitative research, in R. Burgess (ed.), *Studies in Qualitative Methodology: Computing and Qualitative Research*. London: JAI Press.

Higgins, P. and Johnson, J. (eds) (1988) *Personal Sociology*. New York: Praeger.

Hilger, M. (1966) *Field Guide to the Ethnological Study of Child Life*. New Haven: Human Relations Area Files Press.

Hill, M. (1993) *Archival Strategies and Techniques*. California: Sage.

Hobbes, T. (1991) *Leviathan*. R. Tuck (ed.). Cambridge: Cambridge University Press. First published 1651.

Hocking, B. and Thompson, C. (1992) Chaos theory of occupational accidents. *Journal of Occupational Health and Safety*, 8 (2) pp. 99–119.

Holland, N. (1980) Recovering 'the purloined letter': reading as a personal transaction, in S. Suleiman and I. Crossman (eds), *The Reader in the Text: Essays on Audience and Interpretation*. Princeton: Princeton University Press.

Holman, H. (1993) Qualitative inquiry in medical research. *Journal of Clinical Epidemiology*, 46 (1) pp. 29–36.

Horkheimer, M. (1982) *Critical Theory: Selected Essays*, trans. M. O'Connell and others. New York: Continuum.

Huber, G. and Garcia, C. (1993) Voices of beginning teachers: computer-assisted listening to their common experiences, in M. Schratz (ed.), *Qualitative Voices in Educational Research*. London: Falmer Press.

Human Relations Journal (1993) 46 (2). (Special issue on action research.)

Humphreys, L. (1970) *Tea Room Trade: Impersonal Sex in Public Places*. Chicago: Aldine.

Husserl, E. (1931) *Ideas I*, trans. W. Boyce Gibson. London: George Allen & Unwin.

——(1989) *Ideas II*, trans. R. Rojcewisz and E. Schuwer, trans. W. Boyce Gibson. Dordrecht: Kluwer. First published 1969.

Illich, I. (1977) *Limits to Medicine, Medical Nemesis: The Expropriation of Health*. London: Penguin.

Irigary, L. (1973) *Le Langage des Déments Collection*. Approaches to Semiotics. The Hague: Mouton.

——(1974) *Speculum of the Other Woman*. Translated by G. Gill. Ithaca: Cornell University Press.

Iser, W. (1980) Interview. *Diacritics*, 10, pp. 57–74.

Janas, B. and Hymans, J. (1997) New Jersey school nurses' perceptions of school based, prenatal nutrition education. *Journal of School Health*, 67 (2) pp. 62–67.

Jackson, M. (1989) *Paths toward a Clearing: Radical Empiricism and Ethnographic Inquiry*. Bloomington: Indiana University Press.

Jick, T. (1979) Mixing qualitative and quantitative methods: triangulation in action. *Administrative Science Quarterly*, 24, pp. 602–611.

Johnston, D. (1970) Forecasting methods in the social sciences. *Technological Forecasting and Social Change*, pp. 173–187.

Jordan, S. and Yeomans, D. (1995) Critical ethnography: problems in contemporary theory and practice. *British Journal of Sociology and Education*, 16 (3) pp. 389–408.

Josselson, R. (ed.) (1993) *Ethics and Process in the Narrative Study of Lives*, vol. 4. The Narrative Study of Lives. California: Sage.

Josselson, R. and Amia, L. (eds) (1993) The Narrative Study of Lives (series). Newbury Park: Sage.

Josselson, R. and Lieblich, A. (eds) (1993) The Narrative Study of Lives (series). California: Sage.

——(1994) *Exploring Identity and Gender*. The Narrative Study of Lives. California: Sage.

——(1995) *Interpreting Experience*, vol. 3. The Narrative Study of Lives. California: Sage.

Kant, I. (1974) *Critique of Pure Reason*. London: Dent. First published 1781.

Kasper, A. (1994) A feminist, qualitative methodology: a study of women with breast cancer. *Qualitative Sociology*, 17 (3) pp. 263–281.

Kellehear, A. (1993) *The Unobtrusive Researcher: A Guide to Methods*. Sydney: Allen & Unwin.

Kemmis, S. (1994) A guide to evaluation design. *Evaluation News and Comment*, 3, May.

Kemmis, S. and McTaggart, R. (1988) *The Action Research Planner*, 3rd edition. Geelong: Deakin University Press.

Kidder, L. and Judd, C. (1986) *Research Methods in Social Relations*, 4th edition. Tokyo: CBS Publishing.

Kincheloe, J. and McLaren, P. (1994) Rethinking critical theory and qualitative research, in N. Denzin and Y. Lincoln (eds), *Handbook of Qualitative Research*. California: Sage.

King, G., Kochane, R. and Verba, S. (1994) *Designing Social Inquiry: Scientific Inference in Qualitative Research*. Princeton: Princeton University Press.

Kingsley, S. (1988a) *Action Research: Method or ideology*. Wivenhoe: Association of Researchers in Voluntary Action and Community Involvement.

——(1988b) *Human Inquiry in Action*. California: Sage.

Kippax, S., Crawford, J., Benton P. , Gault, U. and Noesjirwan, J. (1988) Constructing emotions: weaving meanings from memories. *British Journal of Social Psychology*, 27, pp. 19–33.

Kitzinger, J. (1994) The methodology of focus groups: the importance of interaction between research participants. *Sociology of Health and Illness*, 16 (1) pp. 103–120.

Kleinman, S. and Copp, C. (1993) *Emotions and Fieldwork*. Newbury: Sage.

Knafl, K. and Breitmeyer, B. (1991) Triangulation in qualitative research: issues of conceptual clarity and purpose, in J. Morse (ed.), *Qualitative Nursing: Research as Contemporary Dialogue*. London: Sage.

Koutroulis, S. (1992) *Memory work: process, practice and pitfalls*. Paper presented to the conference of the Australian Sociological Association (TASA), Adelaide.

Krieger, S. (1983) *The Mirror Dance: Identity in a Women's Community*. Philadelphia: Temple University Press.

——(1985) Beyond 'subjectivity'. the use of the self in social science. *Qualitative Sociology*, 8 (4) pp. 309–324.

Krippendorf, K. (1980) *Content Analysis: An Introduction to Its Methodology*, 4th edition. California: Sage.

Kristeva, J. (1970) *Le Texte du Roman: Approche Semiologique d'une Structure Discursive Transformationnelle*. The Hague: Mouton.

——(1984) *Revolution in Poetic Language*. New York: Columbia University Press.

Krueger, R. (1994) *Focus Groups: A Practical Guide for Applied Research*, 2nd edition. California: Sage.

Kurosawa, A. (1950) *Rashomon* (film and video recording). Japan: Daiei Production.

Lacan, J. (1979) *The Four Fundamental Concepts of Psycho-analysis*. London: Penguin.

Lain-Entralgo, P. (1964) *La Relacion Medico-Enfermo: Historia y Teoria*. Madrid: Revista de Occidente.

Lash, S. (1991) *Post-structuralist and Post-modernist Sociology*. Cambridge: Cambridge University Press.

Lather, P. (1986) Issues of validity in openly ideological research: between a rock and a hard place. *Interchange*, 17 (4) pp. 63–84.

——(1988) Feminist perspectives on empowering research methodologies. *Women's Studies International Forum*, 11 (6) pp. 569–581.

——(1989) *Deconstructing/deconstructive inquiry: issues in feminist research methodologies*. Paper presented at the New Zealand Women's Studies Association Conference, Christchurch, August.

——(1993) Fertile obsession: validity after post-structuralism. *Sociological Quarterly*, 34 (4) pp. 673–693.

Laurie, H. (1992a) Multiple methods in the study of household resource allocation, in J. Brannen (ed.), *Mixing Methods: Qualitative and Quantitative Research*. Avebury: Aldershot.

——(1992b) *Using the ethnograph: practical and methodological implications*. Paper presented at the Qualitative Research Process and Computing Conference, Bremen, Germany, October.

Laurie, H. and O'Sullivan, O. (1991) Combining qualitative and quantitative methods in the longitudinal study of household allocations. *Sociological Review*, 39, pp. 113–139.

Layder, D. (1993) *New Strategies in Social Research*. Oxford: Polity Press.

Le Compte, M., Millroy, W. and Preissle Goetz, J. (eds), *The Handbook of Qualitative Research in Education*. New York: Academic Press.

Le Compte, M. and Preissle Goetz, J. (1982) Problems of reliability and validity in ethnographic research. *Review of Educational Research*, 52 (1) pp. 31–60.

Lee, J. (ed.) (1994) *Life and Story: Autobiographies for a Narrative Psychology*. Westport: Praeger.

Leininger, M. (1985) *Qualitative Research Methods in Nursing*. Philadelphia: W. B. Saunders.

Levi-Strauss, C. (1968) *Structural Anthropology*. London: Penguin.

Lewin, K. (1946) Action research and minority problems. *Journal of Social Issues*, 2, pp. 34–46.

Lewis, M. and Simon, R. (1986) A discourse not intended for her: learning and teaching within patriarchy. *Harvard Educational Review*, 56 (4) pp. 457–472.

Lieblich, A. and Ruthellen, J. (eds) (1994) *Exploring Identity and Gender*. The Narrative Study of Lives. California: Sage.

Lincoln, Y. and Guba, E. (1985) *Naturalistic Inquiry*. California: Sage.

Linde, C. (1993) *Life Stories: The Creation of Coherence*. Oxford: Oxford University Press.

Linden, R. (1992) *Making Stories, Making Selves: Feminist Reflections on the Holocaust*. Columbus: Ohio University Press.

Lofland, J. (1971) *Analysing Social Settings*. California: Wadsworth.

Lonkila, M. (1995) Grounded theory as an emerging paradigm for computer assisted qualitative data analysis, in U. Kelle (ed.), *Computer-Aided Qualitative Data Analysis: Theory, Methods and Practice*. London: Sage.

Lukes, S. (1985) *Emile Durkheim: His Life and Work: A Historical and Critical Study*. California: Stanford University Press.

Lunn, E. (1985) *Marxism and Modernism*. London: Verso.

Lupton, D. (1992) Discourse analysis: a new methodology for understanding the ideologies of health and illness. *Australian Journal of Public health*, 16 (2), pp. 145–150.

Lupton, D. and Chapman, S. (1995) A healthy lifestyle might be the death of you: discourses on diet, cholesterol and heart disease in the press and among the lay public. *Sociology of Health and Illness*, 17 (4) pp. 477–494.

Lyotard, J.-F. (1983) Answering the question: what is post-modernism? in E. Hassan and S. Hassan (eds), *Innovation and Renovation*. Maddison: University of Wisconsin Press.

——(1984) *The Post Modern Condition: A Report on Knowledge*, trans. G. Bennington and B. Massumi. Minneapolis: University of Minnesota Press.

Macann, C. (1993) *Four Phenomenological Philosophers: Husserl, Heidegger, Sartre, Merleau Ponty*. London: Routledge.

MacLachlan, G. and Reid, I. (1994) *Framing and Interpretation*. Melbourne: Melbourne University Press.

Madey, D. (1982) Some benefits of integrating qualitative and quantitative methods in program' evaluation, with illustrations. *Educational Evaluation and Policy Analysis*, 4, pp. 223–236.

Malinowski, B. (1932) *The Sexual Life of Savages in North Western Melanesia: An Ethnographic Account of Courtship, Marriage and Family Life among the Troubriand Islands, British New Guinea*. London: Routledge and Kegan Paul.

——(1967) *A Diary in the Strict Sense of the Term*. Translated by N. Guterman. London: Routledge and Kegan Paul.

Mannheim, K. (1966) *Ideology and Utopia: An Introduction to the Sociology of Knowledge*, trans. L. Wirth and E. Shils. London: Routledge and Kegan Paul. First published 1936.

Manning, P. (1987) *Semiotics and fieldwork*. Qualitative Methods series, 7. Beverley Hills: Sage.

Manning, P. and Cullum-Swan, B. (1994) Narrative, content and semiotic analysis, in N. Denzin and Y. Lincoln (eds), *Handbook of Qualitative Research*. California: Sage.

Manwar, A., Johnson, B. and Dunlap, E. (1994) Qualitative data analysis with hyper text: a case of New York city crack dealers. *Qualitative Sociology*, 17 (3) Research note, pp. 283–292.

Manzo, J., Blonder, L. and Burns, A. (1995) The social and interactional organisation of narrative and narrating among stroke patients and their spouses. *Sociology of Health and Illness*, 17 (1) pp. 307–327.

Marcus, G. (1994) What comes (just) after 'post'? The case of ethnography, in N. Denzin and Y. Lincoln (eds), *Handbook of Qualitative Research*. California: Sage.

Marcus, G. and Fischer, M. (1986) *Anthropology as Cultural Critique: An Experimental Moment in the Cultural Sciences*. Chicago: University of Chicago Press.

Marotta, V. (1996) The status of the 'social' and the individual in the life history approach. *Australian Journal of Social Research*, 2 (1) pp. 129–134.

Marx, K. (1906) *Capital: A Critique of Political Economy: The Process of Capitalist Production*. F. Engels (ed.). Translated by S. Moore and E. Aveling. New York: Modern Library.

——(1971) *Capital: A Critical Analysis of Capital Production*, trans. S. Moore and E. Aveling. London: George Allen & Unwin. First published 1893 and 1894.

Marx, K. and Engels, F. (1974) *The German Ideology*. London: George Allen & Unwin. First published 1887.

Mason, J. (1994) Linking qualitative and quantitative data analysis, in A. Bryman and R. Burgess (eds), *Analysing Qualitative Data*. London: JAI Press.

Mathison, S. (1988) Why triangulate? *Educational Researcher*, March, pp. 13–14.

Maxwell, J. (1992) Understanding and validity in qualitative research. *Harvard Educational Review*, 62 (3) pp. 279–300.

McCoy, M. and Aronoff, M. (1994) Against all odds: revitalisation of local self help alternatives by long term mental health consumers. *Qualitative Sociology*, 17 (4) pp. 365–381.

McGregor, W. (1991) Discourse analysis and intercultural communication. *Australian Journal of Communication*, 18 (1) pp. 13–29.

McKeown, T. (1976) *The Modern Rise of Population*. London: Edward Arnold.

——(1979) *The Role of Medicine*. Oxford: Basil Blackwell.

——(1988) *The Origins of Human Disease*. Oxford: Basil Blackwell.

McKie, L. (1995) The art of surveillance or reasonable prevention? The ease of cervical screening. *Sociology of Health and Illness*, 17 (4) pp. 441–457.

McLaren, P. (1995a) Collisions with otherness, in P. McLaren and J. Giarelli (eds), *Critical Theory and Educational Research*. New York: State University of New York Press.

——(1995b) *Postmodernism, Postcolonialism and Pedagogy*. South Melbourne: James Nicholas.

McLaren, P. and Giarelli, J. (eds) (1995) *Critical Theory and Educational Research*. New York: State University of New York Press.

McRobbie, A. (1994) *Postmodernism and Popular Culture*. London: Routledge.

McTaggart, R. (1994) Participatory action research: issues in theory and practice. *Educational Action Research*, 2 (3) pp. 313–337.

McWilliam, C., Stewart, M., Brown, J., McNair, S., Desai, K., Patterson, M., Del Maestro, W. and Pittman, B. (1997) Creating empowering meaning: an interactive process of promoting health with chronically ill older Canadians. *Health Promotion International*, 12 (2) pp. 111–123.

Mead, G. (1934) *Mind, Self and Society*. Chicago: University of Chicago Press.

Mead, M. (1928) *Coming of Age in Samoa: A Study of Adolescence and Sex in Primitive Societies*. Harmondsworth: Penguin.

——(1963) *Growing up in New Guinea: A Study of Adolescence and Sex in Primitive Societies*. Harmondsworth: Penguin.

Mechanic, D. (1978) *Medical Sociology*, 2nd edition. New York: Free Press.

Meredith, P. (1993) Patient participation in decision making and consent to treatment: the case of general surgery. *Sociology of Health and Illness*, 15 (3) pp. 315–336.

Merleau-Ponty, M. (1943) *The Structure of Behaviour*. Trans. A. Fischer. Boston: Beacon Press.

——(1962) *The Phenomenology of Perception*. Trans. C. Smith. London: Routledge and Kegan Paul.

Merton, R. (1968) *Social Theory and Social Structure: Part One on Theoretical Sociology: Five Essays Old and New*. New York: Free Press.

Merton, R., Fiske, M. and Kendall, P. (eds) (1990) *The Focused Interview: A Manual of Problems and Procedures*, 2nd edition. Glencoe, Illinois: Free Press, Macmillan. First published 1956.

Mies, M. (1990) Women's research or feminist research? The debate surrounding feminist science and methodology, in M. Fonow and J. Cook (eds), *Beyond Methodology: Feminist Scholarship as Lived Research*. Bloomington: Indiana University Press.

Miles, M. and Huberman, M. (1984) *Qualitative Data Analysis: A Sourcebook of New Methods*. California: Sage.

——(1994a) *Qualitative Data Analysis: An Expanded Sourcebook*, 2nd edition. California: Sage.

——(1994b) Data management and analysis methods, in N. Denzin and Y. Lincoln (eds), *Handbook of Qualitative Research*. California: Sage.

Mill, J. (1906) *A System of Logic*. London: Longman. First published 1843.

Miller, K. and Rouse, T. (1995) *CAAAPU: An Evaluation*. Menzies Occasional Papers, 1. Darwin, Northern Territory University: Menzies School of Health Research.

Miller, W. and Crabtree, B. (1994) Clinical research, in N. Denzin and Y. Lincoln (eds), *Handbook of Qualitative Research*. California: Sage.

Minichiello, V., (1992) Gay men discuss social issues and personal concerns, in E. Timewell, V. Minichiello and D. Plummer (eds), *AIDS in Australia: Context and Practice*. Melbourne: Prentice Hall.

Minichiello, V., Aroni, R., Timewell, E. and Alexander, L. (1995) *In-depth Interviewing: Principles, Techniques, Analysis*, 2nd edition. Melbourne: Longman.

Mishler, E. (1984) *The Discourse of Medicine: Dialectics of Medical Interviews*. Cambridge: Cambridge University Press.

——(1986) *Research Interviewing: Context and Narrative*. Cambridge, Massachussetts: Harvard University Press.

——(1990) Validation in inquiry-guided research: the role of exemplars in narrative research. *Harvard Educational Review*, 60, pp. 415–442.

Mitchell, E. (1986) Multiple triangulation: a methodology for nursing science. *Advances in Nursing Science*, 8, pp. 18–26.

Mitchell, T. (1993) *Bridesmaids Revisited: Health, Older Women and Memory Work*. Master's thesis, School of Nursing, Flinders University of South Australia, Adelaide.

Moi, T. (ed.) (1986) *The Kristeva Reader*. Oxford: Basil Blackwell.

Moore, C. (1987) *Group Techniques for Idea Building*. California: Sage.

Morgan, D. (1975) Exploring mental illness. *Archives Européans de Sociologie*, 16, pp. 262–280.

——(1988) *Focus Groups as Qualitative Research*. Qualitative Research Methods, 16. California: Sage.

——(1992) Doctor–care giver relationships: an exploration using focus groups, in B. Crabtree and W. Miller (eds), *Doing Qualitative Research: Multiple Strategies*. California: Sage.

——(1995) Why things (sometimes) go wrong in focus groups. *Qualitative Health Research*, 5 (4) pp. 516–523.

Morgan, O. (1993) Qualitative content analysis: paths not taken. *Qualitative Sociology*, 3 (1) pp. 112–121.

Morris, B. (1991) *Western Conceptions of the Individual*. Oxford: Berg.

Morris, J. (1992) Personal and political: a feminist perspective on researching physical disability. *Disability, Handicap and Society*, 7 (2) pp. 157–166.

Morse, J. M. (1991) Approaches to qualitative–quantitative triangulation. *Nursing Research*, 40, pp. 120–123.

Murphy, J. and Pardeck, J. (1988) Technology in clinical practice and the technological ethic. *Journal of Sociology and Social Welfare*, 15 (1) pp. 119–128.

Murphy-Lawless, J. (1988) The obstetric view of feminine identity: a nineteenth century case history of the use of forceps on unmarried women in Ireland, in A. Todd and S. Fisher (eds), *Gender and Discourse: the Power of Talk*. Norwood, New Jersey: Ablett.

Myerhoff, B. (1992) *Remembered Lives: The Work of Ritual, Storytelling and Growing Older*. Ann Arbor: Michigan University Press.

Myrdal, G. (1970) *Objectivity in Social Research*. London: Duckworth.

Nabakov, V. (1965) *Lolita*. London: Weidenfeld and Nicholson.

Narayan, K. (1993) How native is a 'native anthropologist'? *American Anthropology*, 95, pp. 671–686.

Navarro, V. (1976) *Medicine under Capitalism*. New York: Prodist.

——(1986) *Crisis, Health and Medicine*. London: Tavistock.

Nelson, K. (1992) The emergence of autobiographical memory at age 4. *Human Development*, 35, pp. 172–177.

Newton, K. (1990) *Interpreting the Text*. Hertfordshire: Harvester Wheatsheaf.

North, D., Davis, P. and Powell, A. (1995) Patient responses to benzodiazepine medication: a typology of adaptive repertoires developed by long-term users. *Sociology of Health and Illness*, 17 (5) pp. 632–650.

Nye, A. (1990) *Word of Power: A Feminist Reading of the History of Logic*. London: Routledge.

Oakley, A. (1981) Interviewing women: a contradiction in terms, in H. Roberts (ed.), *Doing Feminist Research*. London: Routledge and Kegan Paul.

——(1990) Who's afraid of the randomised controlled trial? Some dilemmas of scientific methods and 'good' research practice, in H. Roberts (ed.), *Women's Health Counts*. London: Routledge.

O'Brien, K. (1993a) Improving survey questionnaires through focus groups, in D. Morgan, *Successful Focus Groups*. California: Sage.

——(1993b) Using focus groups to develop health surveys: an example from research on social relationships and AIDS-preventive behavior. *Health Education Quarterly*, 20 (1) pp. 361–372.

O'Brien, P. (1978) The Delphi technique: a review of the research. *South Australian Journal of Education Research*, 1 (1) pp. 57–75.

O'Conner, H. (1993) Bridging the gap. *Nursing Times*, 89 (32) pp. 63–66.

O'Connor, J. (1977) *The Fiscal Crisis of the State*. London: St Martins Press.

Offe, C. (1985) *Disorganised Capitalism: Contemporary Transformations of Work and Politics*. Oxford: Polity Press.

Olesen, V. (1994) Feminisms and models in qualitative research, in N. Denzin and Y. Lincoln (eds), *Handbook of Qualitative Research*. California: Sage.

Opie, A. (1992) Qualitative research, appropriation of the 'other' and empowerment. *Feminist Review*, 40, pp. 53–69.

Orum, M., Feagin, J. and Sjoberg, G. (1991). Introduction: the nature of the case study, in J. Feagin, M. Orum and G. Sjoberg (eds), *A Case for the Case Study*. North Carolina: University of North Carolina Press.

Paget, M. (1993) *A Complex Sorrow: Reflections on Cancer and on an Abbreviated Life*. M. de Vault (ed.). Philadelphia: Temple University Press.

Parliament of Victoria Social Development Committee (1986) *Inquiry into Alternative Medicine and the Health Food Industry*. Melbourne: Government Printer.

Parons, H. (1974) What happened at Hawthorne? *Science*, 183, pp. 922–930.

Parsons, T. (1951) *The Social System*. Glencoe: Free Press.

——(1978) Health and disease: a sociological and action perspective, in T. Parsons (ed.), *Action Theory and the Human Condition*. London: Macmillan.

Patai, D. (1988) *Brazilian Women Speak*. New Brunswick: Rutgers University Press.

Paterson, B. and Bramadat, I. (1992) The use of the preinterview in oral history. *Qualitative Health Research*, 2 (1) pp. 99–113.

Patton, M. (1988) Paradigms and pragmatism, in D. Fetterman (ed.), *Qualitative Approaches to Evaluation in Education: The Silent Revolution*, pp. 16–137. New York: Praeger

——(1990) *Qualitative Evaluation and Research Methods*. California: Sage.

Pelto, P. and Pelto, G. (1978) *Anthropological Research: The Structure of Inquiry*. Cambridge: Cambridge University Press.

Personal Narratives Group (ed.) (1989) *Interpreting Women's Lives: Feminist Theory and Personal Narratives*. Bloomington: Indiana University Press.

Peshkin, A. (1985) Virtuous subjectivity: in the participant-observer's I's, in D. Berg and K. Smith (eds), *Exploring Clinical Methods for Social Research*. California: Sage.

Phillips, D. (1987) *Philosophy, Science and Social Inquiry: Contemporary Methodological Controversies in Social Sciences and Related Applied Fields of Research*. Oxford: Pergamon Press.

——(1990) Subjectivity and objectivity: an objective inquiry, in E. Eisner and A. Peshkin (eds), *Qualitative Inquiry in Education: The Continuing Debate*. New York: Teachers College Press, Columbia University.

Piaget, J. (1971) *Biology and Knowledge*, trans. B. Walsh. Chicago: University of Chicago Press.

Platt, J. (1992) Cases of cases . . . of cases, in C. Ragin and H. Becker (eds), *What is a Case? Exploring the Foundations of Social Inquiry*. London: Cambridge University Press.

Plummer, K. (1983) *Documents of Life: An Introduction to the Problems and Literature of a Humanistic Method*. London: George Allen & Unwin.

Poland, B. (1995) Transcription quality as an aspect of rigor in qualitative research. *Qualitative Inquiry*, 1 (3) pp. 290–310.

Polkinghorne, D. (1983) *Methodology for the Human Sciences*. New York: Albany State University.

——(1988) Narrative knowing and the human sciences, in L. Langsdorf (ed.), *Philosophy of the Social Sciences*. New York: State University of New York Press.

Popkewitz, T. (1995) Foreword in P. McLaren and G. Giarelli (eds), *Critical Theory and Educational Research*. New York: State University of New York Press.

Popper, K. (1969) *Conjectures and Refutations: The Growth of Scientific Knowledge*, 2nd edition. London: Routledge and Kegan Paul.

Potter, J. (1996) *Representing Reality: Discourse, Rhetoric and Social Construction*. California: Sage.

Potter, J. and Weatherall, M. (1987) *Discourse and Social Psychology: Beyond Attitudes and Behaviour*. London: Sage.

——(1994) Analysing discourse, in A. Bryman and R. Burgess (eds), *Analysing Quantitative Data*. London: Routledge.

Powdermaker, H. (1966) *Stranger and Friend: The Way of an Anthropologist*. New York: W. W. Norton.

Power, R., Jones, S., Kearns, G. and Ward, J. (1996) An ethnography of risk management amongst illicit drug injectors and its implications for the development of community based interventions. *Sociology of Health and Illness*, 18 (1) pp. 86–106.

Pradilla, R. (1992) *Qualitative and quantitative models of social situations: the case for triangulation of paradigms*. Paper presented at the international symposium on the Qualitative Research Process and Computing, Bremen, Germany, October.

Prein, G. (1992) *Traps of triangulation: what can be done by combining quantitative and qualitative methods?* Paper presented at the international symposium on the Qualitative Research Process and Computing, Bremen, Germany, October.

Preskill, H. (1995) The use of photography in evaluating school culture. *Qualitative Studies in Education*, 8, pp. 183–193.

Prior, P. (1995) Surviving psychiatric institutionalisation: a case study. *Sociology of Health and Illness*, 17 (5) pp. 651–667.

Quine, S. and Cameron, I. (1995) The use of focus groups with the disabled elderly. *Qualitative Health Research*, 5 (4) pp. 454–462.

Rabinow, P. (1977) *Reflections on Fieldwork in Morocco*. Berkeley: University of California Press.

Ragin, C. and Becker, H. (eds) (1992) *What is a Case? Exploring the Foundations of Social Enquiry*. New York: Cambridge University Press.

Ragins, A. (1995) Why self care fails: implementing policy at a low income sickle cell clinic. *Qualitative Sociology*, 18 (5) pp. 331–354.

Ramazanoglu, C. (ed.) (1993) *Up Against Foucault: Explorations of Some Tensions between Foucault and Feminism*. London: Routledge.

Rank, M. (1992) The blending of qualitative and quantitative methods in understanding childbearing among welfare recipients, in J. Gilgun, J. Daly and G. Handel (eds), *Qualitative Methods in Family Research*, pp. 281–300. California: Sage.

Rasmussen, P. (1989) *Massage Parlour Prostitution*. New York: Irvington.

Reason, P. (1988) Whole person medical practice, in P. Reason (ed.), *Human Inquiry in Action: Developments in New Paradigm Research*. London: Sage.

——(1994) Three approaches to participative inquiry, in N. Denzin and Y. Lincoln (eds), *Handbook of Qualitative Research*. California: Sage.

Reichardt, C. and Rallis, S. (eds) (1994) *The Qualitative–Quantitative Debate: New Perspectives*. San Francisco: Jossey Bass.

Reid, J. (1983) *Sorcerers and Healing Spirits*. Canberra: Australian National University Press.

Reinharz, S. (1992) *Feminist Methods in Social Research*. New York: Oxford University Press.

——(1993) Neglected voices and excessive demands in feminist research. *Qualitative Sociology*, 16 (1) pp. 69–75.

Reissman, C. (1990) *Narrative Analysis*. Qualitative Research Methods, 30, P. Manning, J. Van Maanen and M. Miller (eds). California: Sage.

Renaud, M. (1975) On the structural constraints to state intervention in health. *International Journal of Health Services*, 5 (4) pp. 559–572.

Rich, J. (1968) *Interviewing Children and Adolescents*. New York: St Martins Press.

Richards, T. and Richards, L. (1994) Using computers in qualitative research, in N. Denzin and Y. Lincoln (eds), *Handbook of Qualitative Research*. California: Sage.

Richardson, L. (1992) The consequences of poetic representation: writing the other, rewriting the self, in C. Ellis and M. Flaherty (eds), *Investigating Subjectivity: Research on Lived Experience*. California: Sage.

——(1994) Writing as a method of enquiry, in N. Denzin and Y. Lincoln (eds), *Handbook of Qualitative Research*. California: Sage.

Robillard, A. (1994) Communication problems in the intensive care unit. *Qualitative Sociology*, 17 (4) pp. 383–395.

Robrecht, L. (1995) Grounded theory: evolving methods. *Qualitative Health Research*, 5 (2) pp. 169–177.

Robson, C. (1993) *Real World Research: A Resource for Social Scientists and Practitioner-Researchers*. Oxford: Basil Blackwell.

Roethlisberger, F. and Dickson, W. (1964) *Management and the Worker: An Account of a Research Program Conducted by the Western Electric Company, Hawthorne Works, Chicago*. Cambridge: Harvard University Press.

Roman, L. (1992) The political significance of other ways of narrating ethnography: a feminist materialist approach, in M. Le Compte, W. Millroy and J. Preissle Goetz (eds), *The Handbook of Qualitative Research in Education*. New York: Academic Press.

Roman, L. and Apple, M. (1990) Is naturalism a move away from positivism? Materialist and feminist approaches to subjectivity in ethnographic research, in E. Eisner and A. Peshkin (eds), *Qualitative Inquiry in Education: The Continuing Debate*. New York: Teachers College Press, Columbia University.

Ronai, C. (1992) The reflexive self through narrative: a night in the life of an erotic dancer/researcher, in C. Ellis and M. Flaherty (eds), *Investigating Subjectivity: Research on Lived Experience*. California: Sage.

Rosenau, P. (1992) *Post-modernism and the Social Sciences: Insights, Inroads and Intrusions*. Princeton: Princeton University Press.

Rosenhan, D. (1973) Being sane in insane places. *Science*, 179, January, pp. 250–258.

Rosenwald, G. and Ochberg, R. (eds) (1992) *Storied Lives: The Cultural Politics of Self-Understanding*. New Haven: Yale University Press.

Ross, D. and Ross, S. (1984) The importance of type of question, psychological climate and subject set in interviewing children about pain. *Pain*, 19, pp. 71–79.

Rossman, G. and Wilson, B. (1985) Numbers and words: combining quantitative and qualitative methods in a single large-scale evaluation study. *Evaluation Review*, 9 (5) pp. 627–643.

Roszak, T. (1986) *The Cult of Information: The Folklore of Computers and the True Art of Thinking*. New York: Pantheon.

Rowe, G., Wright, G. and Bolger, F. (1991) Delphi: a revaluation of research and theory. *Technological Forecasting and Social Change*, 39, pp. 235–251.

Russell, A. (1994) *Synergetic focus groups: a data gathering method for phenomenographic research*. Unpublished paper.

Sabarino, J., Stott, F. and the Faculty of the Erikson Institute (1987) *What Children Tell Us*. New York: Jossey Bass.

Saint-Germain, M., Bassford, T. and Montano, G. (1993) Surveys and focus groups in health research with older Hispanic Women. *Qualitative Sociology*, 3 (3) pp. 341 367.

Sandelowski, M. (1986) The problem of rigour in qualitative research. *Advances in Nursing Science*, 8 (3) pp. 27–37.

Sarbin, T. (ed.) (1986) *Narrative Psychology: The Storied Nature of Human Conduct*. Westport: Praeger.

Sartre, J.-P. (1960) *Critique de la Raison Dialectique: Questions de Méthode*. Paris: Gallimard.

——(1963) *Search for a Method*. New York: Knopf.

Scambler, G. (ed.) (1987) *Sociological Theory and Medical Sociology*. London: Tavistock.

Schatzman, L. (1991) Dimensional analysis: notes on an alternative approach to the grounding of theory in qualitative research, in D. Maines (ed.), *Social Organisation and Social Process: Essays in Honour of Anselm Strauss*. New York: Aldine de Gruyter.

Schatzman, L. and Bucher, R. (1964) Negotiating a division of labour among professions in the state mental hospital. *Psychiatry*, 27, pp. 266–277.

Scheff, T. (1966) *Being Mentally Ill: A Sociological Theory*. London: Weidenfield and Nicholson.

Scherer, J. (ed.) (1990) *Picturing Cultures: Historical Photographs in Anthropological Inquiry: Visual Anthropology*, special edition. New York: Harwood Academic.

Schratz, M. (1993) *Qualitative Voices in Educational Research*. London: Falmer Press.

Schwartz, D. (1989) Visual ethnography: using photography in qualitative research. *Qualitative Sociology*, 12 (2) pp. 119–154.

Schwartzman, H. (1993) *Ethnography in Organisations*. California: Sage.

Scott, J. (1991) The evidence of experience. *Critical Inquiry*, 17 (4) pp. 773–797.

Scriven, M. (1972) *Goal Free Evaluation in School Evaluation: The Politics and the Process*. E. House (ed.). Berkeley: McCutchan.

Seals, B., Sowell, R., Demi, A., Moneyham, L., Cohen, L. and Guillary, J. (1995) Falling through the cracks: social service concerns of women infected with HIV. *Qualitative Health Research*, 5 (4) pp. 496–515.

Secretariat of the National Aboriginal and Islander Childcare (1996) *Proposed Plan of Action for the Prevention of Child Abuse and Neglect in Aboriginal Communities*. Canberra: AGPS.

Seidel, J. (1991) Method and madness in the application of computer technology to qualitative data analysis, in N. Fielding and R. Lee (eds), *Using Computers in Qualitative Research*. London: Sage.

Seidman, S. (1994) *Contested Knowledge: Social Theory in the Postmodern Era*. Oxford: Basil Blackwell.

Seidman, S. and Wagner, D. (eds) (1992) *Postmodernism and Social Theory: The Debate over General Theory*. Cambridge: Basil Blackwell.

Sells, S., Smith, T. and Sprenkle, D. (1995) Integrating qualitative and quantitative methods: a research model. *Family Process*, 34 (2) pp. 199–218.

Shaffir, W. and Stebbins, R. (eds) (1991) *Experiencing Fieldwork: An Inside View of Qualitative Research*. California: Sage.

Shapiro, J. (1991) Interviewing children about psychological issues associated with sexual abuse. *Psychotherapy*, 28 (1) pp. 55–66.

Shields, C. (1990) *Mary Swann*. London: Fourth Estate. First published 1987.

Shields, L. (1995) Women's experiences of the meaning of empowerment. *Qualitative Health Research*, 5 (1) pp. 25–35.

Shorter Oxford English Dictionary (1973). Vols I and II, rev. and ed. C.T. Onions. Oxford: Oxford University Press.

Sieber, S. (1973) The integration of fieldwork and survey methods. *American Journal of Sociology*, 78, pp. 1335–1359.

Silverman, D. (1987) *Communication and Medical Practice*. London: Sage.

——(1993) *Interpreting Qualitative Data: Methods for Analysing Talk, Text and Interaction*. London: Sage.

——(1997) *Qualitative Research: Theory, Method and Practice*. London: Sage.

Small, W. (1997) 'Keeping emotion out of it': the problem (and promise) of the investigator's feelings in social research. *The Australian Journal of Social Research*, 4 (1) pp. 98–118.

Smith, A. and Louis, K. (1982) Multimethod policy research. *American Behavioral Scientist*, 26, pp. 133–144.

Smith, D. and Smith, P. (1995) *Getting Strength from Country: Report of the Outstation Impact Project Concerning the Delivery of Services to Outstations in the Kimberley Region of Western Australia*. Perth Western Australian Health Department.

Smith, J. and Heshusius, L. (1986) Closing down the conversation: the end of the quantitative–qualitative debate among educational inquirers. *Educational Researcher*, 15 (1) pp. 4–12.

Smith, L. (1990) Ethics in qualitative field research: an individual perspective, in E. Eisner and A. Peshkin (eds), *Qualitative Inquiry in Education: The Continuing Debate*. New York: Teachers College Press, Columbia University.

Smith, M. (1989) *Evaluability Assessment: A Practical Approach*. Norwell: Kluwer.

Sontag, S. (1966) *Against Interpretation and Other Essays*: New York: Dell.

Southern Australia and Community Health Research Unit (1996) *Changing Times: Planning Evaluation and Outcomes in Metropolitan, Community and Women's Health Services*. Adelaide: SACHRU.

Southern Metropolitan Health Advisory Board (1996) *Southern Health Area Priorities*. Adelaide: South Australian Health Commission.

Spradley, J. (1970) *You Owe Yourself a Drunk: An Ethnography of Urban Nomads*. Boston: Little, Brown.

——(1980) *Participant Observation*. New York: Holt, Rinehart and Winston.

Stainback, S. and Stainback, W. (1988) *Understanding and Collecting Qualitative Research*. Reston: Council for Exceptional Children.

Stake, R. (1980) Program evaluation, particularly responsive evaluation, in W. Dockerell and D. Hamilton (eds), *Rethinking Educational Research*. London: Hodder and Stoughton.

——(1995) *The Art of Case Study Research*. California: Sage.

Stange, K., Miller, W., Crabtree, B., O'Connor, P. and Zyzanski, S. (1994) Multimethod research: approaches for integrating qualitative and quantitative methods. *Journal of General Internal Medicine*, 9, pp. 278–282.

Stanley, K. (1992) *The Autobiographical I: The Theory and Practice of Feminist Autobiography*. Manchester: Manchester University Press.

Stanley, L. (ed.) (1990) *Feminist Praxis, Research, Theory and Epistemology in Feminist Sociology*. London and New York: Routledge.

Stanley, L. and Temple, B. (1995) Doing the business? Evaluating software packages to aid the analysis of qualitative data sets, in R. Burgess (ed.), *Studies in Qualitative Methodology: Computing and Qualitative Research*. London: JAI Press.

Stanley, L. and Wise, B. (1990) Method, methodology and epistemology in feminist research processes, in L. Stanley (ed.), *Feminist Praxis:*

Research, Theory and Epistemology in Feminist Sociology. London: Routledge.

Star, S. (1991) The sociology of the invisible: the primacy of the work of Anselm Strauss, in D. Maines (ed.), Social Organisation and Social Process: Essays in Honour of Anselm Strauss. New York: Aldine de Gruyter.

Starr, P. (1982) The Social Transformation of American Medicine. New York: Basic Books.

Steckler, A., McLeroy, K., Goodman, R., Bird, S. and McCormick, L. (1992) Toward integrating qualitative and quantitative methods: an introduction. Health Education Quarterly, 19 (1) pp. 1–8.

Stevenson, O. and Parsloe, P. (1993) Community Care and Empowerment. York: Joseph Rowntree Foundation, with Community Care.

Stewart, D. and Shamdasani, P. (1990) Focus Groups: Theory and Practice. Newbury Park: Sage.

Stoecker, R. (1991) Evaluating and re-thinking the case study. Sociological Review, 39 (1) February, pp. 88–112.

Straughan, P. and Seow, A. (1995) Barriers to mammography among Chinese women in Singapore: a focus group approach. Health Education Research, 10 (4) pp. 431–441.

Strauss, A. (1987) Qualitative Analysis for Social Scientists. London: Cambridge University Press.

Strauss, A. and Corbin, J. (1990) Basics of Qualitative Research. California: Sage.

Strauss, A., Fagerhaugh, S., Suczek, B. and Weiner, C. (1985) The Social Organisation of Medical Work. Chicago: University of Chicago Press.

Straw, M. and Marks, K. (1995) The use of focus groups in program development. Qualitative Health Research, 5 (4) pp. 426–443.

Stringer, E. (1996) Action Research: A Handbook for Practitioners. California: Sage.

Suczek, B. (1993) Chronic renal failure and the problem of funding, in B. Glaser (ed.), Examples of Grounded Theory: A Reader. California: Sociology Press.

Sudnow, D. (1972) Studies in Social Interaction. New York: The Free Press, Macmillan.

Summers, A. (1996) 'For I have ever so much more faith in her ability as a nurse': the eclipse of the community midwife in South Australia 1836–1942. PhD, Flinders University of South Australia, Adelaide.

Taylor, S. and Ashworth, C. (1987) Durkheim and social realism: an approach to health and illness, in G. Scambler (ed.), Sociological Theory and Medical Sociology. London: Tavistock.

Taylor, S. and Bogdan, R. (1984) Introduction to Qualitative Research Methods: The Search for Meanings, 2nd edition. New York: John Wiley.

Tesch, R. (1990) Qualitative Research: Analysis Types and Software Tools. New York: Falmer Press.

Theobold, M. (1993) Writing the Lives of Women Teachers: Problems and Possibilities. Studies in Education, L. Yates (ed.). Melbourne: Melbourne University.

Thompson, B., Fries, E., Hopp, H., Bowen, D. and Croyle, R. (1995) The feasibility of a proactive stepped care model for worksite smoking cessation. Health Education Research, 10 (4) pp. 455–465.

Thompson, C., Thompson, B. and Hocking, B. (1992) Application of chaos theory to the management of occupational health and safety. Journal of Occupational Health and Safety, 8 (2) pp. 99–119.

Thompson, H. (1967) Hells Angels. Harmondsworth: Penguin.

Thompson, P. (1978) The Voice of the Past: Oral History. Oxford: Oxford University Press.

Tixier, Y., Vigil, Y. and Elassasser, N. (1976) The effects of ethnicity of the interviewer on conversation: a study of Chicano women, in B. Dubois and I. Couch (eds), Sociology of the Language of American Women. Texas: Trinity University Press.

Todd, A. and Fisher, S. (eds) (1988) Gender and Discourse: The Power of Talk. Norwood, New Jersey: Ablett.

Tong, R. (1989) Feminist Thought: A Comprehensive Introduction. Boulder: Westview Press.

Toolan, M. (1988) A Critical Linguistic Introduction. London: Routledge.

Tosh, J. (1991) The Pursuit of History: Aims, Methods and New Directions of Modern History, 2nd edition. London: Routledge.

Traylen, H. (1989) Health Visiting Practice: An Exploration into the Nature of the Health Visitors' Relationship with Their Clients. Master's dissertation, School of Management, University of Bath, Bath.

Trinh, T. Minh-ha (1989) Woman, Native, Other: Writing Post Coloniality and Feminism. Bloomington: Indiana University Press.

Trost, J. (1986) Statistically non-representative stratified sampling: a sampling technique for qualitative studies. *Qualitative Sociology*, 9 (1) Spring.

Turnbull, E. (1992) *Storytelling and selfmaking: writing the quality of becoming*. Paper presented at the TASA Conference, Adelaide, November.

Turner, B. (1984) *The Body and Society: Explorations in Social Theory*. Oxford: Basil Blackwell.

——(1987) *Medical Power and Social Knowledge*. London: Sage.

——(1994) *Orientalism, Postmodernism and Globalism*. London: Routledge.

Turner, T. (1992) Defiant images in the Kayapo appropriation of video. *Anthropology Today*, 8 (6) pp. 5–10.

Van Dijk, T. (1985) *Handbook of Discourse Analysis*, 4 vols. London: Academic Press.

Van Loon, A. (1995) *What Constitutes Caring for the Human Spirit in Nursing*. Master's thesis, School of Nursing, Flinders University of South Australia, Adelaide.

Van Maanen, J. (1988) *Tales of the Field: On Writing Ethnography*. Chicago: University of Chicago Press.

Van Manen, M. (1984) Practising phenomenological writing. *Phenomenology and Pedagogy*, 2 (1) pp. 36–39.

——(1989) By the light of the anecdote. *Phenomenology and Pedagogy*, 7, pp. 232–253.

——(1990) *Researching Lived Experience*. New York: State University of New York Press.

Vaughn, S., Shay Shum, J. and Sinagub, J. (1996) *Focus Group Interviews in Education and Psychology*. California: Sage.

Wagner, J. (1979) *Images of Information: Still Photography in the Social Sciences*. California: Sage.

Waitzkin, H. (1981) The social origins of illness: a neglected history. *International Journal of Health Sciences*, 11 (1) pp. 77–103.

Wajcman, J. (1991) *Feminism Confronts Technology*. Sydney: Allen & Unwin.

Walker, A. and Moulton, R. (1989) Photo albums: images of time and reflections of self. *Qualitative Sociology*, 12 (2) pp. 155–182.

Walker, B. (1993) Computer analysis of qualitative data: a comparison of three packages. *Qualitative Health Research*, 3 (1) pp. 91–111.

Walker, R. (1993) Finding a silent voice for the researcher: using photographs in evaluation and research, in M. Schratz (ed.), *Qualitative Voices in Educational Research*. London: Falmer Press.

Wallis, R. (1977) The moral career of a research sociologist, in C. Bell and H. Newby (eds), *Doing Sociological Research*. London: George Allen & Unwin.

Walton, J. (1980) *Talking with Patients: A Teaching Approach*. London: Nuffield Provincial Hospitals Trust.

Wang, C., Burris, M. and Ping, X. (1996) Chinese village women as visual anthropologists: a participatory approach to reaching policy makers. *Social Science and Medicine*, 42 (10) pp. 1391–1400.

Wasserfall, R. (1993) Reflexivity, feminism and difference. *Qualitative Sociology*, 16 (1) pp. 23–41.

Wearing, M. (1996) Medical dominance and the division of labour in the health professions, in C. Grbich (ed.), *Health in Australia: Sociological Concepts and Issues*. Sydney: Prentice Hall.

Weber, M. (1949) *The Methodology of the Social Sciences*, trans. E. Shils and H. Finch. New York: Free Press.

——(1966) *The Theory of Social and Economic Organisation*, trans. M. Henderson and T. Parsons. New York: Free Press. First published 1947.

——(1968) *Economy and Society: An Outline of Interpretive Sociology*, trans. E. Fischof. New York: Badminter Press. First published 1915.

Weber, P. (1985) *Basic Content Analysis*. California: Sage.

Webler, T., Levine, D., Rakel, H. and Renn, O. (1991) A novel approach to reducing uncertainty: the group Delphi. *Technological Forecasting and Social Change*, 39, pp. 253–263.

Webster, S. (1986) Realism and reification in the ethnographic genre. *Critique of Anthropology*, 6 (1) pp. 39–62.

Weedon, C. (1987) *Feminist Practice and Post Structuralist Theory*. Oxford: Basil Blackwell.

Weiler, K. (1992) Remembering and representing life choices: a critical perspective on teachers' oral history narratives. *International Journal of Qualitative Studies in Education*, 5 (1) pp. 39–50.

Weitzman, E. and Miles, M. (1995) *Computer Programs for Qualitative Data Analysis: A Software service book*. California: Sage.

Wexler, P. (1987) *Social Analysis of Education: After the New Sociology*. London: Routledge and Kegan Paul.

White, G. and Thomson, A. (1995) Anonymized focus groups as a research tool for health professionals. *Qualitative Health Research*, 5 (2) pp. 256–261.

White, K. (1991) The sociology of health and illness. *Current Sociology*, 2, Autumn Trend Report.

Whiting, J., Child, I. and Lambert, W. (1966) *Field Guide for a Study of Socialisation*. New York: John Wiley.

Whyte, W. (1955) *Street Corner Society: The Social Structure of an Italian Slum*. Chicago: University of Chicago Press.

——(1984) *Learning from the Field: A Guide from Experience*. California: Sage.

——(1991) *Participatory Action Research*. Newbury Park: Sage.

Wicks, D. (1992) *Nurses and doctors and discourses of healing*. Paper presented at the Australian and New Zealand Sociology Conference (TASA), Adelaide.

Williams, D., Best, J., Taylor, D. and Gilbert, J. (1990) A systematic approach for using qualitative methods in primary prevention research. *Medical Anthropology*, 4 (4) pp. 391–409.

Williams, N. (1994) *An evaluation of the C.A.R.P.A. Standard Treatment Manual*. Master's dissertation, School of Medicine, Flinders University of South Australia, Adelaide.

Williams, R. (1976) Symbolic interactionism: the fusion of theory and method? in D. Thorns (ed.), *New Directions in Sociology*. Newton Abbot: David and Charles; New Jersey: Rowman and Littlefield.

Willis, E. (1989) *Medical Dominance: Division of Labour in Australian Health Care*. Sydney: Allen & Unwin.

Wilson, H. and Hutchinson, S. (1991) Triangulation of qualitative methods: Heideggerian hermeneutics and grounded theory. *Qualitative Health Research*, 1, pp. 263–276.

Winter, R. (1987) *Action Research and the Nature of Social Inquiry: Professional Innovation and Educational Work*. Aldershot: Gower.

——(1989) *Learning from Experience: Principles and Practice in Action Research*. Lewes: Falmer Press.

Wolcott, H. (1979) Criteria for an ethnographic approach to research in schools. *Human Organisation*, 34 (2) Summer, pp. 111–127.

——(1990) On seeking and rejecting validity in qualitative research, in E. Eisner and A. Peshkin (eds), *Qualitative Inquiry in Education: The Continuing Debate*. New York: Teachers College Press, Columbia University.

Wolf, D. (ed.) (1996) *Feminist Dilemmas in Fieldwork*. Boulder: Westview Press.

Wolf, M. (1992) *A Thrice Told Tale: Feminism, Post Modernism and Ethnographic Responsibility*. California: Stanford University Press.

Wolff, B., Knodel, J. and Sittitrai, W. (1993) Focus groups and surveys as complementary research methods: a case example, in D. Morgan (ed.), *Successful Focus Groups: Advancing the State of the Art*. California: Sage.

Women's Health Statewide (1996) *Evaluation of Women's Healthline: Health Information and Counselling Services*. Adelaide: Southern Australia and Community Health Research Unit.

Wrong, D. (1961) The oversocialised conception of man in modern sociology. *American Sociological Review*, 26 (2) pp. 183–193.

Wuest, J. (1995) Feminist grounded theory: an exploration of the congruency and tensions between two traditions in knowledge discovery. *Qualitative Health Research*, 5 (1) pp. 125–137.

Wyllie, A. (1997) Evaluation of a New Zealand campaign towards reduction of intoxication on licensed premises. *Health Promotion International*, 12 (3) pp. 197–207.

Yin, R. (1984) *Case Study Research: Design and Methods*, 1st edition. California: Sage.

——(1993) *Applications of Case Study Research*. California: Sage.

——(1994) Case Study Research: Design and Methods, 2nd edition. California: Sage.

Zadeh, Z. (1988) Fuzzy logic. *Computer*, 21 (4) pp. 83–93.

Ziller, R. (1990) *Photographing the Self: Methods for Observing Personal Orientations*. Newbury Park: Sage.

Ziller, R., Vera, H. and de Santoya, C. (1989) The psychological niche of children of poverty and affluence through auto-photography. *Children's Environmental Quarterly*, 6, pp. 186–196.

Zimmerman, H. (1991) *Fuzzy Set Theory and its Applications*. Boston: Kluwer Academic.

Zimmerman, H., Zadeh, L. and Gaines, B. (eds) (1984) *Fuzzy Sets and Decision Analysis*. New York: Elsevier Science.

Znaniecki, F. (1934) *The Method of Sociology*. New York: Farrer and Rinehart.

Zola, I. (1978) Pathways to the doctor: from person to patient, in D. Tuckett and J. Kaufert (eds), *Basic Readings in Medical Sociology*. London: Tavistock.

Index